The Men's Health
GYM BIBLE

INCLUDES HUNDREDS OF EXERCISES FOR
WEIGHTLIFTING AND CARDIO
Plus Everything You Need to Get the Most
from Your Gym Membership

MYATT MURPHY, C.S.C.S.
and MICHAEL MEJIA, M.S., C.S.C.S.

RODALE.

D1089585

RODALE *wellness*

Live happy. Be healthy. Get inspired.

Sign up today to get exclusive access to our authors, exclusive bonuses,
and the most authoritative, useful, and cutting-edge information on health,
wellness, fitness, and living your life to the fullest.

Visit us online at RodaleWellness.com

Join us at RodaleWellness.com/Join

Rodale books may be purchased for business or promotional use or for special sales. For information, please write to:
Special Markets Department, Rodale Inc., 733 Third Avenue, New York, NY 10017.

Printed in the United States of America

Rodale Inc. makes every effort to use acid-free ♾, recycled paper ♻.

Book design by Christina Gaugler

Photographs on page 189 by Matt Rainey (top) and page 296 Matrix Fitness (bottom).
All other photographs by Mitch Mandel/Rodale Images.

Library of Congress Cataloging-in-Publication Data is on file with the publisher.

ISBN: 978–1–62336–811–1 paperback

Distributed to the trade by Macmillan

2   4   6   8   10   9   7   5   3   1   paperback

 RODALE.

Follow us @RodaleBooks on

We inspire health, healing, happiness, and love in the world.
Starting with you.

CONTENTS

ACKNOWLEDGMENTS

WHEN I WAS ASKED TO COWRITE the sequel to *The Men's Health Home Workout Bible* back in 2005, it was truly an honor. Michael and I felt the pressure to truly "raise the bar"—pardon the gymspeak—and the fact that it has remained an important informational tool so many years later tells me that we managed to do exactly that. Which is why bringing this mainstay book up to speed through this updated second edition has been just as much of a privilege.

For us, that means we managed to create the perfect tool for guiding you through every gym, every piece of fitness equipment you might experience within a gym, every possible health club scenario—but most important—every fitness goal you have today, tomorrow, and for the rest of your life.

I want to thank every editor who has—in one way or another—allowed me to deliver my take on exercise and fitness to millions of readers worldwide for so many years. I've been blessed to write more than 1,000+ pieces for 50+ international magazines now and work with some of the best health, fitness, and nutrition editors in the magazine business. Hopefully, I haven't left anyone off this list—but here goes: Rochelle Udell, Lucy Danziger, Gabrielle Studenmund, Stephen George, Bobby Lee, Mike Carlson, Carol Brooks, Pamela Miller, Jennifer Fields, Kimberly Papa, Laura Gilbert, Jeff Csatari, Rosie Amodio, Duane Swierczynski, Lara McGlashan, Ed Dwyer, Liz O'Brian, Jennifer Walters, Trevor Thieme, Nicole Dorsey, Albert Baime, Alex Strauss, Beth Bischoff, Gordon Bass, Diane Hart, Stephanie Young, Lorie Parch, Meaghan Buchan, Rachel Crocker, Scott Quill, Phillip Rhodes, Steve Perrine, Nichele Hoskins, Mary Christ, Su Reid, Gail O'Connor, Abigail Walch, Dana Points, Lisa Delany, David Kalmansohn, Jerry Kindela, Nina Willdorf, and Alison Ashton.

And, to the hundreds of personal trainers, exercise physiologists, nutritionists and sports psychologists I've studied under, interviewed, trained with—and ghostwritten for—I want to say thank you as well. It's been a pleasure to work with nearly every top fitness professional in the business, and as I say in each and every book I write—there's no greater education than that.

I also want to thank everyone at Rodale who took our words and turned them into the book you're about to use for a lifetime, including Mark Weinstein, Franny Vignola, Christina Gaugler, Nancy Bailey, Sean Sabo, Mitch Mandel, Troy Schnyder, and Andy Speer.

Finally, thanks, Dad, for teaching me about exercise when I was young. If you hadn't shared everything that you knew about fitness with me, I never would have been able to share everything I know about fitness with the readers in this book.

—*Myatt*

INTRODUCTION

Fitness center.　　**Aerobics studio.**
Health club.　　　**Box.**
Sports center.　　**Gym.**

THERE SURE ARE A LOT OF different expressions for the places we're willing to pay to sweat, lift, and stretch in, aren't there? All in the desperate pursuit to build up and chisel out the perfect physique. With so many names for some silly building we essentially shell out membership dues to use for exercise, it's no wonder the whole process of choosing—and using—any of the above is so difficult for so many people.

Deciding to make exercise a regular part of your lifestyle is a major step that takes a certain level of serious commitment on its own. Add joining a gym to that picture—and for the sake of consistency, we'll be using the term "gym" to refer to all of the above for the rest of this book—and you create a whole new level of confusion.

We know how you feel. A gym—no matter what its size, location, or clientele—can be intimidating for so many reasons. Wading through the daunting and intentionally confusing contracts. Wondering if you're somehow breaking any of the "unspoken" rules of gym etiquette by saying or doing the wrong thing. Staring at rows and rows of exercise equipment you simply have no clue how to use—or what they even do! Questioning if you should waste dough paying one of their personal trainers to show you.

The whole idea of a gym membership can leave you feeling as helpless as trying to invest in real estate or the stock market without knowing what you're doing. Just another thing you *know* could make a huge difference in your life—if only you could figure out how to get the most from it.

Well, problem solved.

After all, that's why you're here, right? If you're reading this book, then either you're planning to start going to a gym or you already belong to one and want to get even more from the membership you have.

It doesn't matter in which of the two situations you find yourself. In fact, it doesn't even matter what your fitness goals are—whether you want to lose weight and burn fat, build strength, develop firmer, leaner muscles, improve your sports performance, or just turn back the clock by staying fit and healthy. It doesn't matter if you're male or female, young or old. We all want to avoid the same three things when it comes to joining a gym.

- You don't want to look foolish or like an amateur.
- You don't want to waste your money.
- You don't want to fail at reaching your individual fitness goals.

We hear you loud and clear. That's exactly why we've designed this book—to make sure that none of the above ever happens to you on our watch—no matter what type of gym eventually becomes *your* gym.

HOW TO USE THIS BOOK

Before you begin trying this guide on for size, it helps to know a few basic facts first.

According to recent research performed by the International Health, Racquet & Sportsclub Association (IHRSA) health club membership has grown by 22 percent from 2009 to 2015, with the total number of club visitors increasing by 24 percent. In fact, when the first edition of this book came out in 2006, there were 26,830 health clubs in the United States alone. Ten years later, that number has risen to more than 36,000. IHRSA's statistics have also shown that for over two decades, the total number of people belonging to gyms and health clubs in the United States has continued to rise by at least 1,000,000 every year.

In 2006, we first reported that a staggering 41.3 million active health club members were out there, paying their dues and sweating it out in gyms throughout the country. Just a decade later, there are now 55.3 million (and more than 64 million health club visitors), with nearly half of those individuals visiting their health club for at least 100 days per year. In fact, as of 2015, nearly one out of five Americans belonged to at least one type of health club or gym. So hearing these numbers, we had to design this updated book with each and every one of you out there in mind.

You see, if you step into enough gym facilities, as we have over the years, something becomes painfully clear. Every single gym or health club—even those that belong to a chain with hundreds of facilities worldwide—is uniquely different when it comes to its layout, available exercise equipment and classes, and everything else it may offer its members.

With more than 36,000 possible gyms in the United States alone to choose from—and many thousands and thousands more worldwide—this book had to be structured to be easy to use to work in any type of gym, no matter how much or how little "your" gym has to offer. That's why the exercise chapters are divided according to specific types of equipment you're likely to encounter.

Even the most basic gym has dumbbells and/or barbells lying around to lift. So we'll start you off with an array of the best body- and free-weight exercises imaginable. From there, subsequent chapters will teach you hundreds of other exercises you can use, depending on whatever amenities your gym may have (including cable machines): a variety of moves for the weight bench, plus sandbags and kettlebells, battle ropes, TRX systems, power sleds, power racks, and squat cage exercises; we also include a full chapter covering the most common weight-stack and cardiovascular machines.

To make all of these chapters even more user-friendly, all of the exercises in each chapter are divided by muscle groups—chest, back, arms, shoulders, legs, abs, and so on—so you can locate exactly what moves you need—instantly! If you're not as savvy at picking the right combination of moves to create the best possible workout, just turn to page 309 to find sample routines to help you reach your fitness goals, no matter what they are and regardless of your level of exercise expertise—beginner, intermediate, or advanced.

If you're ready to go from being gym illiterate to maximizing every penny of your health club membership, then we've got everything you need right here.

PART ONE

MEMBERSHIP YOUR MUSCLES

CHAPTER ONE

THE OFF-SITE ADVANTAGE

SO YOU'RE FINALLY READY TO INVEST in a gym membership, eh?

Welcome to the club . . . literally.

Here are the facts: Exercising at home may be more convenient, but the day you decide to put a few bucks down and take advantage of everything a gym has to offer, you're truly making a serious investment in yourself. And there's no better way to get a return on that investment than joining a gym that has everything your body needs to get the job done.

Those in the know about exercise already understand the difference that the right gym can make in helping them achieve every single one of their fitness goals. But if that's not you, then you may be one of the few who's not completely sold on everything joining a gym has to offer.

We know why you may have your doubts. A lot of people think of health clubs as being modern-day snake oil salesmen, peddling the promise of better bodies and perfect abs, yet never seeming to deliver results. There are a few shady gym owners out there looking to take your money, and in Chapter Three we'll show you what to watch for before signing a contract.

Others fall under the impression that joining a gym means they'll instantly get in shape as soon as the ink's dry on the contract. When that doesn't happen, they assume it must have been the gym's fault for not having the right equipment or enough "trendy" exercise classes. To be honest, the average gym typically does have every-thing your body needs to reach its fitness goals. The real reason some people get less than they bargained for from a gym membership is usually because they don't spend enough time using it in the first place.

To get the best results from exercise—and your gym—experts recommend that you work out a minimum of 20 minutes a day, three times a week. But according to research from IHRSA, the average gym membership owner only goes to the gym twice a week! To make matters worse, statistics also show that about two-thirds of people with a gym membership (67 percent) never use them. The final straw? According to many surveys, 50 to 60 percent of people quit within 6 months of starting an exercise regime. With those kinds of numbers, it's no wonder so many people never see a single change after they sign up.

But that's not going to be you, now, is it?

Knowing the real reasons why most people don't achieve their goals or see results when they join a gym is exactly why you won't be one of them. Armed with that knowledge, along with the hundreds of gym exercises, workout routines, and practical information in this book, you—and your body—will get your money's worth from your membership and a whole lot more.

Need a little more reassuring before making any serious commitment to your workouts? Here are just a few reasons why working out away from home is truly worth your body's time.

IT'S NOT AS EXPENSIVE AS YOU THINK

Do you cringe at the thought of actually paying a monthly fee? Then do yourself a favor and put a gym membership cost in honest perspective. According to IHRSA, the median annual dues paid across all club types in 2014 was $828 (roughly $69 a month). And in smaller fitness-only facilities, those dues were even lower, averaging around $52 a month.

Think about that for a second. What other place can you essentially "use" and spend time in "all day long" for two bucks? Break down how much it costs per hour to sit in a coffee shop or a bar, watch a movie, or get your hair cut. All of the above are not only far more expensive, but none of them improve your appearance, overall self-confidence, and health simultaneously.

MONEY IS ALWAYS THE BEST MOTIVATOR

If the thought of signing your life away on the dotted line frightens you, then stop worrying. In fact, be grateful you feel that way.

It's only a blow to your wallet if you quit or decide not to go often enough to get your money's worth. Deciding to invest in exercise equipment for your home instead still carries financial risk if you don't stay committed to working out. However, paying for membership fees every month can serve as a constant reminder that you're spending money on something that you'd better start using. To ease your concerns on paying too much, though, we'll show you a few tips in a later chapter on how to get a better break on your total membership cost.

THERE'S LESS RISK OF BEING FOOLED

Take a closer look around any health club and you'll notice that many of the cheesy infomercially hawked, "twenty-four easy payments of $29.95" products you constantly see on TV are strangely missing from the picture. There's a reason for that. Gym owners aren't as easily tricked into purchasing fitness products for their facility that don't work. For the exercise novice, that can mean more protection from wasting time—and money—on buying and using fitness equipment that simply don't get the job done properly.

IT'S EASIER TO STAY FOCUSED ON YOUR GOALS

Hey, we're not going to tell you that exercising at home isn't convenient. But it can also be inconvenient if too many priorities are constantly interfering with your workout. At the gym, there are no ringing phones or screaming kids or annoying neighbors dropping by or unfinished house projects vying for your undivided attention. That's why for many people it can be a lot easier to take the time to focus on themselves at a gym, where they're not surrounded by other responsibilities or distractions.

THERE'S MORE VARIETY FOR YOUR MUSCLES

Guess what? Your muscles get bored from exercise just like you do. Studies have shown that your muscles can adapt to an exercise after performing it just five or six times. To keep them interested enough to change and grow, you need to consistently experiment with increasing the poundage of the weights you lift, as well as trying different exercises as often as possible.

Work out at home and you're limited by money and space. Unless you have an extra 4,000 square feet in your house that's loaded wall-to-wall with every piece of exercise equipment known to man, odds are your home gym pales in comparison to what even the most bare-bones gym can offer your muscles. Joining a gym gives your muscles access to a much wider assortment of equipment, so you can mix things up as often as necessary for nonstop results.

IT'S MORE OF A TIME-SAVER THAN YOU REALIZE

Unless the gym you're planning to join is tripping distance from your home or workplace, odds are you'll have to tack on a few extra minutes of travel time to get there. That may seem like a time eater when compared to the beauty of exercising at home, but if you plan on capitalizing on everything a gym has to offer, it may actually save you precious time. That's because even the easiest-to-use, multi-exercise home gyms still typically require you to waste time readjusting them to set up each and every exercise. Plus, remember what we said about it being harder sometimes to focus at home because of everyone vying for your attention? Well, every distraction at home can add more and more unnecessary minutes to your workout.

In a gym, you jump on whatever machine you want to use, do your thing, wipe off your sweat, and move on. Less setup time means less wasted time in between sets, making your overall workout time much shorter than you might expect in the long run. Plus, your consideration of another gym goer's turn on the machine you're using will eliminate any tendency you have to linger longer than you need to.

YOU MAY LEARN MORE ABOUT YOUR BODY

Some gyms—not all, but a fair share—offer fitness testing to their clients, sometimes for free or for a certain fee. Just a few of those services can include getting a body mass index and fat test, having your heart rate and blood pressure checked, receiving a measurement to determine the size of your lungs, or having a postural analysis to see if your spine is in alignment, for example.

Some higher-end clubs may even offer the means to measure your VO_2 max, considered one of the best indicators of a superior cardio respiratory system and the potential to excel in aerobic or endurance sports. The 8- to 15-minute test requires exercising on a piece of cardio equipment (typically a treadmill or bike), starting at a low intensity, then gradually increasing the resistance and/or workload while wearing a lightweight breathing mask that measures the amount of oxygen you consume during each minute of exercise.

YOU CAN TAKE YOUR WORKOUTS ON THE ROAD

Convenience is one of the top factors that can affect whether you exercise regularly or not. Add a busy work schedule, a few fun vacations, or any other excuse to travel, and you can pretty much count out "not" exercising if you typically work out at home. Joining a larger gym chain, however, can sometimes give you a form of freedom no home gym setup can ever touch, and that's being able to exercise from a multitude of different locations—either for free or with a substantial discount. For you, that means never letting being on the road bring your workouts to a screeching halt. That's also why we made sure every possible gym exercise you may find in your travels is in this book. That way, you won't be confused by any random machine or exercise you may encounter when taking your workout out of town.

YOUR MUSCLES MAY RECOVER BETTER

Once your workout's over, it's what you do afterward that can oftentimes decide what your performance will be like the next time you exercise. Being in a gym means you may also have access to a number of passive and active ways to help your muscles recuperate immediately afterward, such as a swimming pool, foam rollers, ice baths, saunas, an area for stretching, and possibly the means to get a massage directly on-site.

THERE IS STRENGTH IN NUMBERS

There's a certain inspiring camaraderie that being a member of a gym can bring to your workouts. Many people tend to work themselves harder when they know other people are watching them. Plus, it lets you silently expand your exercise repertoire as you casually watch what others are doing to stay in shape. Even the group exercise classes that many gyms offer can be highly motivating and fun. But inspiration and education aren't the only two perks you'll get from having other gym members around you.

If reshaping your muscles is on your list of goals—and it should be, regardless if your primary concern is just to burn fat, reduce stress, increase your energy levels, or improve your total health—then having a few extra hands nearby can make accomplishing that goal even easier. See, to get your muscles to change, you need to challenge them beyond what they're used to so they have a reason to grow stronger and larger. Being able to rely on other gym members' assistance as you exercise—from letting them help you get a few extra repetitions from a set to making sure you don't drop the weight—can let you push your muscles as hard as they need to be pushed, with less risk of injury to your muscles or yourself.

INSTANT ACCESS TO THE EXPERTS

Toil away in your own home gym and your ability to pick the brains of those who may know more about exercise than you do is limited to whomever is living under the same roof with you. But being a gym member means you're most likely surrounded by personal trainers working with clients and putting them through their paces.

All that expertise around you works to your advantage in several ways. One, it makes it easy to watch what they're doing, see who looks like they know their thing, and eventually ask for some guidance. (And when that day comes, make sure you read Chapter Twenty first to know what to look for in a trainer.) Two, even if hiring a personal trainer isn't in your future, looking over at (or even eavesdropping) one every once in a while may give you a few free pointers on what to do—and what never to do.

CHAPTER TWO

HOW TO PICK THE RIGHT GYM FOR YOU

JOINING A HEALTH CLUB MAY BE one of the best ways to get the results you're looking for, but joining the wrong one still remains one of the best ways to waste your hard-earned dough. With more and more clubs springing up with dollar-saving offers that seem a little too good to be true, it makes it hard to know which one's up your alley. Or which one is perfectly matched to meet your personal exercise and fitness goals.

With all of the clubs to choose from, it can be hard to evaluate whether you're joining the right one. These tips can save you from choosing the wrong gym instead of the right one for you.

TIME YOUR DRIVE TO THE GYM

Run a search for health clubs and the town you live and write down only those within a 15-minute radius from where you live. The rule of thumb is to invest in a gym or health club that's no more than 15 minutes from where you live. Why? Most experts agree that picking a gym that's any farther than that reduces your chances of staying committed to exercise considerably. If you typically spend more time at work than at home and figure you'll be leaving for the gym from work, then choose a gym that's 15 minutes away from your workplace instead.

GO ON TOUR

Some clubs will list dozens of features that they offer to make them seem like the best choice. But just because the club's ads or literature says it's fully loaded with the best equipment doesn't mean all those things actually exist. Do yourself a favor and make sure to get a list of everything the club claims it has to offer, then demand to check out each area personally. During your tour, ask yourself these three important questions:

1. *Do I really need this area?*

   Just because you have no interest in using their fancy Olympic-size pool or free childcare service doesn't mean you're not indirectly paying for them in the total cost of your yearly membership fee. If more than half of the services they offer aren't really what you need, there may be a different club that offers more of what you need and less of what you don't . . . at a much cheaper membership price.

2. *Is this area really as impressive as their literature or salesperson claims?*

   You're told they have a juice bar and a special area for stretching. But all you see is a vending machine and some mats thrown down in the darkest corner of the gym. The point: If they aren't being honest about things you can easily recognize, keep in mind that some of the features you may not see or quite understand (such as their claim that they have state-of-the-art equipment and hundreds of exercise classes) may also be exaggerations of the truth.

3. *Will I be charged separately to use this area or is this service free?*

Some gyms show you everything they provide, but forget to tell you that many of the services may be à la carte or part of a more expensive "gold," "platinum," "enhanced," or "upgraded" membership plan. If you see any class, service, etc., that you're interested in, ask if it's included in the membership, and if not, find out what it will cost. Then, estimate how many times you'll need to pay extra for that in a given year. Finally, remember to add that price to the total membership cost before comparing the fees with other local clubs.

TAKE A TEST DRIVE

Insist on getting a free one-day pass to check out the facilities for yourself. Some gyms will even offer you up to three days—or even a full week—to try them on for size. But if they don't let you experience their facility for free, then don't bother and walk out—that alone should clue you in on their poor business practices right from the start.

Once you get a pass, you may think the smartest plan would be to check out the gym during its busiest hours (5 to 7 p.m.) to see how crowded it gets. That's fine, if that's the time you would normally go, but not if you plan on exercising at a different time during the day. Instead, go at the time you would normally work out each day.

Don't just keep track of how crowded it gets, but also pay attention to the atmosphere. It's the atmosphere that can make or break your future workouts down the road, since the mood of a gym can be the deciding factor in how often you use the facilities and how motivated you are to exercise when you're there. Because the atmosphere of any club changes every hour, depending on the classes, the clientele, and so on, just be sure that you feel the environment is as motivating during that time as you need it to be.

HUNT AROUND FOR SOMEONE WHO LOOKS LIKE YOU

If you don't see anyone around that's your age or body type, there may be a reason for that. Certain gyms cater to specific communities, such as hardcore bodybuilders, serious aerobic junkies, or the over-50 crowd. If you do manage to find someone like you, ask them—when you're trying out the gym for free—a few questions like,

"Does this place always look this good?" "Is the staff always this friendly?" or "Does the equipment break down a lot?" Members have a great sense of history and can clue you into the weaknesses of the club before you encounter them yourself—after the ink is already dry on the contract.

WATCH HOW THE STAFF TREATS THE PAYING CUSTOMERS

Don't be fooled by all the extraordinary attention you might get when checking out a new gym. If you're walking around with the gym manager, the rest of the trainers and staff know you're most likely a potential client, so trust us, they are on their best behavior. Instead of being fooled by having the staff shower you with niceties, look around to see how they treat the rest of the people exercising around you. Watching if the staff is just as attentive to the regular gym members can tell you what to really expect from them down the road.

CHECK THE LEGROOM

In an effort to pack the gym with as much equipment as possible, some gyms leave out one important thing: room to breathe. Look at how close machines and benches are to one another. Extra equipment is useless if you have to wait constantly for someone to finish on the machine next to you. Also, look for cleanliness. You may feel awkward taking a tour of the locker room, but it can be the best place to visit if you're curious about cleanliness. This area isn't usually in a high-visibility area, which is why it's typically a great barometer of how clean the rest of the gym may be on a regular basis.

DO THE MATH

Don't be afraid to ask how many members they currently have and what their capacity is. If it's a new gym—or you're joining a gym in the summertime when more people tend to forsake the gym for the out-of-doors—you may only be looking at half of the members. In 6 months, the gym could be twice as crowded.

QUESTION THEIR LONGEVITY

Ask how long they've been in business if you don't already know the answer. If it's a gym that's been around for a while, odds are, you won't have any problems with them suddenly shutting their doors down the road. If they're new, ask about their history. Sometimes, a gym or club may have had a change in ownership and are considered "new." The problem: You may be joining a gym that changed hands because it wasn't making any money, which could increase the odds of it closing down sooner or later. If that's the case, try to get a sense of how busy it seems to be—if it's new and always empty, you may be investing money in a membership that could turn south.

CHECK OUT THEIR TOP TRAINERS' CREDENTIALS

Any gym can buy the right equipment if they have enough cash, but a health club is only as good as its instructors. The problem is, anyone can also hang out a shingle and claim to be a personal trainer, massage therapist, or aerobics instructor. If you want to truly gauge how good the classes or personal instruction may be, ask about the background of their staff. Seeing any of the following acronyms either on their certification certificate or after their name—ACE, ACSM, AFAA, AFB, CIAR, CSCS, IFPA, NASM, NFPT, NSCA, NSCA-CPT, NIRSA—means they're certified with some of the more reputable exercise and fitness organizations, instead of some fly-by-night company.

INVEST IN YOURSELF

After you've picked your gym, try having a physical profile done either at the club—if they offer that service—or through your family doctor. Then, have another profile done after 3 months and compare the results. This way, you can see if your investment is truly paying off. If you don't, it's like throwing money into a stock portfolio and never getting a statement to tell you how you're doing.

CHAPTER THREE

WHAT TO LOOK FOR IN A CONTRACT

WHO WOULD EVER HAVE GUESSED THAT a piece of paper could be so scary?

Whether you're confronted with a 1-page sheet or a 15-page opus for a contract, it doesn't take away the unnerving feeling that somewhere, somehow, buried deep within all the legalese mumbo-jumbo are a few clever tricks meant to rip you off.

Not all gyms have contracts. And of the many that do, not all are out to get you. Sure, some are written in a way that may have you forfeiting your right to sue them if one of their trainers injures you. Or they could have a clause that lets them strip away services they promised you. Or worse yet, they could keep charging you—legally—long after your membership expires.

But that's okay. Now that you're reading this chapter, they can try all they want, but they won't succeed. Knowing the ins and outs of gym contracts won't just prevent you from being a victim of bad health clubs, but it can also make it easier to find the good health clubs that offer more than you would expect.

Here's how to dissect that contract—and get everything you deserve.

STEP ONE: LOOK FOR THE OBVIOUS TRICKS

They know you're interested when you walk in, but they also know you could change your mind the moment you step out their door. Or they know the competition down the street has more to offer you. Before you even ask to see a contract to take home and read, here are a few common tricks some gyms use to seal the deal before you have time to think straight. Watch out for these.

"Today-Only" Deals

Some gyms may offer you what they claim is a cheaper rate if you sign a contract that day. If that's the offer being presented to you, then walk away from the table. The price should always be the same for you today as it is for you tomorrow, so ask to take the contract home with you. In fact, in most cases, the longer you wait to sign their contract, the greater your odds of seeing a better break on your total membership costs. That's because—just like a used car salesman—they know that the longer you linger, the more likely you are to check out their competition in town.

Lifetime Memberships

Although not as common of a price ploy as they once were, lifetime memberships—where a club offers you a lifetime membership to their club for a "special" higher one-shot price—can still be found, and may seem like a great way to save money long-term. Not only is this a colossal waste of your money should you ever decide to quit, move away, or just not like working out there anymore, but the real catch is how they define "lifetime." These types of memberships are generally good for the lifetime of the club, not you! That means they could pack it up tomorrow and legally take all your money with them.

To protect yourself, check with your state Attorney General to see what your rights are—should any gym or club go belly-up where you live—by heading over to naag.org. In some states, such as Wisconsin, California, and Washington—lifetime contracts are illegal. However, in other states, the law may demand that a gym or health club post a bond for a certain amount of time. That way, if it goes belly-up within a certain period of time, you'll get your money back.

Rebates of Any Kind

Some gyms may offer you hundreds of dollars in "special rebates" for joining their facility. However, it's not cash they plan on giving you back, but coupons for services in their facility that you perhaps wouldn't use in the first place, such as discounts on personal training, massages, and nutritional consulting.

Any Asterisks in Their Ads

Many gyms try the ol' bait-and-switch when it comes to their ad prices. If you see an asterisk, chances are there's something wrong with the "terrific" deal they are presenting to you. That "special" price could be the cost of their "no-frills" package, it could apply only if you're willing to use their gym during their off-hours, and so on.

Believe it or not, some gyms presell memberships before their gym is even built. The benefit to you is that the club will offer a much lower rate for getting in on the ground floor. The risk is that you may not get what you pay for once the cement dries and the walls go up. You may be told how nice the club will look when it's done, but there's never a guarantee that it will have everything it promised.

Upfront Money Requests

No gym should ever ask you for your credit card information or a deposit before you've even had a chance to read the contract. It's entirely unnecessary, so if they do, there's your first clue that they are probably shady in many other areas as well. In that case, let your conscience be your guide, break for the door, and find another facility without wasting any more of your time.

STEP TWO: GIVE THE CONTRACT THE ONCE-OVER . . . AT HOME

Mortgage contracts. Marriage certificates. Those annoying agreements you say yes to whenever you download software updates onto your phone.

It's amazing how many things we say "yes" to without reading all the fine print, isn't it? But we have news for you. When it comes to a gym contract, you had better know what you're agreeing to before you even think of signing it. That means saying "no" to signing anything before you have the chance to take it home and read it over.

Unfortunately, there really isn't any standard gym contract; every contract is different, depending on the facility and what they have to offer. But we know what tricks—or perks—the one you bring home is most likely to have tucked inside it. Here are the big ones to pay attention to.

Bad Words to Watch For
FINANCE CHARGES

You may think you're paying only $600 to $700 total for the year, but if there are hidden finance charges buried in the contract, you could be liable for a lot more than you bargained for. Some gyms can whack you with up to

GET A PASS INSTEAD!

Don't feel like bothering with contracts? Hate being tied down to one gym or club? The American Health and Fitness Alliance (health-fitness.org) has what they call Fitness PassBooks. These voucher books cost less than $100 and give you hundreds of free admission passes to select health clubs in Chicago, Houston, Los Angeles, or New York for one full year. Every pass is good not just for one, but two visits, with some usable for an entire month. They also offer Yoga PassBooks and Pilates PassBooks that allow similar access to studios throughout each city.

18 to 20 percent extra when all is said and done. If you see any finance charges, do the math—the gym may not be as cheap over the long run as it seems to be in the short term.

AUTOMATIC TRANSFERS AND ROLLOVER POLICIES

Typically, when you join a club for a period of at least 12 months, the gym will set up your membership so they can either pull from your checking account or bill your credit card—unless you're rich enough to pay the membership in full on the first day, of course.

What gets tricky is that many contracts have an automatic renewal—or rollover—feature in them. Instead of ending your membership after the length of a contract, it gives the health club the right to automatically renew your membership and keep charging your account on a month-to-month basis until you finally tell them to stop.

Don't just assume that letting your membership run its course will leave you free and clear. Most gyms require that you provide written notice 30 days before the end of the contract—just like a landlord—but the rules can vary from place to place. If you don't see or understand the rules in the contract, ask specially about their "rollover" policy so you don't end up paying long after you've left the building.

Final tip: Even if everything looks good and you end up signing a contract with an automatic transfer in place, don't use your debit card—use your credit card, or pay month-to-month with a check—instead. Not only does that option offer more personal identity protection, but if there's ever an issue, you can ring the credit card company to have them either hold payment or reverse charges, a process that can be a lot more difficult to do with a bank.

Your odds of having to fight for money back are minimized even more if you just stick with doing something that may sound entirely archaic—and that's paying with checks. Will it probably get a laugh out of the twenty-something clerk you hand it to each month? Absolutely! But, that silly piece of paper protects you big-time. After all, your gym or club can't take your money if they don't have access to it, which means you'll never need to deal with your bank or credit card company if you're ever overcharged.

ANNUAL MEMBERSHIP FEE

Just like your cable or phone company, many gyms usually charge an initial activation fee in addition to the monthly fee you'll be paying each month. Sometimes, these fees are due at signing, stretched out through tacking them onto your monthly fee, or added in every few months at certain times.

It's normal, but since that fee can vary from gym to gym, you may want to ask yourself if that fee is a bit over-inflated. Even worse, some gyms try to get you to pay that same fee every year, calling it an "annual membership fee." If you see this, ask them what it's for—usually the excuse is routine maintenance, which is ridiculous.

In some instances, a high annual fee and maintenance fees are what allow a gym or club to advertise a relatively low month-to-month rate. It's the ol' bait-and-switch I mentioned above, where you're given a monthly price that seems reasonable, then told about the maintenance fees at the end of signing. Once added in, your "new" monthly fee may not be a bargain anymore, so remember what role it plays before you sign.

RESERVATION OF RIGHTS

What would you do if that "open 24 hours a day" gym that works well with your late-night schedule decided to limit its hours? Or what if you joined a gym for its free babysitting service while you worked out, and all of a sudden they canceled the program? This little phrase—when attached to any of the amenities the gym is promising to offer you—gives them the right to change its services later on. The problem is, you can't use those changes as an excuse to cancel.

WAIVER AND RELEASE

A lot of gyms ask that you sign a waiver when joining, which prevents you from finding them liable if you injure yourself using their equipment or you get hurt working with their personal trainers. It's not necessarily a bad word, since it's not uncommon to sign similar waivers for other activities, like using a climbing wall, going skydiving, or even joining a sports team, for example. But check this clause carefully to make sure it applies only to the equipment and services you're willingly going to use.

There are a few unscrupulous gyms that word their contracts in a way that prevents them from being sued for other injuries that aren't directly related to their equipment. You could be signing something that protects them from being sued if you injure yourself anywhere inside the gym—which could leave you powerless in court if you fall in their shower or get hit in the head by a piece of their ceiling. Even worse, it might even extend outside of the gym within a certain perimeter—which means you could be agreeing not to sue if you slip on ice in their parking lot, for example.

"BIG NUMBERS"

The last thing to look for has nothing to do with words, but relates to numbers—especially anything exceeding 3 years. By law, no gym or health club contract can obligate you for any longer than that.

Good Words to Watch For
BONDING

We discussed this earlier in this chapter when referring to lifetime memberships, but seeing that a gym has posted a bond—which is when they let the government hold a certain amount of money to protect gym members in case of fraud—is reassuring if you're thinking of signing up long-term (year to year). That way if they close up, you get a refund.

If the gym doesn't have a bond on file, there should still be a disclosure statement in the contract that advises you of that fact, so you're aware that you're taking a risk buying a long-term contract. If that's the case, and you still want to join, opt for a month-to-month plan in case they close up suddenly.

BUYER'S RIGHT TO CANCEL

Legally, you are typically entitled to 3 days—which can vary up to 5 days, depending on the state you live in—to change your mind after signing and end the contract without question. In some places, such as British Colum-bia, you have up to 10 days upon receiving a contract to cancel your membership for any reason.

In most places, a gym or club is then required by law to refund your money within 30 days of that date. If you cancel within that window, there should be no fee, although canceling after that deadline typically means you'll be paying a cancellation fee.

Just know that there are other rights that can be attached to this clause as well. A good contract should entitle you to be able to cancel should you move a certain distance away from the gym and you can't transfer the contract to a comparable facility—the average distance being around 25 miles—or if they forfeit offering all of the services they promised you at the start of the contract.

TRANSFER MEMBERSHIP

This option isn't as common to discover in the fine print, but seeing this phrase generally means you probably have the right to pass on whatever months are left of your paid membership to someone else. If you move or decide to leave the gym for some reason, you can either give the balance away to a friend or sell it off to someone else. To pull it off, just bring your friend (the buyer) to the gym and work with a manager to settle the details. But don't be surprised if there's a fee—sometimes there isn't one, but it could run as much as $50.

CANCELLATION UPON DEATH OR DISABILITY

If you care about your loved ones, then this clause is a must. That's because these five words protect your family from having to pay off your membership should something ever happen to you. It also protects you by letting you cancel your membership if you're ever injured and

BEFORE YOU SIGN . . . INVESTIGATE THOROUGHLY

We told you in the previous chapter that any reputable gym will allow you to test-drive their facility with a free day pass, right? That's not just your opportunity to exercise; it's also your chance to pick a few brains. Don't be afraid to use your free day in the gym to ask other members about their own experiences with the gym. Then, go home and check with your local chapter of the Better Business Bureau or your state attorney general's office to see if any complaints have ever been filed against the gym by unhappy former members. These agencies can also tell you all the laws regulating health club memberships in your state, so you can double-check to see if they match the contract.

have a doctor's excuse that orders you not to exercise for a certain amount of time.

STEP THREE: GO BACK TO THE GYM PREPARED

So, the contract has passed your home inspection and you're ready to take it back to the gym to sign it. Smart plan, but you're not done yet.

Don't just give it to whomever is staffing the front desk that day. Instead, ask to see the manager of the gym or a staff member who's capable of explaining fees, contractual issues, etc. Then you need to ask them these important questions if you couldn't find the answers on the contract itself.

What's My Cool-Off Period Once I Sign?

If you couldn't find anything in the contract about the "buyer's right to cancel," which gives you a certain number of days after you sign to cancel, no questions asked, come right out and ask what their policy is. Every state is different, but by law, you should be able to get a refund and cancel your contract within 3 to 5 days. Once you know their policy, ask for it to be written on the contract.

Can I Freeze My Membership?

Many states require gyms and health clubs to extend a consumer's membership if they can't use it due to a temporary injury, disability, or pregnancy. That means that some gyms may allow you to suspend your membership, so that you either pay less each month—or no monthly fee whatsoever—for the months it's frozen. That "freeze period" can range from an average minimum of 1 to 3 months, although in the case of pregnancy, it may extend as long as 9 months. Every club is different, so taking the time to see where they stand may help you save money in the future.

Can I Use My Membership Anywhere Else?

Certain memberships may let you use different clubs when you travel. Bigger gym chains that have several locations throughout the state—or country, depending on their size—may let you use any of their gyms for free once you're a member. Others may only offer you a "member discount" when using a facility somewhere else. Still, there are still a handful of chains—usually privately owned—that may not work that way. It's best to ask

if that matters to you, so you don't walk away assuming your membership works everywhere.

What Classes and Services Cost Extra?

Don't believe your eyes! In some gyms, not everything you see is available when you sign up. That interesting exercise class you walked past on the tour may be something you have to pay for à la carte, or that lap pool may cost an extra few bucks a month to use. The "financial policy" portion of the contract may not state it, but some gyms may charge more money for their more popular fitness classes or require an additional fee just to have a locker. To get them to reveal the "full" cost, act rich and just tell them that you want to have access to everything, then watch the numbers start to add up if there are additional fees they aren't telling you about.

Are You Running Any Special Promotions?

Thank everyone's New Year's resolution to get in shape, because January is typically the month many gyms offer discounts on membership specials. According to the International Health, Racquet & Sportsclub Association (IHRSA), 11 percent of all memberships are sold on average in January, but that doesn't mean they aren't running other deals throughout the year. That's because for the other 11 months of the year, most gyms only see single-digit sales in memberships, ranging from 8.9 percent to as low as 7.1 percent according to IHRSA. So when things slow down, that's when gyms and health clubs love to boost their numbers with deals that are harder to pass up.

If you come into the gym and don't mention a deal you saw in the paper, chances are they may not tell you about what specials they're running other times unless they feel they need to. If they don't have any current deals, but have one planned for a few months away, don't be afraid to ask them for that deal that day. If they say no, you can always opt to come back when the promotion finally begins.

How Often Do Your Rates Go Up?

Be sure to ask how much their rates have gone up over the past few years to make sure it's nothing too shocking. Then ask if your contract locks you into a certain monthly fee until your contract runs out.

Some contracts let you lock in a monthly rate for the length of your membership, while others have an "exceptions" clause that lets them increase dues whenever they feel the need, making your old monthly agreement obsolete.

GO BACK TO SCHOOL—SORT OF!

If you're a college grad and still live close by to your alma mater, being a former graduate could grant you access to your former college or university's gym for far less than joining a traditional health club. Most higher education institutions grant a discount to their alumni for a year-round membership, or allow alumni to purchase day passes to use certain facilities at certain times.

This little "exceptions" clause can generally be taken out before you sign up—if they know it's a deal breaker for you.

What Happens If I Decide to Quit?

As we mentioned earlier in this chapter, you should be allowed to cancel your membership if you end up moving more than 25 miles away (on average) or suffer an injury that prevents you from exercising. There are even a few facilities that will let you terminate your contract if you lose your job. But unfortunately, a few gyms out there aren't so accommodating. Some gyms charge a cancellation fee if you need to break the contract. That's why you need to know what the worst-case scenario is, should you ever decide to call it quits.

In your contract, there should be something related to "Cancellation" or "Termination" that spells out exactly what you have to do. Most clubs ask for at least a 30- to 60-day notice in writing to cancel, but this differs from place to place. And if you're wondering why they need 1 to 2 months notice, just like a landlord, there's no justification behind it—it's all about the money. See, making you wait that long after you've decided you're done means they get an extra month or two of fees from you, and odds are, you won't even be there using their gym during that time—it's a win-win.

The key is to find out "exactly" what you need to do in order to leave. Sometimes a gym or club won't accept your cancellation unless it's sent by certified mail. Or it may require you to meet with someone face-to-face—like a manager—which essentially gives them one last opportunity to woo you back and keep you on board. In some cases, you may need to present proof of relocation (such as a utility bill, a lease, or even a letter from human resources where you're employed) to prove you've moved. They may even require a letter from your physician, should your reason for cancelling be for medical reasons. Just be sure all the rules are spelled out on the contract

and that you're comfortable with them before you sign.

Final note: Some gyms and clubs may let you cancel your membership at any time, and that may sound fantastic and effortless, but ask if there's a charge and how that fee works. Most implement a prorated fee where you're charged a percentage of your monthly dues, while being allowed access to the gym for a certain amount of days.

How Long Have You Been in Business?

It's important to know that the gym you're joining isn't going to have an "office space for rent" sign on it the next month. Knowing how long they've been in business can give you some peace of mind that the owners know how to make ends meet. But don't think this question just applies to the smaller, individually owned gyms. Owners of larger brand-name gyms—like a Gold's Gym or a Planet Fitness, for example—pay a fee to buy into a major gym franchise. That doesn't always mean their gym will be successful enough to stay afloat.

Which Day of the Month Are My Dues Owed?

Even if you're using an automatic payment system to handle your fees each month, knowing the exact day the gym expects to be paid for next month's changes is helpful. Why? Because some gyms charge you extremely high late fees and/or may deny you access if you're a day late and a dollar short.

Whom Would I Speak to If I Had a Problem?

It's nice to know ahead of time how complaints are typically handled. Some facilities require you to speak with the owner, who may conveniently never be around. Other chains may ask you to file a complaint online or call a customer service number, which could lead you to a dead end that doesn't resolve your issue. So don't be afraid to ask who handles any issues that might arise.

That way, you'll know exactly whom to go to if/when they do or if the process is so convoluted that it may be smarter to go with the gym or club on the next block.

Can I Get a Month-to-Month Contract?

Paying month to month is almost always more expensive than signing up for a year-long contract, but you could end up saving money in the long run if you're still on the fence about your commitment to exercise and/or that particular gym. If the gym doesn't work out, you can cut your losses without owing them for months on end. If you stick with it for 6 months without fail, it'll have cost you roughly $40 to $70 more than if you had signed a 1-year deal, but at least you'll know it's the right gym for you.

Can I Sleep on It?

Even if the manager has jumped through every hoop for you, answered every single one of your questions, and has presented you with every answer you were hoping to hear—tell them you'll be back tomorrow. Reason being: There may be one final question you forgot to ask or you may be more aware of something you didn't like but neglected to notice right away. In any case, waiting a day or two to sign a contract is always a smart move and may put you in a better position to negotiate when you come back.

STEP FOUR: GET THE LAST LAUGH

The contract is perfect. You're absolutely certain you want to join. But that doesn't mean they have to know that, so you can strike a better deal. They will never tell you this, but many gym membership rates are negotiable. Just like a car salesman, the manager typically has approval to charge any price to sign you up, so long as they don't go lower than a certain predetermined rate. They may even eliminate your startup fee, give you an extra month for free, or even offer you services that you typically pay extra for—if you know how to play them.

Here's how to always land the best deal every time.

Show No Interest In Anything

The less they know about what you really need from a gym, the harder you are for them to read. For example, if they know you're a swimmer and they have the only pool in town, they know you're not really shopping around and have an edge over you. Instead, be smart and don't show any personal interest in anything as you take the tour of the gym and see what they have to offer. It can give you a slight edge when it's time to negotiate later on.

Bring Some Numbers

To prepare yourself, call other gyms to compare prices, or ask other members what they paid to join when you take your one-day test-drive—whatever tactic gives you a few cheaper prices to throw at them when it's time to sign. Then try using those numbers at the very end of talking with the manager as a way to negotiate the price down just a little. The more they know you're aware of what other options you have—meaning the other gyms and clubs they compete against—the more likely you'll be to strike a better deal with them.

Know Their Competitors

They could try to convince you that you won't get the same amenities and services at other gyms. Remember when we told you to call other clubs to find out their fees? Do yourself a favor and also ask them what services and amenities they offer and have that list with you—that way, you'll know when they're throwing you a line, and you can call them on it.

Get It in Ink

Sure, you've got the manager making you all sorts of promises today, but what happens when he's working somewhere else tomorrow? Before you sign your name to

AFTER YOU SIGN . . . KNOW YOUR RIGHTS

If your gym decides to ignore the terms of your contract, take it directly to the gym's manager. If they can't—or won't—help you, then contact your state attorney general's office and/or file a complaint against them with the Federal Trade Commission (877-FTC-HELP or ftc.gov).

a contract because of the promise of a better deal, make sure that deal is in writing first.

Look for the Handouts

That gym manager wants your business and knows you probably have options—so don't be afraid to ask for a few free guest privileges that may not be part of your contract. It never hurts to inquire about seeing if the manager can throw in something right then and there, such as a free personal training session, a few specialized classes that aren't part of your package, or a limited-time pass to areas of the gym you won't be able to access later. Just tell them that if they throw in a few bonuses, it's a done deal—plus, experiencing these perks now may motivate you to bump up your membership later.

Go Food Shopping Before You Sign

You know the numbers. You've struck the best deal. Now, excuse yourself and head to a Costco, Sam's Club, or any local bulk retailer to see if they can beat it. Believe it or not, these type of stores actually sell 1- or 2-year gym memberships to major gym/club franchises (such as 24 Hour Fitness, Planet Fitness, or World Gym) at a price well below—many times between 25 percent to 70 percent below—what you may get by signing up directly at the gym.

CHAPTER FOUR

LITTLE THINGS MEAN A LOT

THERE'S MORE TO A GYM THAN just big, expensive machines.

When you first walk into a commercial gym, there's an awful lot of stuff to take in. Endless rows of cardio equipment, a bunch of expensive-looking machines, and free weights as far as the eye can see. From barbells, dumbbells, and kettlebells to a bevy of other strength-training equipment that doesn't end in "bell," such as sandbags, power sleds, suspension equipment, and battle ropes.

Throw in some of the beautiful bodies you're bound to see prancing around, and it's easy to miss some of the finer details. Things like weight collars and stability balls don't usually garner much attention when there's so much more impressive visual stimuli to focus on. The truth is, these and some of the other less glamorous things you'll find lying around the gym can often have a huge impact on your workout.

So, before we teach you about all of the state-of-the-art equipment you might encounter, we're going to make sure you know how to use all the little stuff. Because even though some of it may seem pretty insignificant now, down the road this is the kind of information you're going to be glad you have. Nothing can interrupt the flow of a workout more than wondering what a certain handle is for or trying to figure out how to adjust a bench to the appropriate level. It's like they say: The devil is in the details. And the quicker you figure out those details, the faster your results are going to come.

WEIGHT COLLARS

They're the little clamps that fit onto a barbell to secure weights in place. Why are they important? Well, for one thing, they keep the weights on the bar, which is helpful if you would like to avoid any embarrassing and potentially dangerous accidents if you lose your balance during a lift.

Collars come in a variety of shapes and sizes, each attaching to the bar by twisting, clamping, or bolting onto it. But the basic premise is that they're for keeping weight plates on the barbell where they belong and not all over the floor or worse, on someone else's foot. Besides their safety implications, losing your balance on a lift like

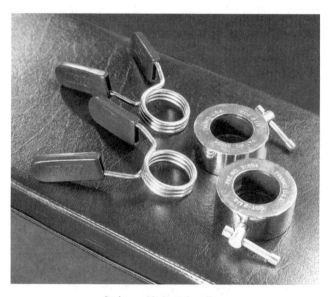

Spring and bolt-style collars

a squat or bench press without collars on the bar can cause the weights to fall suddenly off one side and then the other. This sudden weight shift can easily cause you to become injured, to say nothing of the indignity you'll suffer if the weights do end up falling off the bar. Nothing screams "geek" like a bunch of weights crashing to the floor.

Your gym may have one (or a combination) of the following styles:

- **The classic spring collar:** This looks exactly as it sounds—like a spring. Simply squeeze its two handles together to loosen the spring, then once it's in place, you let go and it clamps around the bar. It weighs practically nothing and is fairly easy to take on and off.

- **Threaded collar:** This kind spins around the bar like a nut around a screw as you turn it. However, it only works with a bar that is threaded as well, so don't expect it to work on a smooth bar.

- **Bolt-style collar:** This type uses an adjusting knob sticking out from the collar. As you turn it, the bolt presses into the bar—or tightens the collar around the bar, depending on the style.

- **Clamp-style collar:** As advertised, once you slide this collar on the bar, you push down on a small piece of plastic that snaps it onto the bar—think of how a ski boot snaps into a ski.

WEIGHTED VESTS

No, it's not a life jacket—and if it was, you would sink pretty quickly to the bottom of the pool. These vests allow you to add resistance to your body that can range in increments of 10 pounds, 20 pounds, up to 40 pounds. Why would you want to do that? Well, there's only one problem with building bigger muscles while blasting fat. The leaner and stronger you get, the easier it becomes to perform body-weight exercises such as pullups, chinups, dips, squats, and lunges, to mention a few. These vests let you work out at a heavier body weight than you're currently packing, which can let you train your muscles in a progressive fashion.

They're also adjustable, allowing you to increase or decrease the amount of resistance from 1 to 20 pounds or 1 to 40 pounds using ¼- to 1-pound weighted rods or sacks, depending on the model of the vest. To keep one in place,

they rely on fully adjustable Velcro straps that wrap around your waist. Some even allow other portions of the vest to adjust via Velcro for a customized fit along your torso. No matter which brand your gym has, they all are designed to hug your body without restricting your range of motion.

PLYO BOXES

Available in multiple heights that can range from as little as 6 inches up to 42 inches (they generally increase in height by increments of 6 inches, so think 12 inches, 18 inches, 24 inches, 30 inches, and 36 inches), plyo boxes are more commonly found in gyms or clubs that are more sports-minded. Why? Because these elevated platforms allow you to pull off a variety of jumping exercises that help build leg strength, boost your vertical jumping ability, increase foot speed, and improve your cardiovascular endurance.

They are typically stackable (nesting into each other to save space), made from metal or wood able to sustain at least 300 pounds, and have a nonslip rubber surface so they stay put as you leap.

STABILITY BALLS

These brightly colored orbs can usually be found in the core/stretching area, or perhaps even corralled up in the area reserved for exercise classes. Don't let this fool you though—these babies can be used all over the gym. In addition to enabling you to perform a multitude of different core exercises, stability balls can also be used during dynamic warmups, to help improve flexibility, and even in place of a bench on certain strength exercises like dumbbell bench presses and flies. You'll find a bunch of really unique and challenging exercises you can do with stability balls in Chapter Seven.

To make sure you're working with the appropriate-size ball, sit on it and check your knee angle. If the ball is fully inflated and you have an approximately 90-degree bend in your knees, it's the right size for you. Using a ball that's either too big or too small can end up causing faulty exercise execution and may lead to injury.

Another way to eyeball it is to read the side of the ball for its dimensions. More than likely, that measurement will be in centimeters, so when you're picking out a ball, here are the numbers to know about:

- **If you're below 4 feet 6 inches tall:** Look for a 30 cm ball.

- **If you're between 4 feet 6 inches and 5 feet:** Grab a 45 cm ball.
- **If you're between 5 feet and 5 feet 6 inches:** Pick a 55 cm ball.
- **If you're between 5 feet 6 inches and 6 feet 2 inches:** Choose a 65 cm ball.
- **If you're 6 feet 2 inches or taller:** You need a 75 cm ball.

MEDICINE BALLS

Back in the old days these were big, hulking leather spheres stitched together with shoelaces that only the biggest guys in the gym dared pick up. Today they come in far more user-friendly sizes and colors and have a wide variety of uses. They're great for adding resistance to core exercises and for getting your body limbered up prior to training. You can also use them for all sorts of throwing exercises to develop explosive power—that is, provided you have adequate room and someone willing to catch for you.

Medicine balls can range in weight between as little as 1 pound up to 50-plus pounds, but which size you should choose depends entirely on the exercise you're doing, how many reps you're hoping to perform, and your individual strength level. No matter what the situation, what's most important is that you can handle the ball comfortably with both hands.

Just don't be shocked to see a medicine ball with built-in handles. These dual-grip medicine balls make it easier to pull off either one- or two-hand exercises, although one of the benefits of a traditional med ball—sans handles—is that they work your hands and forearms indirectly just to maintain a grip. The handled variety are also trickier to perform throwing and/or

catching exercises with, since your fingers can sometimes get jammed when trying to catch one, and the handles make it harder to predict where the ball will rebound if thrown against the floor or a sturdy wall.

WRIST ROLLERS

This short bar with a rope attached to its middle may look unassuming, but it's essential if your goal is building impressive Popeye-like forearms and a vise-like grip. By adding weight to the end of the rope—either a weight plate or even a dumbbell, depending on the attachment at the end of the rope—all you do is stand up on a box or bench, hold the bar down by your waist, then roll it so that the weight rises up to meet the bar. This simple tool strengthens both your forearm flexors and extensors (see Chapter Five for more details about these mighty muscles), along with the muscles throughout your hands.

ADJUSTABLE FREESTANDING BENCHES

Without question, these are amongst the most useful pieces of equipment in the entire gym. These benches allow you to do any number of exercises from a wide array of angles. All it takes is the pull of a pin or the adjustment of a simple lever for you to go from a flat to an incline or decline position. You can usually find these over in the free-weight section near the dumbbell racks, but most have wheels and can easily be transported across the gym floor for use inside of cable stations, squat racks, and power cages.

PLATE MATES

Not every gym has them, but these little magnetized discs certainly have

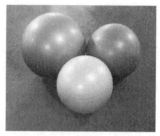
Stability Balls

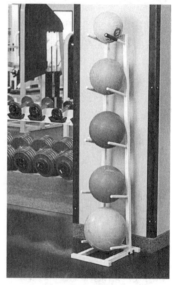
Medicine Balls

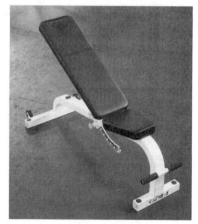
Adjustable Freestanding Bench

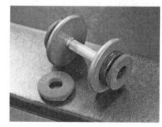
Plate Mate

a lot to offer. In most cases, once the dumbbells get past 20 pounds, they start increasing by 5 pounds instead of by 2½-pound increments. Sometimes, you're just not ready to make that kind of jump. If you just barely got your last rep with the 50-pound dumbbells, for instance, going all the way up to 55 pounds per side represents a 10 percent increase in weight. For some people, that might just be too much. So what can you do if you still want to increase the load a little bit without overtaxing yourself?

By simply attaching a couple of plate mates to the end of the dumbbells, you can go up by 1¼ to 2½ pounds per side. It may not sound like much, but this more manageable increase in load just might be enough to allow you to continue to progress, rather than give into the frustration of being stuck continuously lifting the same amount of weight week after week. It's called microloading, and as any serious lifter will tell you, it's the key to big-time gains. Even if you're not into increasing strength per se, plate mates can still be an incredibly valuable training tool in your arsenal.

BAR PADS

Usually found over by the squat rack or Smith machine, these padded tubes are for wrapping around the bar to make squats and other exercises where you rest the bar on your upper back more comfortable. Believe it or not, not everyone enjoys the feeling of a loaded barbell digging into their upper trapezius muscle. Another option to consider, if your gym has one, is called the Manta Ray. To use it, simply snap the bar into the groove and then step under it as you rest this oddly shaped blue wedge on your upper trapezius. It gives you a much more biomechanically correct feel than placing a pad on your back.

BODY BARS

In case you're a little intimidated by the iron barbells, these foam-coated bars offer a kinder, gentler way of adding some resistance to your workouts. Ranging in weight anywhere from 4 to 27 pounds, these color-coded bars are covered in a soft foam padding, making them much more comfortable for both gripping and resting on your upper back during various lower-body exercises. They're particularly great for women and teens and a great learning tool for advanced barbell exercises like squats and deadlifts.

WOBBLE BOARDS, DYNA DISCS, AND BOSUS

If your gym is really well stocked, you may notice some people balancing on various types of boards and air-filled discs. Or maybe you've seen others doing different types of core drills and balancing exercises on a bright blue orb with one flat side. While some of the exercises may look more like something you see in a circus rather than a commercial gym, rest assured that these devices aren't without merit. All of them can help you improve balance and coordination in slightly different ways.

Physical therapists use balance boards for rehabbing lower-body injuries, but they can also make some staple gym lifts much more challenging. Doing a squat on a wobble board, for instance, requires you to use your core a lot more and forces all those little stabilizing muscles in the legs to snap to attention to keep you from losing your balance. Be sure to try these without weight at first, though. Dyna Discs work much the same way, except for the fact that since they're filled with air, the surface is that much more unstable. This causes the muscles of the lower leg and foot to fire like crazy to hold your position as you perform the exercise. It's great for those of you with chronically weak ankles.

BOSUs are probably the most popular of the lot because they share some of the properties of both the balance boards and the discs. Place the flat side down and you can do an endless array of core exercises, along with various types of lunges and step-overs. Flip it over and it becomes a real challenge to balance on when doing pushups and squats. With that kind of versatility, it's no wonder you see entire classes built around this unique training device.

AB WHEELS

At first you might be surprised to see such a rudimentary training device in a fully equipped gym. Give it a try, though, and you'll soon find why many gym owners consider it an absolute must (pun intended). All you do here is kneel down and grab hold of the handles as you allow the wheel to roll forward, straightening out your torso as you go. How far out you get depends on the strength and stability of your torso and shoulders. After reaching your farthest point, you then use those same muscles to roll the wheel back into the starting position. You really adventurous types who have the strength can even try it on your feet instead of your knees. Be careful though, since this is an extremely advanced version.

TRACTOR TIRES

If your gym looks like it's storing a few extra tires for John Deere, it's probably a gym that enjoys having a few unconventional strength building tools within its inventory. Tractor tires are great for building functional power, explosive strength, and serious endurance by performing primarily tire flips or tire drags or by hitting one with a sledgehammer. The weight can range from as little as 100 pounds up to 500 pounds. (We've seen them lower and higher than those numbers, but that range is fairly consistent with most gyms on average.)

FOAM ROLLERS

Look closely in whatever part of your gym has been designated as the stretching area and you're likely to spy a series of different-size round tubes that look more like pool toys than exercise equipment. These cylindrical pieces of foam make it possible to pull off a technique known as self-myofascial release—a fancy name for self-massage. In layman's terms, they let you apply pressure to your muscles by gently rolling specific body parts back and forth overtop of the tube, which helps make them as pliable as possible. This technique also aids in recovery after a hard workout by improving circulation to your muscles and breaking up knots and scar tissue.

WEIGHT-LIFTING CHAINS

And by chains, we mean actual heavy-duty chains that you could purchase at a hardware store—although some manufacturers do make variations that attach to a weight bar. Why would a gym have something that looks more helpful for towing a boat or pulling a trailer? Because they help add what's known as "linear variable resistance" throughout the range of an exercise.

You see, with certain exercises—such as bench presses, military presses, deadlifts, or squats using a barbell, for example—the easiest portion of the movement is always at the top (when your arms or legs are straight). Looping over or attaching a heavy chain over each end of the bar (letting the balance of each chain rest on the floor) changes all that. As you straighten your arms or legs and raise the bar, you end up pulling more and more of the chain off the floor, which adds more weight as you go.

As you can see, taking the time to familiarize yourself with some of the lower profile pieces of equipment in the gym can be well worth the effort. Treadmills and stair-climbers and elaborate machines may get all the attention, but it's often the little things that will have the biggest impact on your workout. These are not exactly the kind of stuff they show you when you first sign up, but the sooner you become acquainted with some of these indispensable training aids, the better off you'll be.

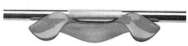

Manta Ray

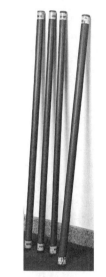

Body Bar

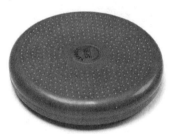

Dyna DISC

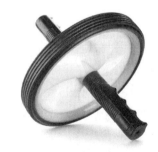

Ab Wheels

PART TWO

GYM RESISTANCE PROGRAMS

CHAPTER FIVE

THE WHERE, WHAT, AND HOW GUIDE TO YOUR MUSCLES

EVERYONE KNOWS WHICH MUSCLES THEY WANT to improve, but being in shape isn't about picking favorites.

To be in the best shape possible—and please, if that's not why you're reading this book, then you're obviously in deep denial—you can't leave a single stone unturned. It doesn't matter to us if your goal is losing 10, 20, or 100 pounds or adding 10, 20, or 100 pounds to your bench press, or whether your aim is improving your backhand or trying to get back the body you once had. Focusing on every muscle group in your body from head to toe—and not just the random body parts that you want to change—is the smartest and fastest way to reach your fitness objective.

Not sure which stone to start with first? That's okay. Read this chapter and you'll begin to understand why every exercise and routine we've laid out for you later in this book is exactly what you need to maximize your gym experience.

MIDSECTION

Everyone could use a smaller, leaner middle, but your body is more concerned about the strength of your waistline and not just the amount of fat around it. How hard or fast you can pull, swing, or throw all depends on the transferred power that occurs whenever you twist your torso.

Conditioning the abdominal and lower back muscles together—affectionately known as your core muscles or "core musculature"—helps your waist deliver more twisting power whenever you need it. More important, it lowers your risk of injury by realigning your spine, a postural perk that helps all of your muscles work more efficiently with each other, preventing unnecessary stress on overused joints or muscles.

If you're more concerned about your looks—and who isn't?—then sculpting a strong, flat stomach still takes the right diet and cardiovascular exercise to shave off excess calories and fat. However, conditioning your core muscles can help them look more impressive once you've lost the weight. Plus, the stronger these muscles are, the easier it is for them to prevent you from the slouching that makes your stomach look bigger by pushing it outward.

Unfortunately, most people typically leave their core muscles out of balance, either from spending too much time doing crunches for their abs or running to lose weight (which tightens up the lower back muscles). Strengthening both muscle groups equally can correct this muscular imbalance. That's exactly what the exercises recommended in Part Two will do for you, but knowing which muscles you're working and why will help you get more from them when the time comes.

Rectus Abdominis

Where you'll find it: The truth is, despite its name, the "six-pack" muscles aren't six muscles at all, but one long sheet of muscle called the rectus abdominus. This broad, thin group of fibers extends vertically between your pubis and your ribcage.

What it does: It's this muscle that's responsible for flexing your spinal column, bringing the rib cage and the pelvis toward each other. To picture that, it's what you're doing when you perform a crunch. This muscle also assists in bending your body to the side and stabilizing your trunk when your head is raised when lying down.

Something to keep in mind: If you're wondering how some people have a six-pack when this muscle is really just one muscle, there's a reason for that. You have three strips of tendons that run across the rectus abdominus that protect and stabilize it over your intestines. There's also another tendon that goes down the rectus abdominus. These horizontal and vertical tendons cross over each other and create lines overtop your rectus abdominus—dividing it into the six-pack you're hoping to see one day.

Obliquus Abdominis

Where you'll find them: Most people know these muscles, but call them by their other nickname—the love handles. Attached to your rib cage down to your pelvis, your "handles" are actually a pair of muscles called the external and internal obliques. Your external obliques lie diagonally down from your lower ribs to your pelvis and pubic bone, while your internal obliques are tucked below your external obliques, lying diagonally to them.

What they do: Together, your internal and external obliques are the muscles that let you rotate from side to side. They also assist in lateral flexion, which is a big word that means bending to the side.

Something to keep in mind: No matter what you've read or what you've been told, you can't burn off your love handles by just doing a lot of the rotation and twisting exercises that work them. These types of moves are terrific for improving your core stability and developing the muscles beneath any fat you may have—as you'll discover when we show you some of the best ways to do so in this book—but if one of your goals is losing your love handles, watching your diet and burning excess calories using the routines in this book is the most effective way to get them to disappear for good.

Transverse Abdominis

Where you'll find it: This thin muscle layer runs deep below the rest of your abdominal muscles, stretching from your lower ribs to your pubic bone.

What it does: It's the muscle that helps you look good on command. Its official job is to contract your abdominal wall in toward your spine—basically, to suck your gut in. It also protects your internal organs from injury and helps you push out air.

Something to keep in mind: Despite how often we count on this muscle to pull in our bellies in front of the mirror, it's also the hardest abdominal muscle to focus on. But don't worry. We'll show you how to target it while working other muscles, using techniques we'll teach you in later chapters.

Erector Spinae

Where you'll find them: The erector spinae—or spinal erectors—are two deep muscles that run along both sides of the spinal column, starting at the back of the occipital bone (the back part of the skull) to the pelvis.

What they do: Together, both erectors extend your spine—or in other words, straighten your body back up whenever you bend it forward. They also let you arch your spine backward. When you're not busy leaning forward or bending backward, they help support your spinal column on a continual basis.

Something to keep in mind: How hard or fast you can pull, swing, or throw all rely on transferred power that comes from twisting your torso. Shoring up your lower back muscles can reinforce your core so your waist can deliver more twisting power when you need it.

CHEST AND UPPER BACK

Throughout this book, you'll notice we've paired up the muscles of the chest with the muscles that make up your back. Why would we do something like that? To make sure you develop the best body possible, that's why!

You see, most people stay true to the muscles they see in front of them and ignore the ones the mirror doesn't reveal. It's this kind of neglect that can lead to muscular imbalance. Developing your back muscles can help accentuate the chest muscles that lie in front, making all parts involved appear more impressive from all sides instead of just from one angle. But it's not just about how your muscles look, it's more about how they work together to prevent problems down the road that's important.

Not working your back as often as your chest leaves one side stronger than the other. This can cause overdeveloped fibers to pull against underutilized ones, setting you up for tendonitis, impingement, postural problems, and exercise-related injuries over time. It's this muscular unevenness that can hold you back performance-wise as well.

Thinking of your chest and back as two areas that both deserve equal attention may help you remember to work both sides of your body evenly. But don't worry. If you forget, the programs in this book will always train your back and chest equally.

Pectoralis Major

Where you'll find them: You probably already refer to your chest as a pair, which is exactly what it is, since it's composed of two separate muscle groups. The pectoralis major stretches across your chest in a fan shape, starting wide at the center of your body, then tapers together at the side of your body to attach into the top of the humerus (the bone in your upper arm). The pectoralis minor—a thinner, more triangular muscle that lies beneath your pectoralis major—starts along your ribs and also connects to your humerus.

What they do: Together, the pectoralis major and pectoralis minor are responsible for rotating your upper arms and moving them across your body horizontally, as well as flexing your shoulder joints.

Something to keep in mind: To really work your chest, you have to use a variety of exercises that position your arms at different angles above and across your chest. That's why you'll notice this book recommends a wide range of chest exercises—from moves that require you to lie on flat, incline, and decline benches (which change the angle of your arms), as well as various fly moves, cable crossovers, and dip moves.

Latissimus Dorsi

Where you'll find them: Located on both sides of your body, the latissimus dorsi—the largest muscles of your back—are a set of fan-shaped muscles that start from the upper end of the humerus (upper arm bone) and run down to attach low on your vertebral column and pelvic girdle.

What they do: The "lats," as they are commonly called, play a huge role in how your body functions. The main job is to pull your arm down toward your pelvis—

which is what you're doing whenever you perform any rowing motion. But, when your arm is fixed (for example, when you do a chinup), your lats work to bring your body up toward your arm. The lats also help stabilize your torso during many other exercises, plus help to rotate your upper arm internally, which plays a big part in giving you that extra snap of power whenever you punch or throw. Each of these jobs gets a little help from the teres major—a smaller muscle that runs from the outer edge of the scapula (shoulder blade) to the humerus.

Something to keep in mind: Nearly all of the exercises that work your lats also involve your biceps to some degree. That can be a problem for some people, especially if your biceps tire out before your back muscles get a chance to get a good workout. Whenever you use any of the exercises in this book that work your lats, try wrapping your thumbs on the same side as your fingers so that your hands "hook" the handles instead of grab them. This variation makes it harder for the biceps to get involved and can be used with any pulling or rowing exercise for the back.

Trapezius

Where you'll find it: The trapezius is a long, triangle-shaped muscle that starts at the base of the skull and attaches itself to the back of the collarbone and shoulder blades. If you've ever given anyone a neck massage, it's the meaty part that's easier to knead between the neck and shoulders.

What it does: This muscle is behind many of the movements you do all day long, including scapular elevation (a fancy term for shrugging your arms up), scapular depression (which means pulling your shoulder blades down), and scapular adduction (pulling your shoulder blades together).

Something to keep in mind: Underneath your trapezius muscle are the rhomboids, a set of tinier muscles that also help with scapular adduction. Giving them equal attention—either by strengthening them on their own or tweaking certain rowing exercises to get them involved—can keep them strong and supportive and your shoulder pain-free.

SHOULDERS AND ARMS

Having an amazing back and a powerful chest may seem ideal, but without a strong set of shoulders and arms to work with first, you'll never build either to their full potential. Because of their connection with other muscles, a set of strong shoulders can give you extra strength in almost every exercise you use to train your chest and back, along with moves that build your triceps and biceps.

But their importance doesn't just stop there. The broader your shoulders, the smaller your waist looks in proportion, creating the illusion that you have a smaller stomach than you actually have. Your shoulders also share the responsibility for pulling your arms back behind your body, giving you extra power when you're swimming, rowing, and performing other activities.

The muscles of your upper arm are equally important, but not just so you can have impressive muscles popping out under your sleeves. The biceps and triceps are both secondary muscle groups that assist during other multijointed exercises that work larger muscle groups. That's why your biceps also feel fatigued whenever you train your back, and your triceps get a workout whenever you train your chest and shoulders. Keeping the muscles in your upper and lower arms equally strong can prevent them from giving up on you before they should, bringing you even better gains when training your chest, back, and shoulders.

Deltoids

Where you'll find them: These are the muscles that create the round shape of your shoulders. What you may not know is that this one muscle is divided into three separate parts—anterior, medial, and posterior. The anterior and medial deltoids begin at your collarbone, while the posterior deltoid starts on your shoulder blade (otherwise known as your scapula). All three come together and attach themselves to your upper arm bone (also known as the humerus).

What they do: Together, all three muscles help move your arms away from your body. However, each deltoid also has its own distinct job. The anterior deltoid (located in the front) raises your arms up in front of you. The medial deltoid (the muscle that makes up the sides of your shoulders) lifts your arms up and out to your sides. Finally, the posterior deltoid (located in back of your shoulder) raises your arms up and behind your body.

Something to keep in mind: The reason most people don't have a set of impressive shoulders is that they overtrain—and undertrain them—simultaneously. The

reason: Most people tend to do a lot of exercises for their chest—which also works the front and sides of your shoulders—while they ignore doing any exercises at all for the back of their shoulders. To build a perfect set of shoulders, you need to use a variety of exercises that hit all three of the deltoids equally.

Rotators

Where you'll find them: The rotator cuff muscles—the teres minor, the infraspinatus, the supraspinatus, and the subscapularis—are a small series of muscles found deep below your deltoid.

What they do: Their main job is to stabilize your shoulder joint by keeping tension on your upper arm bone. But they're also the muscles that let you rotate your arms inward and outward. They even take part in helping your deltoids raise your arms out from your sides.

Something to keep in mind: Even though they're not mirror muscles that people train for appearance' sake, the rotators are a crucial area to pay attention to, especially if you want to forsake any shoulder problems in the future. One of the most common causes of shoulder trauma usually comes from straining or tearing the rotator cuff muscles. Keeping all four healthy can keep shoulder pain at bay, letting you lift more and perform at your best.

Biceps Brachii

Where you'll find them: C'mon now! Even the most exercise illiterate person knows this instantly flexible muscle. But in case your memory's a bit foggy, it's the muscle right in front of your upper arm. If you've ever wondered where it got its name, that's because your biceps actually have "two" heads, which is where the prefix "bi" comes from.

What they do: Your biceps bend your arm at the elbow and they also supinate your forearm. In other words, the biceps rotate your forearm so that your palm faces up.

Something to keep in mind: Your biceps aren't meant to work all by themselves, which is why using only exercises that isolate them—like barbell or dumbbell curls, for example—only go so far to help reshape them. If you really want to see results, the smarter plan is to also combine compound exercises—like pullups and rows—which use your biceps as supporting muscles. But don't worry, the routines we recommend in this book have your biceps's best interests in mind.

Triceps Brachii

Where you'll find them: The triceps—which make up the back of your upper arm—is made up of three separate muscles: the lateral head, the long head, and the medial head. The lateral head forms the outside of your triceps and makes up most of the horseshoe shape of your triceps. The long head forms the inside of your upper arm, while the medial head rests underneath the long head and adds to its shape.

What they do: All three heads work together to extend the elbow, which is what you're doing every time you straighten your arm from a bent position.

Something to keep in mind: It doesn't matter if you're looking to make your triceps bigger and stronger or just to keep them from jiggling back there—you still need to give each of the three heads their due. You see, there are many exercises that work your triceps, but most don't work all three heads. Sticking with a mix of moves that train all three heads equally can help you get better results in a shorter amount of time.

Brachialis

Where you'll find it: This broad, flat tendon is wedged between your upper arm bone and your biceps.

What it does: It assists your biceps whenever you move your forearm toward your shoulder, but only when your palms are facing in toward your body or downward.

Something to keep in mind: Just because you can't see it doesn't mean giving this tiny muscle its due isn't worth your time. Building up your brachialis leaves it no choice but to push against your biceps, making them look larger and more cut than they actually are.

Forearm Muscles

Where you'll find them: They're all the muscles that make up your forearms, the area between your elbow and your hand. The forearm extensors are on the outside of your forearm (where hair grows) while the forearm flexors are on the inside of your forearm. The last muscle in the mix is the brachioradialis, found up around your elbow.

What they do: The extensors extend your wrist backward, while the flexors curl your wrist forward. Meanwhile, the brachioradialis assists your brachialis in curling your arm up.

Something to keep in mind: You're only as strong as your weakest link, which is why strengthening these oft-neglected muscles can play a huge role in helping you build up other larger muscles.

LOWER BODY

These muscles decide how high you jump, how fast you can run, and how good you'll look when it's time to break out the shorts. With all that pressure riding on your legs, it's easy to see why the muscles below your waist require as much attention as the ones above it. Although a lot of the exercises and machines we'll show you in this book can target specific muscles within your legs, many of these moves also recruit other muscle groups within your legs to help out.

Just as we've grouped the muscles of your back and chest together to help you understand muscular balance, it's equally important to train both sides of your legs evenly. Overtraining one side more than the other can cause the stronger, tighter muscles of that side to pull your knees out of balance, as well as affect your stride. This may not seem like a big deal, but if fat loss is also on your agenda, the slightest imbalance in your stride is the #1 reason most people experience unnecessary aches, pains, and injuries that cut their aerobic workouts short. The programs in this book will keep your aerobic routine from being victimized, training all of your lower-body muscles equally so you can exercise longer and pain-free.

Quadriceps Femoris

Where you'll find them: These four individual muscles—or heads—make up the front of your thighs. The vastus lateralis forms the outer portion of your upper thigh, while the vastus medialis sits inside your thigh and is responsible for stabilizing your kneecap. The vastus intermedius covers much of the front and sides of your thigh, but it's not visible since it's underneath the rectus femoris, the largest of the four heads.

What they do: The quadriceps are mainly responsible for extending your knees—in other words, straightening your legs—but they also help to support the inner and outer sides of your knee joints.

Something to keep in mind: The constant side-to-side lateral movements that many sports and activities require really challenge the quadriceps from the outside to the inside of the muscle. That's why keeping them strong and resilient from a variety of exercises can keep them from tiring out faster or sustaining an injury.

THE MUSCLE MOST PEOPLE BREAK . . . BUT NEVER WORK

It may not be as much fun to flex, but many people tend to forget that their heart is, yes indeed, also a muscle. And, just like every other muscle within your body, your heart also gets stronger the more you exercise it. Train it often and hard enough—two things we'll show you how to do in a later chapter—and your heart has no choice but to grow larger and stronger. For you, that means building a more efficient heart capable of pumping even more blood with every single beat. Blood helps deliver even more oxygen to your muscles, letting you exercise even longer with less fatigue.

Still, there's a far more important reason to train what is single-handedly the most important muscle in your body. The more blood your heart can pump with each beat, the less often your heart has to beat throughout the day. The less often it has to beat, the lower your blood pressure drops, reducing your risk of strokes, heart attacks, heart failure, or kidney failure in the future.

Most people have a hard time pulling off and sticking to the whole "home cardio" routine. Unless you have a few thousand dollars to drop on a new treadmill or other home cardiovascular machines, your options are limited to workout DVDs, online videos, or exercising outside, and that's weather permitting!

That's the beauty of joining a gym or health club. Having that pass means having a wider variety of exercise options that you—and your heart—can finally take advantage of. More machines and more exercise classes to choose from means FINALLY finding the right aerobic option—perfectly suited for YOUR body—that's guaranteed to strip away fat and improve your cardiovascular endurance and your overall health. More options also lower your odds of getting bored too soon, and your chances of tossing in the towel when things start getting old too fast.

If that sounds right up your alley, you're in luck. The upcoming chapters may deal with a lot of strength-training machines and equipment, but trust us, we'll also be guiding you through all of the aerobic options most gyms have to offer. We'll get you started by showing you the basics, so you can show off the body-sculpting results of your newfound knowledge in just a matter of weeks.

Hamstrings

Where you'll find them: Located on the back of your thighs, your hamstrings are made up of three separate muscle groups—the biceps femoris (located on the outer rear portion of your thigh) and the semitendinosus and semimembranosus (the two muscles that make up the bulk of your inner rear thigh).

What they do: Separately, these three muscles help turn your knees inward and turn your feet outward. But together, they have two major functions: knee flexion (which is when you bend your knees) and hip extension.

Something to keep in mind: Many hamstring exercises are also stability-challenging moves that can improve your center of gravity. Plus, your anterior cruciate ligaments (ACLs) rely on your hamstrings to help them stabilize your knees whenever your knee is bending

while decelerating. Having a strong set of these muscles can help them do their job and lower your risk of injury.

Gluteals

Where you'll find them: You may refer to these as the "butt" muscles, but the three muscle groups that make up your backside go by entirely different names altogether. The gluteus maximus is the largest and strongest muscle in your body—it's also what's responsible for creating the rounded shape of your butt. Two other muscles—the gluteus medius and gluteus minimus—lie directly below the gluteus maximus, along the outside of your hips.

What they do: Besides providing convenient padding every time you sit down, your gluteus maximus's main job is hip extension—which is what happens whenever you kick your leg back behind you. The gluteus medius and minimus work together to extend your leg out to the side—otherwise known as hip abduction.

Something to keep in mind: Your "glutes"—as they are more commonly called—are major players when it comes to your overall mobility—especially at your hips. They also help you extend and rotate your legs, two important movements that decide just how flexible and powerful they are. Luckily, many hip-dominant exercises that train your hamstrings also work your glutes simultaneously.

Hip Flexors

Where you'll find them: Attached to the front of your pelvis—directly on the opposite side of your glutes—are the psoas major and iliacus (the two muscles that make up your hip flexors).

What they do: When standing, it's these muscles that help raise your thigh up. When lying flat, these muscles also lift your legs toward your torso and/or lift your torso up into a situp position.

Something to keep in mind: Strengthening your hip flexors isn't a problem since they tend to be strong enough from everyday use. The problem is making sure they stay loose and flexible. Sitting down for long periods of time keeps them in a flexed position. The end result: a set of tight muscles that can limit your ability to fully straighten your hip. Tight hip flexors also pull down on your pelvis, causing it to tilt forward and compress the lower back. Doing certain stretches helps to loosen them up and keeps them from messing up your posture.

Calves

Where you'll find them: Along the back of your lower leg are the two muscles that make up your calves. The gastrocnemius is the larger of the two and the one that's visible. Below it lies the soleus. When fully developed, both muscle heads combine to form the diamond-shaped muscle that extends from the back of your knee to your ankle.

What they do: The gastrocnemius's job is plantar flexion, or elevating your heel—which is what you do whenever you go up on your toes. The soleus does exactly the same thing, but only when your knees are bent.

Something to keep in mind: Many of the exercises that hit the quadriceps also use your gastrocnemius and soleus muscles at the same time.

CHAPTER SIX

A PLAN FOR ALL REASONS

Learning How to Put What You've Got to Good Use

JUST BECAUSE YOU NOW HAVE a fully equipped gym at your disposal doesn't mean you're guaranteed to get the kind of results you're looking for. This has nothing to do with effort, mind you—you can actually end up pushing your body to the brink and still not see an appreciable change in size, strength, or cardiovascular function. How can this be, you ask? Is it really possible to surround yourself with a bunch of state-of-the-art equipment and not get into great shape? The somewhat surprising answer is a resounding yes! If it were as simple as showing up at the gym and just breaking a sweat, we'd all have the body of our dreams.

Unfortunately, it doesn't work that way. So, if you thought you could just hop onto one of those high-end cardio machines and watch the fat miraculously melt away, or blast out a few reps on the bench press and have your chest swell up à la Arnold back in his heyday, you've got another thing coming. If you're really serious about making this whole fitness thing a permanent part of your life and not just some seasonal rite of passage, you're going to have to put a little effort into mapping out a game plan. Without one, you'll just end up like the countless others who join a gym each year only to see their money go wasted on monthly membership dues long after they've stopped going.

If you're worried because you have absolutely no idea how to get started, don't sweat it—that's what this chapter is for. We're going to show you exactly what you need to do to reach your goals, regardless of what they might be. It doesn't matter if you want to lose weight, bulk up a bit, or lower your cholesterol by twenty points. There's a right way and a wrong way to go about things. Our objective is to teach you the right way right now and save you a whole lot of time and frustration in the process. So for a little while at least, we want you to suppress that urge to go running toward the equipment like a kid to his gifts on Christmas morning. By simply exercising a little foresight right now, you'll be able to reap large dividends down the road.

GET "IN THE KNOW"

Before you can even begin worrying about getting a good workout, you first need to know what comprises one. Although it may not look that complicated, an awful lot goes into a typical trip to the gym.

Besides trying to find an empty locker, or fighting over a treadmill, you need to know things like how to warm up effectively, how many exercises to do, and which exercises to do, as well as about a dozen other things that will significantly impact your workout. You've also got to figure out how much weight to use, as well as give at least some consideration to things like reps, sets, and how much recovery time you should take between them. All of this and we haven't even touched on cardio yet!

When it comes to working the old ticker, you'll have a whole other list of concerns. Which machines burn the most calories? Which ones are easier on the joints? Not to mention figuring out the best intensity for burning fat and improving cardiovascular function. And while you're at it, learning how to gauge said intensity would probably be a good idea. This is where knowing things like your target heart rate zone, or how to make sense of an RPE scale (Rating of Perceived Exertion) will come in pretty handy (see next page).

KNOW THE TERMINOLOGY

In addition to being able to gauge your exercise intensity, part of your exercise education involves learning gym lingo. To help you out, we've included the handy glossary below. Study this handy little guide, and by the time you finish reading this section of the book, you'll be well versed in the art of composing a workout based on your specific goals and needs. There'll be no more walking into the gym and wandering aimlessly about. No more copying what others are doing and hoping for similar results. From here on out, you're going to have a set game plan for getting what you want out of your gym membership. You'll know exactly what to do, how long and hard to do it, and when to change it up so your gains don't plateau. Not a bad trade-off for reading one measly chapter.

1. **Repetition (rep):** one single complete movement of an exercise from start to finish.

2. **Set:** A group of repetitions performed in succession until completion.

3. **Recovery interval:**

   - **Strength training:** The amount of rest you take between sets. Usually changes depending on the amount of weight you're using.

   - **Cardiovascular conditioning:** During an interval workout, an active recovery period will follow a brief, intense bout of exercise to help ensure that you are adequately recovered to attempt the higher intensity again.

4. **Intensity:**

   - **Strength training:** Simply refers to the amount of weight being lifted.

   - **Cardiovascular conditioning:** Refers to how hard you're working as indicated by heart rate, RPE, or both.

ANATOMY OF A WORKOUT

To keep things as simple as possible, we're going to divide your training into three distinct segments: strength training, cardiovascular conditioning, and flexibility. Not that we necessarily want you to think of these various components of fitness as separate entities—quite the contrary; they're all interrelated in terms of the way you call upon them during the course of daily living.

Few activities outside the gym rely exclusively on one of these properties without the others being present to some extent. You couldn't, for instance, sprint to catch your morning train, viewed by many as primarily a cardiovascular endeavor, without sufficient strength and flexibility to propel your body forward. We're merely grouping them this way to keep things from getting too confusing.

In terms of strength training, your first step will be deciding which exercises you should do. Regardless of what your goals may be, your best bet here is to stick mainly with large muscle group, compound exercises (exercises that involve action at more than one joint). We advocate this because exercises like squats, deadlifts, bench presses, rows, and overhead presses not only recruit more muscle mass than single joint isolation exercises (think biceps curls and leg extensions), but in doing so they also require a greater caloric expenditure. So they're a great choice whether you're interested in burning fat or building muscle. And for those of you interested in improved performance, sticking primarily with the free-weight version of these lifts will have tremendous carryover to your favorite sport and leisure activities.

HEARTFELT CONCERNS

Shifting the focus to cardio, your three biggest concerns here will be the exercise modality, intensity, and duration. Or, in other words, what you're going to use, how hard you're going to push yourself, and for how long.

THE RATING GAME: GAUGING YOUR EXERCISE INTENSITY

Target Heart Rate: Refers to a range in which your heart rate should fall to ensure that you're working at the proper intensity. A heart rate that falls below the range would indicate that you aren't pushing hard enough, while one that exceeds the upper limits of the range is a signal you may be overdoing it a bit. Although not entirely accurate, it can help you at least get a handle on your overall exercise intensity.

To figure out your target heart rate, simply subtract your age from 220 and then multiply that number by .60 and .85 respectively. The numbers you get represent the lower and upper limits of your "training sensitive zone," meaning that this is the optimal range for you to work in to bring about improvements in aerobic metabolism and/or body fat reduction. In order to check if your heart rate falls within the range, simply place your first two fingers on the thumb side of your wrist, just below the palm of your hand, and feel for your pulse. Once you've found it, count the number of beats you get in 10 seconds and multiply by 6. This will give you your heart rate in beats per minute (bpm). You then simply compare to see whether or not this number falls within the range and alter your workout intensity accordingly.

FOR EXAMPLE:

A 28-year-old male would have an age-predicted maximal heart rate of 192 bpm (220−28 = 192).

To set his range, we then multiply 192 x .60 and .85 respectively to yield a target heart rate zone of 115 to 162 bpm.

While checking his pulse during his workout he counts 23 beats in 10 seconds.

6 x 23 = 138 bpm, indicating that this individual is working within his target heart rate zone.

Figuring out your Rating of Perceived Exertion, or RPE, is decidedly less technical than calculating heart rate. This method, which is based on Borg's scale of perceived effort, asks you to select a number between 6 and 20 to help indicate how hard you're working (the numbers run that way because they're supposed to represent the range between a typical resting heart rate—approximately 60—and a typical maximal heart rate—approximately 200). These numbers then correspond to different levels of effort (see the accompanying chart). It's somewhat more subjective than heart rate, but it can at least help you get an idea of just how hard you're working.

WHAT THESE NUMBERS CAN MEAN:

9 corresponds to "very light" exercise. For a healthy person, it's like walking slowly at his or her own pace for a few minutes.

13 on the scale is "somewhat hard" exercise, but it still feels okay to continue.

17, or "very hard," is very strenuous. A healthy person can still go on, but really must push. This type will feel very heavy, making the person very tired.

19 on the scale is an extremely strenuous exercise level. For most people, this is the most strenuous exercise they have ever experienced.

BORG'S SCALE

YOUR NUMBER	PERCEIVED EFFORT
6	No exertion at all
7	Extremely light (7.5)
8	
9	Very light
10	
11	Light
12	
13	Somewhat hard
14	
15	Hard (heavy)
16	
17	Very hard
18	
19	Extremely hard
20	Maximal exertion

Taking these in order, let's talk choice of equipment first. Based on your goals, current fitness level, and personal injury history, you'll probably find certain cardio machines to be more attractive options than others. Treadmills, for example, although extremely popular, aren't great for heavier individuals due to all the jarring and pounding they inflict on the body. In this instance, a more joint-friendly option like an elliptical machine or stationary bike would be a much better choice.

Besides orthopedic concerns, you could also base your choice here on which machines burn the most calories. Whether your goal is weight loss or getting the best cardiovascular workout possible, machines that require the use of both the upper and lower body tend to require a greater energy expenditure than those that just use one or the other. A rowing machine, for instance, will typically burn far more calories than a stationary bike or even a treadmill, assuming all are being used at similar levels of intensity.

Speaking of intensity, this brings us to one of the most important considerations of your cardio workouts: knowing how hard to work!

This is crucial because it basically determines your exercise duration. Simply put, the harder you push, the shorter your workout will be. The question is, is it better to work harder for a shorter period of time (10 to 20 minutes) or take things down a couple of notches and go for a longer duration (30 to 60 minutes)? This is a question that has plagued gym goers for years and has caused many heated debates amongst personal trainers far and wide. Without going into some long, drawn-out explanation, we're going to attempt to demystify this controversial topic.

We generally tend to favor shorter, more intense cardio workouts for a couple of reasons.

1. Since they result in a greater caloric expenditure, they're great for burning fat—not just during the workout itself, but for hours afterward, due to the large elevations in metabolism they bring about.

2. Because they're shorter in duration, they offer a much more time-efficient way to get in your cardio training.

3. Their higher intensity also makes them a more potent cardiovascular training stimulus than the slow, steady type of cardio work most people tend to

favor. That said, we realize that working at high intensities may not be the best approach for everyone.

Those of you who are deconditioned, for instance, may find the types of workouts we're advocating here too difficult initially. It can be pretty tough to work at a winding pace, either intermittently or steadily, for 10 to 20 minutes at a clip. Or perhaps you're an endurance athlete who needs to train for long durations to get better at your sport. Whatever the case, it's perfectly fine if you decide to opt for lower intensity, longer duration forms of cardio exercise. Just know going in that they don't "burn more fat" than interval workouts (brief bouts of intense exercise interspersed with active recovery periods), or high-intensity forms of training like sprinting and jumping rope.

Last but not least, you'll also need to give some consideration to how often you need to be doing cardio work for best results. Once again, this is completely dependent on your individual situation. Someone looking to maintain cardiovascular health might be able to get by with two intense interval workouts per week, whereas someone on a hardcore fat-loss program might require as many as four weekly training sessions. The chart on the next page will help you determine the optimal frequency, intensity, and duration of your cardio workouts based on your current goals and needs.

STRETCHING: THE TRUTH

If we had to pick one area that's lacking in most fitness programs, it would undoubtedly be flexibility. When it comes to getting in shape, most people are quick to lift weights and do cardio, but few place any real emphasis on improving their basic ability to move efficiently. That's too bad, because increasing the range of motion around key joints like the ankles, knees, hips, and shoulders can not only help you move better, but it can also make it easier to build muscle, burn fat, or meet any other goals you might have. Got your attention with that one, didn't we?

Think about it for a second; if you increase the range of motion that a muscle or group of muscles can move through, you're basically increasing their work capacity. Lifting a weight through a larger range, or using a longer stride or stroke during cardio exercises like running and rowing, is going to force you to work harder. You'll build more muscle and burn more calories than you would

COMPOUND INTEREST

Dumbbell Sumo Squat (page 72)

Deadlift (page 41)

Lunge—forward, reverse, or lateral (page 40)

Dumbbell Flat Bench Press (page 121)

Dip (page 38)

Seated Row (page 95)

Military Press (page 61)

Pullup or Lat Pulldown (page 40/180)

Once you've narrowed down your list of exercise choices, your next step is determining how many you should do per workout. The following are some basic guidelines based on your goals and level of training experience.

NUMBER OF EXERCISES PER WORKOUT

GOAL	BEGINNER	INTERMEDIATE	ADVANCED
Size and strength	4–6	4–6	3–5
Fat burning/general fitness	8–10	8–10	6–8

Note: The lower number of exercises for advanced trainees is due to the fact that they'll be doing more sets per exercise and working at higher intensity than both beginners and intermediates.

Next up comes figuring out how much weight you should use, which will in turn dictate how many sets and repetitions you'll end up doing. Here's where those of you in the strength/muscle-building crowd and the fat-burning/general fitness crowd will really begin to part company. Generally speaking, those of you interested in developing strength and muscle mass will opt for heavier loads, performing fewer repetitions for a larger number of sets. The ones looking to burn fat and improve general fitness will lean more toward lighter loads, higher reps, and fewer sets. For instance:

SETS, REPS, AND LOADS

GOAL	BEGINNER/INTERMEDIATE			ADVANCED		
	Sets	Reps	Loads	Sets	Reps	Loads
Size and strength	2–3	6–8	Mod–Hvy	3–5	4–6	Hvy
Fat burning/general fitness	1–2	12–15	Lt–Mod	2–3	10–12	Mod

Note: The loading here is subjective—meaning that it is not expressed as a percentage of 1 RM (the maximal amount of weight a person can lift one time) as in most programs, but rather should just be sufficient to bring about fatigue in the desired number of repetitions.

GOAL	FREQUENCY	INTENSITY	DURATION
Fat loss	3–5 days per week	Steady Paced [70–80% MHR/RPE = 15–17] Interval [Work = 80-90% MHR/RPE 17–19] 30 seconds [Recovery = 55–60% MHR/RPE 12–14] 60 seconds	30–40 minutes 12–20 minutes
Improved cardiovascular (CV) health	3–4 days per week	Interval [Work = 75–85% MHR/RPE 16–18] 90 seconds [Recovery = 60–70% MHR/RPE 14–15] 90 seconds	15–25 minutes
Maintenance of CV fitness	1–2 days per week	Interval [Work = 85–95% MHR/RPE 18–20] 15 seconds [Recovery = 70–75% MHR/RPE [16–17] 45 seconds	10–12 minutes
Increased endurance	4–6 days per week	Steady Paced [65–80% MHR/RPE 14–16]	40–60 minutes

have doing these same activities through a more restricted range of motion. Not to mention the fact that your improved movement efficiency will also show itself in lots of ways outside the gym. Things like running around and playing with your kids, or reaching up to place something on a high shelf will suddenly feel a whole lot easier.

Now keep in mind, when we advocate stretching we're not necessarily talking about static stretching—the kind where you place a muscle, or group of muscles, in a stretched position and then hold the position without any movement for at least 15 to 20 seconds at a time. That's all well and good at the end of your workout, when you're trying to wind down and return those muscles to their preworkout length.

As a means of warming up, however, or when done between sets of strength training exercises, static stretches really aren't much help at all and might even prove detrimental. That's because the overriding signal they send your muscles to relax is the last thing you want when you're either getting ready to, or in the process of, exercising vigorously.

A far better choice would be engaging in what are known as dynamic stretching exercises. These are basically stretches you do while in motion. Various forms of squatting, lunging, reaching, and twisting are all excellent ways to get your muscles limbered up and ready for activity. Unlike static stretches, which cause your muscles to relax and reduce their potential to generate force, dynamic stretches increase both body temperature and bloodflow and also get your central nervous system fired up and ready for work.

Of course, static stretches are not completely without merit. They can be done both at the end of a tough workout after your muscles have been repeatedly contracting, and at times when you're not exercising to help restore your muscles to a more relaxed state. In the next chapter you'll find a wide array of both dynamic and static stretches that you can incorporate into your workouts based on the guidelines we've just established.

USE IT OR LOSE IT

Now that you have a better understanding of what makes up a workout, you should have a much easier time constructing one that will help you reach your goals. The information contained in this chapter will give you a distinct advantage over most of your fellow gym goers. Just do yourself a favor and make sure you take advantage of it. Don't make the mistake of thinking you can just walk into the gym and wing it and expect to see results. You might make some initial gains, but they won't be anything near what you'll be able to accomplish by following a more structured approach.

In the chapters that lie ahead, you're going to learn a lot about various types of equipment and have access to more exercise pictures and descriptions than you ever knew existed. We've even provided you with a variety of premade workout plans you can follow if you so choose. This is the only place in the book, though, where you get the chance to completely individualize your workouts—and we're urging you to use it. One of the biggest reasons most people get frustrated and quit the gym is because they failed to make the kind of improvements they were hoping for. And one of the most common reasons for that is that they never took the time to map out a plan. You're already one step ahead of the game.

CHAPTER SEVEN

BODY OF WORK

Your Body: The Ultimate Workout Machine

SEEING HOW THIS BOOK IS CALLED the Gym Bible, you're probably wondering why we've decided to devote an entire chapter to body-weight exercises. With high-tech machines and free weights as far as the eye can see, why even bother covering a bunch of stuff you can do in your own home at no added expense? We admit it may seem a bit odd, but rest assured, many of the drills featured here can add some much-needed diversity to the typical gym workout. Let's face it. What sense does it make to lie on a bench or sit in a machine and push a bunch of weight if you can't even move your own body weight efficiently?

Besides just building strength, though, many body-weight exercises can also help improve flexibility. By allowing you to put your body into extreme ranges of motion it might not otherwise be able to reach while loaded with weights, many of these exercises can bring

about significant changes in movement efficiency. And speaking of moving better, let's not forget that most stretches require the use of little more than your own body. Add a stability ball into the mix and the exercise options increase exponentially. As you'll soon see, even though it may lack some of the glitz and glamour of those expensive machines out on the gym floor, your body is really the ultimate training aid.

BASIC BODY-WEIGHT EXERCISES

Before you blow these off, realize that they can come in awfully handy in a crowded gym. Think about it. Would you rather wait several minutes for a bench or chest machine to free up, or keep the flow of your workout by dropping down for a quick set of pushups? There's more to body-weight exercises than mere convenience, however. As we're sure you'll find from trying some of these drills, they're not all as easy as they look. In fact, a few of them, like the Unilateral Deadlift and Russian Twist, can be downright difficult—reason enough why they merit some consideration in your overall plan.

CORE

BEGINNER/ INTERMEDIATE	ADVANCED
Unanchored Situp Russian Twist Side Bridge	Hanging Leg Raise

UNANCHORED SITUP

(MUSCLES TRAINED: ABDOMINALS)

Lie on the floor with your knees bent about 90 degrees and your feet flat. Keeping your arms at your sides or folded across your chest, use your abdominals to pull yourself up to a seated position. Hold for a second and lower yourself back down under control.

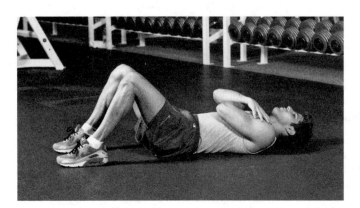
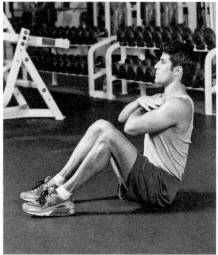

RUSSIAN TWIST

(MUSCLES TRAINED: ABDOMINALS, OBLIQUES)

Sit on the floor with your knees bent about 90 degrees and feet flat on the floor. Next, extend your arms and lean back until your wrists line up over your knees. Hold this same trunk angle as you twist as far as possible to one side and then the other.

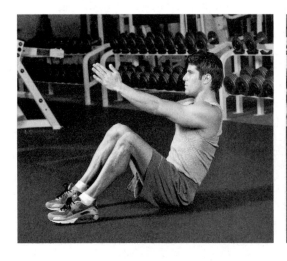
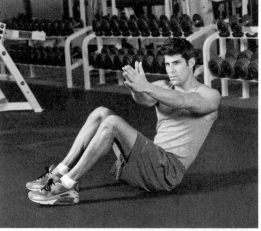

SIDE BRIDGE

Lie on your side with your forearm lined upright beneath your shoulder, perpendicular to your torso. Keeping your body totally straight, contract your abdominals and obliques as you raise your lower torso, hips, and legs off the floor. In the top position your body should form a diagonal line from your feet to your head.

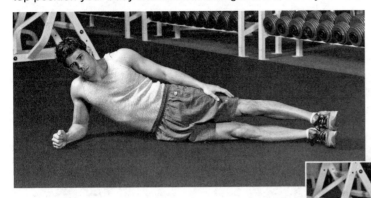

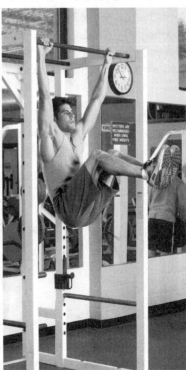

HANGING LEG RAISE

(MUSCLES TRAINED: ABDOMINALS, HIP FLEXORS)

Hang on a chinup bar using an overhand grip with your arms straight and shoulder-width apart. Bend your legs about 15 degrees and keep them bent and relaxed during the entire exercise. Then, use your abdominal muscles to raise your feet upward in an arc until they are a bit higher than a point level with your hips. Pause, lower, and repeat.

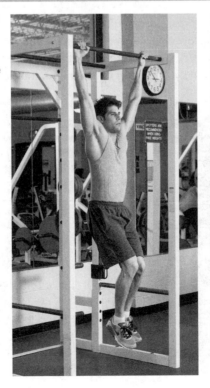

CHEST AND UPPER BACK/ SHOULDERS AND ARMS

	BEGINNER/ INTERMEDIATE	ADVANCED
CHEST	Pushup	T-Pushup
	Dip	
BACK	Chinup	Pullup

PUSHUP

(MUSCLES TRAINED: CHEST, SHOULDERS, TRICEPS)

Place your hands on the floor slightly wider than shoulder-width apart and prop yourself up on your feet. Keeping your back straight, bend your elbows and lower yourself until your chest is within a couple of inches of the floor. Pause and then press back up to the starting position.

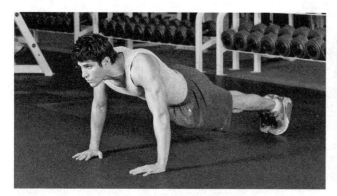
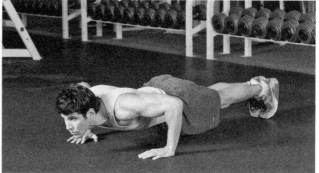

DIP

(MUSCLES TRAINED: CHEST, SHOULDERS, TRICEPS)

Grab the handles of a dip station and press yourself up until your arms are straight. With your ankles crossed beneath you, begin by bending your arms and lowering yourself until your upper arms are parallel to the floor. Pause for a second and then press back up. Keeping your torso more upright and your elbows close to your body will work your triceps a bit more; leaning forward and allowing your elbows to bow out to the sides will make more work for your chest.

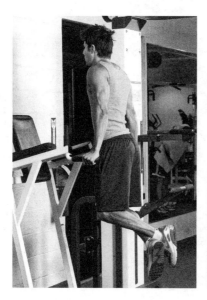
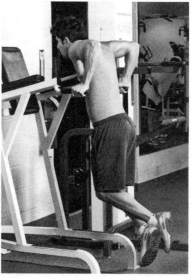

T-PUSHUP

Begin by getting in a pushup position with your feet placed slightly wider than hip-width apart. Start as you would a normal pushup, then, as you reach the top, use your core musculature to rotate your torso toward the ceiling. In the end you should be balancing on one arm with the other extended up toward the ceiling and balancing on the sides of your feet. Lower and repeat on the other side.

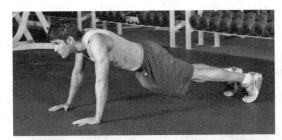
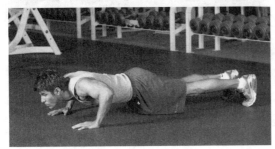
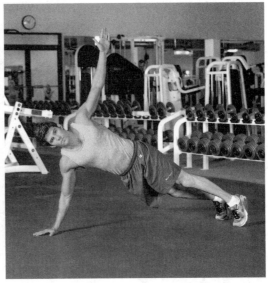

CHINUP

Grab a chinup bar with a shoulder-width, underhand grip, cross your ankles, and hang. Pull yourself up as high as you can. Pause, then slowly return to the starting position.

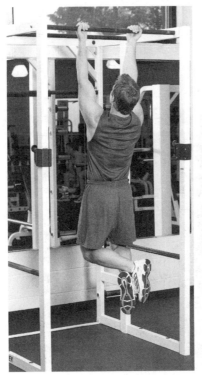
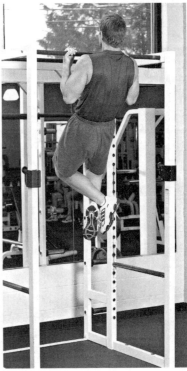

PULLUP

Hang from a pullup bar using an over-hand grip that's just beyond shoulder-width. Cross your feet behind you. Pull yourself up as high as you can—your chin should go over the bar. Pause, then slowly return to the starting position.

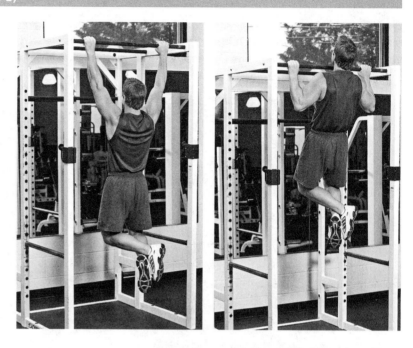

LOWER BODY

BEGINNER/ INTERMEDIATE	ADVANCED
Lunge	Unilateral Deadlift
	Unilateral Romanian Deadlift

LUNGE

(MUSCLES TRAINED: QUADRICEPS, GLUTES, HAMSTRINGS)

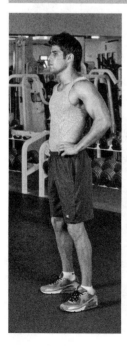
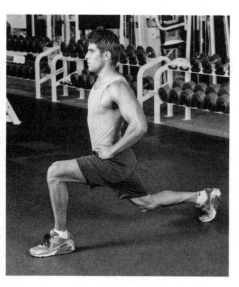

Stand with your feet hip-width apart. Step forward with your nondominant leg (your left if you're right-handed) and lower your body until your front knee is bent 90 degrees and your rear knee nearly touches the floor. Your front lower leg should be perpendicular to the floor and your torso should remain upright. Push yourself back up to the starting position as quickly as you can, and repeat with your dominant leg. That's one repetition. Repeat for the desired number of reps before switching to the other side.

UNILATERAL DEADLIFT

(MUSCLES TRAINED: GLUTES, HAMSTRINGS, QUADRICEPS, LOWER BACK)

From a standing position, bend one leg at a 90-degree angle and hold it up behind you. Begin by dropping your hips back and then bending your knee as you lower your hips toward the floor. Your back is allowed to round since you're not under load. Once your shin grazes the floor, press back up to the starting position. Repeat on the other side.

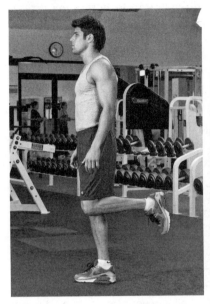 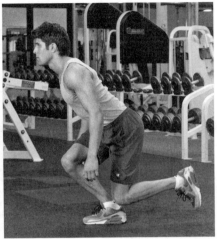

UNILATERAL ROMANIAN DEADLIFT

(MUSCLES TRAINED: GLUTES, HAMSTRINGS)

From a standing position, lift one foot an inch or two off the ground, while maintaining a slight bend in your support knee. Next, drive your hips back as you begin to lean forward until your torso is as close to parallel to the floor as possible. Be sure your support knee doesn't bend any more, or your back rounds as you lower yourself forward. Keep a slight bend in your knee and a slight arch in your lower back. Repeat on the other side.

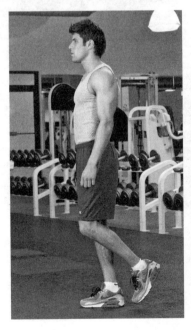 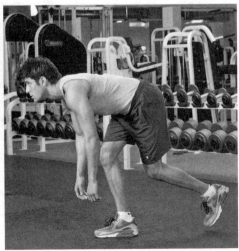

STABILITY BALL EXERCISES

Believe it or not, stability balls can be used for more than just doing crunches. We realize that may be hard to fathom, since that's probably all you ever see them being used for. Besides substituting as a bench for various upper-body movements, they can also be used on their own to perform some rather challenging exercises for your core, legs, and upper body.

Whatever you use them for, their unstable nature makes them great for strengthening all those little stabilizing muscles that often go neglected. Whether it's the muscles of your rotator cuff working harder to help stabilize you during a pushup, or your core firing like crazy to keep you on the ball during a set of stability ball leg curls, you're bound to notice the different training environment they offer.

CORE

BEGINNER/ INTERMEDIATE	ADVANCED
Stability Ball Crunch	Jackknife
	Pike
Stability Ball Pass-Off	

STABILITY BALL CRUNCH

(MUSCLES TRAINED: ABDOMINALS)

Lie on a stability ball with your back and hips in contact with the ball and your feet on the floor. Keeping your knees bent and hips still, place your hands behind your head and use your abdominals to lift your head, neck, and shoulder blades off the surface of the ball. Pause for a second before lowering yourself back to the starting position.

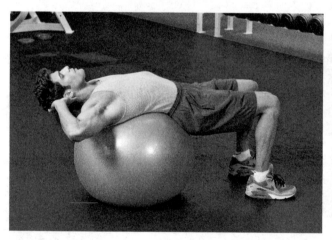 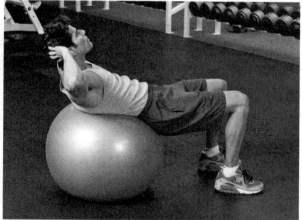

STABILITY BALL PASS-OFF

(MUSCLES TRAINED: ABDOMINALS)

Lie on your back holding a stability ball in your hands with your arms stretched over your head. With your legs raised over your hips, use your abdominals to lift the ball up toward your legs as you place the ball between your feet. Once there, hold your shoulders up off the ground and keep your lower back pressed flat into the floor as you lower your legs as far as you can. Pause, then reverse the direction and pass the ball back to your hands and back down to the floor.

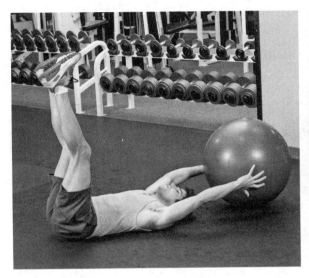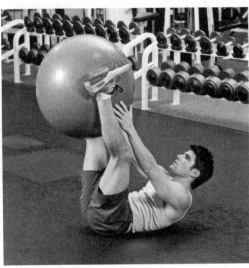

JACKKNIFE

(MUSCLES TRAINED: ABDOMINALS)

Position yourself on a stability ball with your hands on the floor about shoulder-width apart and your shins and feet on the ball. In this position keep your abdominals braced tight and avoid excessively arching your lower back. Begin by slowly pulling the ball toward you using your abdominals and hip flexors. As you do this, your butt should raise up in the air as your knees pull in toward your chest. Once you've pulled it in as far as possible, reverse directions and slowly return the ball to the starting position.

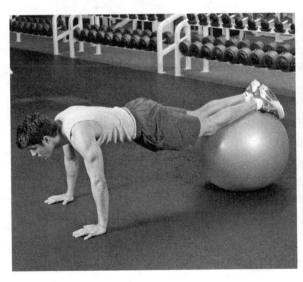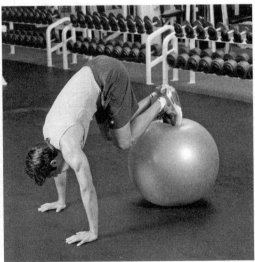

PIKE

Execute these the same way as you would the Jackknife, only this time keep your legs completely straight.

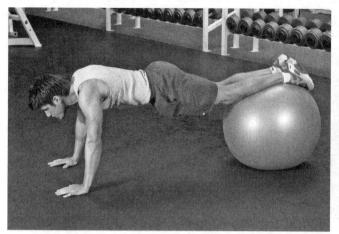

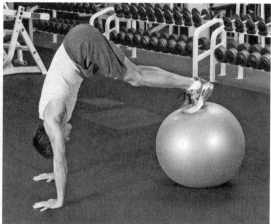

CHEST AND UPPER BACK

BEGINNER/ INTERMEDIATE	ADVANCED
Stability Ball Pushup	Stability Ball Press-Up

STABILITY BALL PUSHUP

(MUSCLES TRAINED: CHEST, SHOULDERS, TRICEPS, CORE)

Get into pushup position—your hands set slightly wider than and in line with your shoulders—but instead of placing your feet on the floor, rest your shins on a stability ball. With your arms straight and your back flat, your body should form a straight line from your shoulders to your ankles. Lower your body until your chest nearly touches the floor. Pause, then push yourself back up to the starting position.

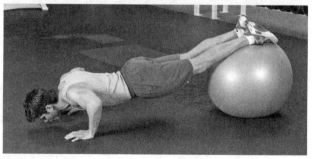

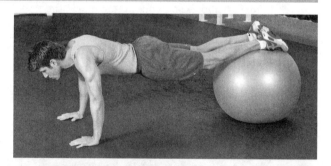

STABILITY BALL PRESS-UP

(MUSCLES TRAINED: CHEST, SHOULDERS, TRICEPS, CORE)

Position your feet as you would during a pushup and place your hands approximately shoulder-width apart on a stability ball placed in front of you. Keeping your body straight and abdominals braced tight, begin by bending your elbows and lowering your body down toward the ball, chest first. Pause at your lowest point and then press back up to the starting position.

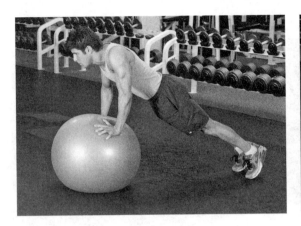 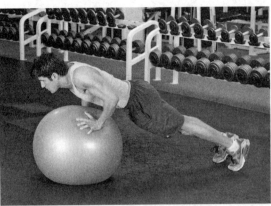

LOWER BODY

BEGINNER/ INTERMEDIATE	ADVANCED
Stability Ball Leg Curl	Unilateral Stability Ball Leg Curl

STABILITY BALL LEG CURL

(MUSCLES TRAINED: HAMSTRINGS, GLUTES, LOWER BACK, CORE)

Lie on your back with your heels and lower calves on a stability ball. First lift your hips up until your body forms a ramp, then pull the ball in toward you by bending your knees and extending your hips. Pause for a second and then slowly reverse the sequence.

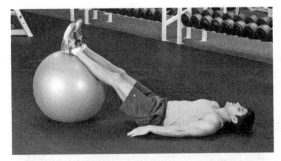 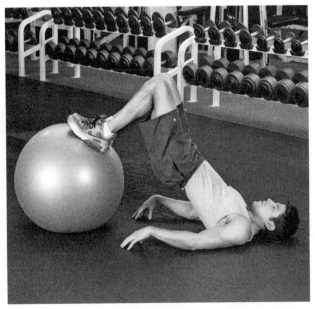

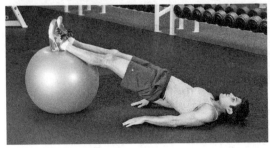

UNILATERAL STABILITY BALL LEG CURL

(MUSCLES TRAINED: HAMSTRINGS, GLUTES, LOWER BACK, CORE)

Perform these as you would the regular Stability Ball Leg Curl, except with one leg held up over your hips and using the other to bring the ball toward you.

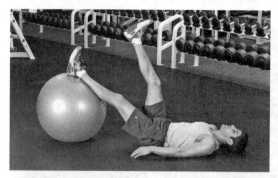

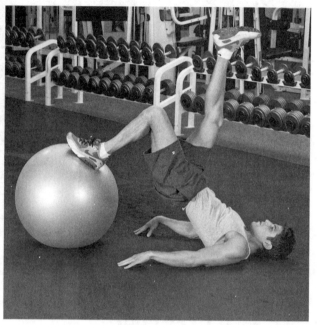

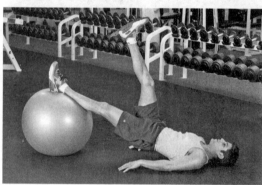

CHAPTER EIGHT

LAND OF THE FREE

The Many Benefits of Training with Free Weights

PUMPING IRON

The mere phrase alone is enough to instill fear in the heart of any novice trainee. And why not? Working with free weights can be a pretty intimidating proposition to the uninitiated. The cold, hard steel, the clanging noises they make when you bang them together, not to mention the fact that all of the biggest, baddest-looking dudes in the gym always seem to be using them. Add in the unwarranted stigma they carry of being "dangerous," and it's no wonder more and more people shy away from barbells and dumbbells as a means of reaching their fitness goals.

Assuming you can get past all of that, though, you just might find that free weights are your best, most time-efficient option for getting in a good workout. For starters, they're extremely versatile, allowing you to alter the way exercises are done to better accommodate the way your body moves.

They also force you to balance and stabilize the weight in addition to lifting it. This not only improves coordination, but it also makes training with free weights more applicable to life outside of the gym. Things like lifting your kids and carrying heavy objects up or down a flight of stairs are just a couple of examples of activities you can't prepare for by training exclusively on machines.

Need more? How about the fact that training with free weights can also help you build more muscle and increase strength to a greater degree than other forms of training. Because they require more muscles to work to stabilize the weight, free weights not only create a greater stimulus for muscle growth, but also impose a greater demand on your central nervous system. This is a good thing, because the better your central nervous system gets at recruiting your muscle fibers to contract, the faster and more efficiently you'll be able to meet physical demands both in and out of the gym.

Finally, a lot of the safety issues concerning the use of free weights are completely blown out of proportion. True, because they require more balance and stabilization to control the weight, free weights are at least potentially dangerous. To be fair, though, the same could be said for just about anything else you might do in a gym. Besides, free weights pose a threat only when people choose to use them irresponsibly. People who use sloppy form and/or attempt to lift more weight than they can handle are really the only ones who need to worry about becoming injured. As long as you stick to the advice provided in the pages to follow, you should be just fine.

Versatility, effectiveness, and safety make the case for using free weights a pretty strong one. The only thing left to address is the difference between the two types. So, which one is better, dumbbells or barbells? In truth, it's not easy, nor is it necessary, to pick just one. You'd be much better served learning the many nuances offered by the two types. That way you can pick and choose which exercises best suit your needs and, in the process, avoid the plight of your fellow gym goers by being stuck doing set after set of bench presses and biceps curls.

WHO YOU CALLIN' DUMB?

We're not sure who it was that gave dumbbells their name, but we can tell you that they were way off base. Simply put, dumbbells are one of the greatest innovations the training world has ever seen. Their compact design means they require very little room to use. This can come in awfully handy when the gym is crowded and space is at a premium. They also allow you to tailor exercises specifically to meet your individual needs. Say, for instance, you have an old shoulder injury that makes barbell bench presses difficult to do. With dumbbells, you can turn your palms to face toward each other and tuck your elbows in a bit closer to your body to take the strain off your shoulders.

The other big selling point with dumbbells is that they allow you to address strength imbalances more effectively. When you work with a barbell, if one of your limbs is stronger than the other, there isn't too much you can do about it. With dumbbells, however, you can specifically target that weak limb by having it do extra sets to catch up with the stronger side. This isn't something that can be easily achieved with a barbell and is just one of the many reasons dumbbell training has become increasingly popular in recent years among both the regular gym population and those in physical rehabilitation settings.

BELLY UP TO THE BAR

Because dumbbells are so great, you might wonder why it's even necessary to train with barbells at all. Well, for starters, it's the preferred way to measure your strength against others. The standard 7-foot Olympic barbell is the tool of choice for bench presses, squats, deadlifts, and any other lift you can think of that guys have used to compare their strength throughout the years. Guaranteed, you walk up to any guy in your gym and ask him what he benches and he'll know. He might not remember his wedding anniversary or his kids' birthdays, but he'll know how much weight he can press upward while lying on his back.

Even if you're not into the whole "I'm stronger than you are" thing, there are still other times when using a barbell is worth your time and effort. One such instance is when doing lower body lifts. Oh sure, you can work your legs with dumbbells, just not as effectively or conveniently as you could with a bar. Barbells just make it a whole lot easier to carry weight for different types of squatting and lunging movements. Ever try doing a front squat with dumbbells? Trust us—it ain't fun! There simply isn't any comfortable way to get a couple of heavy dumbbells up on your shoulders.

Of course, you could always opt to hold the weights in your hands down along your sides as you perform various lower body movements—the only trouble there is that your grip may give out before your legs do, causing you to end the set prematurely. It's so much easier to just step under a loaded barbell that's waiting for you on the supports of a squat rack, load it on your back, and have at it. To tell you the truth, the same could also be said for various types of upper-body pressing movements. One of the only drawbacks with dumbbells is getting them into the "up" position when starting off a set of presses. The stronger you get, the harder this becomes to do—even with the aid of a spotter.

In the end, whether you choose to use one type instead of the other or a healthy mix of both, the most important thing is that you're doing the exercises correctly. The pictures and exercise descriptions that follow will assure you that you're doing just that. Before we get started, though, a word about the way this chapter and the ones that follow it are set up.

The exercises featured here are ones that you can do with no additional equipment beyond some simple free weights. In the next chapter, we'll show you another array of ground-based exercises you can do with just your body and a cable station. That will be followed by all of the exercises you can do using a bench and finally a squat rack, or power cage in successive chapters. And, of course, there'll be a large section to follow on the proper usage of both resistance and cardiovascular machines.

Why set things up this way? Because our aim is to help you build an impressive exercise arsenal based on whatever equipment you have available to you. This way, your whole workout isn't ruined simply because you were unable to secure a certain piece of equipment, or because other members unintentionally interrupted what you were trying to accomplish. For instance, why wait for the bench press machine to free up when you know about eight other ways to work your chest? The bottom line is: The more well versed you become in how to use various types of equipment, the more options you'll have at your disposal to help ensure that your workouts deliver the desired results.

JUST WEIGHT

Stand-alone exercises using only barbells and dumbbells follow.

For easy referencing, we've broken these exercises up into the following five categories: core, chest and upper back, shoulders and arms, lower body, and integrated lifts—the last of which includes nontraditional lifts that target multiple muscle groups at once. Besides offering a nice challenging change of pace, exercises that fit into this category will also have even greater carryover to real-world activities outside of the gym.

CORE

BEGINNER/ INTERMEDIATE	ADVANCED
Weighted Crunch	Saxon Side Bend
Weighted Russian Twist	Barbell Rollout (on knees)
Woodchopper	Barbell Rollout (on feet)
Reverse Woodchopper	

WEIGHTED CRUNCH

(MUSCLES TRAINED: ABDOMINALS)

Lie on your back with your knees bent and feet flat on the floor. Holding a dumbbell against your upper chest, begin by lifting your shoulder blades up off the floor. When you've gone as high as you can without your feet moving, pause for a second and then lower back down to the starting position.

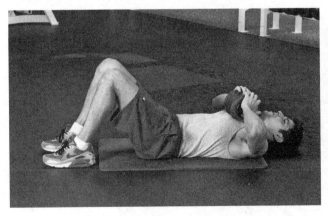
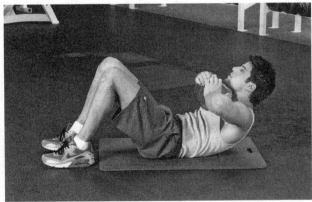

WEIGHTED RUSSIAN TWIST

(MUSCLES TRAINED: ABDOMINALS, OBLIQUES)

Sit on the floor with your knees bent and your feet flat. Hold a light dumbbell at arm's length in front of your chest. Lean back so your torso is at a 45-degree angle to the floor. Twist to the left as far as you can, pause, then reverse your movement and twist all the way back to the right as far as you can.

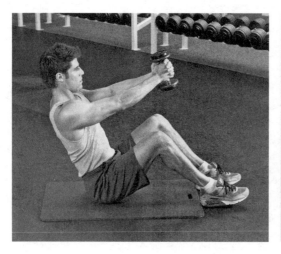 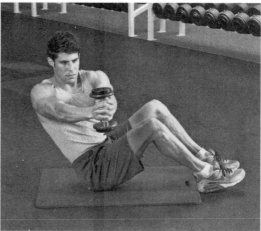

WOODCHOPPER

(MUSCLES TRAINED: ABDOMINALS, OBLIQUES)

Stand with your feet shoulder-width apart and knees slightly bent holding a light dumbbell with both hands, with your arms outstretched over one shoulder. Begin by using your core muscles to "chop" the weight down across the front of your body in an arcing motion, finishing when your hands are outside your opposite leg, midway between your knee and ankle. Pause for a second, then raise back up and repeat.

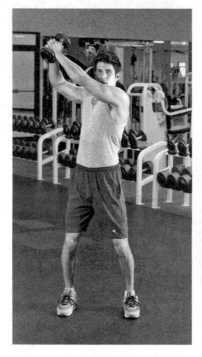 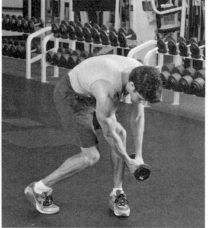

REVERSE WOODCHOPPER

This time you simply reverse the movement by starting in the down position and chopping the weight in a wide arc upward until the weight is above one shoulder.

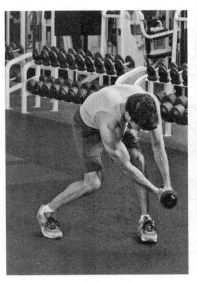
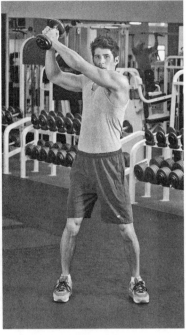

SAXON SIDE BEND

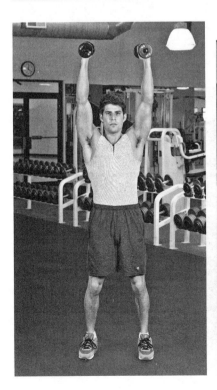
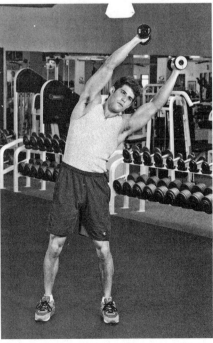

Stand holding a pair of dumbbells over your head with your knees slightly bent and arms straight. Begin by leaning to one side as far as you can, making sure that you keep the same distance between the two dumbbells. Avoid twisting your body as you do this. When you reach your lowest point, pause for a second before returning back to the starting position and repeating to the other side.

BARBELL ROLLOUT (ON KNEES)

(MUSCLES TRAINED: CORE, SHOULDERS)

Kneel on the ground holding a barbell with two small plates on the ends of it with a shoulder-width grip. Keeping your back flat, allow the bar to roll out in front of you as you extend your arms and torso to follow it. Go out as far as you can without arching your back, then use your abdominals to drag the bar back to the starting position.

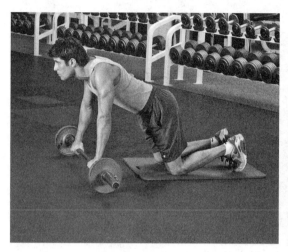 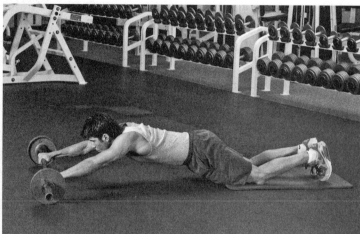

BARBELL ROLLOUT (ON FEET)

(MUSCLES TRAINED: CORE, SHOULDERS)

A much more advanced version of the Barbell Rollout. This time start on your feet instead of your knees and follow the same instructions as above.

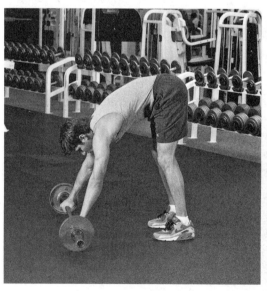 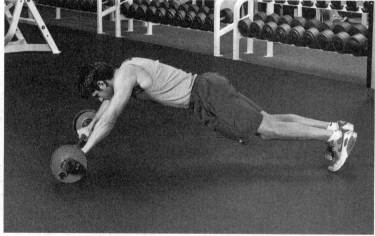

CHEST AND UPPER BACK

	BEGINNER/ INTERMEDIATE	ADVANCED
CHEST	Pushup Position Row	T-Pushup
BACK	Reverse Fly (3 grips)	Dumbbell Bent-Over Row (3 grips)
		Barbell Bent-Over Row (3 grips)

PUSHUP POSITION ROW

(MUSCLES TRAINED: CORE, UPPER BACK, BICEPS)

Grab a pair of dumbbells (hexagonal dumbbells work best for these, but regular round ones will suffice) and position yourself as if to do a set of pushups with your feet slightly wider than shoulder-width apart. Keeping your lower back flat and abs braced tight, row one dumbbell up by drawing your elbow past your torso, as you support your body weight on the other side. Pause at the top for a second, then lower and repeat with the other side. Try to keep your hips as still as possible the entire time you're rowing.

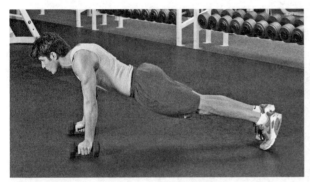

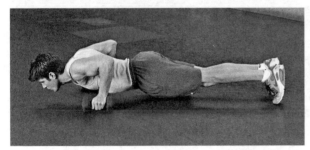

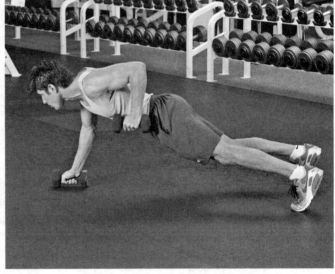

T-PUSHUP

Hexagonal dumbbells work best here. Get into a pushup position with your hands on the handles of a pair of dumbbells that have been placed shoulder-width apart. Do a pushup, and as you come up, rotate your body so that you raise your right arm and the dumbbell straight up over your shoulder and your body forms a T. Lower the dumbbell and yourself, and repeat to the other side.

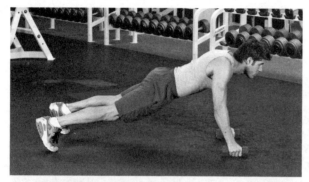

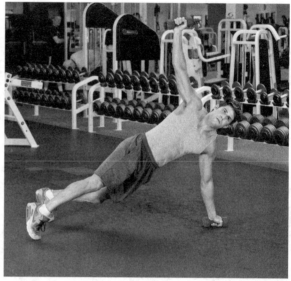

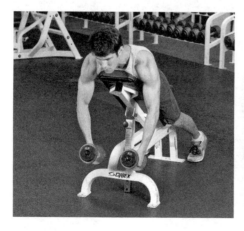

REVERSE FLY (3 GRIPS)

(MUSCLES TRAINED: UPPER BACK, REAR SHOULDERS)

Position yourself prone on an incline bench set to a 45- to 60-degree angle holding a pair of light dumbbells in your hands at arm's length. With your palms facing each other and a slight bend in your elbows, pinch your shoulder blades together as you work the weights up in a wide, arcing motion, pausing when your arms are parallel to the ground. Pause for a second, then lower them back down to the starting position. Keeping your palms facing each other will emphasize the entire upper back, while doing the exercise with your thumbs facing each other and pinky side of your hand rising upward will target the rear shoulders a bit more. Finally, rotating your palms outward so your thumb side of your hand leads the movement will bring the external rotators more into play.

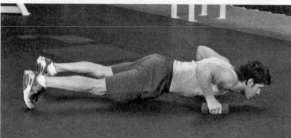

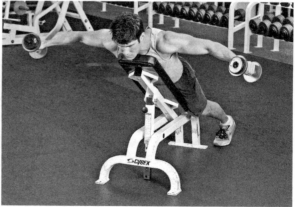

DUMBBELL BENT-OVER ROW (3 GRIPS)

(MUSCLES TRAINED: UPPER BACK, BICEPS)

Grab a pair of dumbbells and hold them at arm's length in front of you. Stand with your feet shoulder-width apart and knees slightly bent. Bend at the hips, lowering your torso about 45 degrees, and let the dumbbells hang straight down from your shoulders. Pull the weights up to the sides of your torso, pause, then slowly lower them. Using a pronated (palms facing you) grip will work to emphasize scapular retraction (pulling the shoulder blades together) and increase the involvement of the rhomboids, middle trapezius, and rear shoulders. A neutral grip where your palms face each other will bring the lats more into play, and a supinated grip (palms facing outward) will increase biceps and lat involvement.

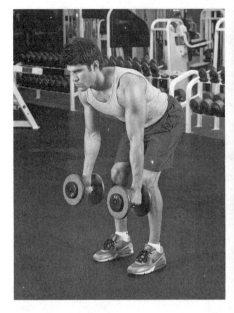 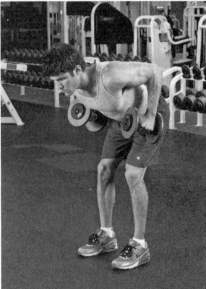 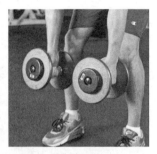 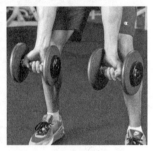

BARBELL BENT-OVER ROW (3 GRIPS)

(MUSCLES TRAINED: UPPER BACK, BICEPS)

Grab a barbell with an overhand grip that's just beyond shoulder-width and hold it at arm's length. Stand with your feet shoulder-width apart and knees slightly bent. Bend at the hips, lowering your torso about 45 degrees, and let the bar hang straight down from your shoulders. Pull the bar up to your torso, pause, then slowly lower it. The same holds true here in terms of muscle involvement for both the pronated and supinated versions of the row.

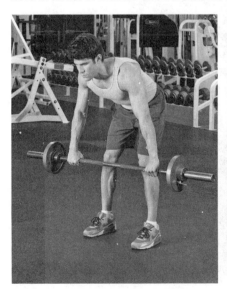 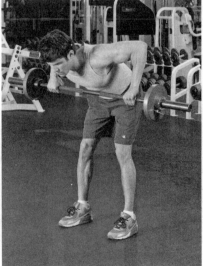 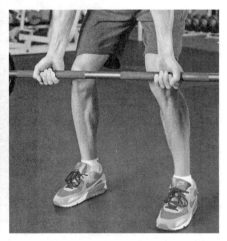

SHOULDERS AND ARMS

	BEGINNER/INTERMEDIATE	ADVANCED
SHOULDERS	Dumbbell Shoulder Press	Dumbbell Rotational Press
	Arnold Press	Dumbbell Overhead Shrug
	Lateral Raise	Dumbbell Hang Clean
	Front Raise	Dumbbell Cuban Press
	Dumbbell Shrug	Barbell Hang Clean
	Dumbbell Upright Row	Barbell Front Raise
	Dumbbell Scarecrow	Barbell Overhead Shrug
	Barbell Upright Row	Bradford Press
	Barbell Shrug	
	Military Press	
TRICEPS	Overhead Dumbbell Triceps Extension	Close-Grip Bench Press
	Lying Dumbbell Triceps Extension	
	E-Z Bar Overhead Triceps Extension	
BICEPS	Standing Dumbbell Curl	Zottman Curl
	Standing Barbell Curl	Barbell Curl Plus
	Standing Concentration Curl	
	E-Z Bar Reverse Grip Curl	
	Standing Barbell Wrist Curl	

DUMBBELL SHOULDER PRESS
(MUSCLES TRAINED: SHOULDERS, TRICEPS)

Stand holding a pair of dumbbells just above your shoulders with your knees bent and back straight. Begin by pressing the dumbbells up overhead until your arms are straight. Pause and lower the weight back down to the starting position. Using a neutral grip with your palms facing your head can take some strain off your shoulders. This exercise can also be done by alternating lifting one dumbbell at a time.

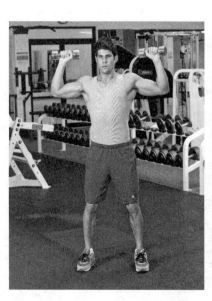 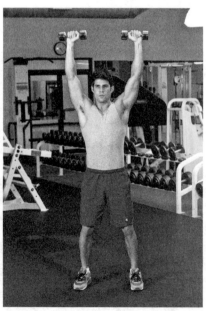

ARNOLD PRESS

Adopt the same starting position as you would when doing the Dumbbell Shoulder Press, only this time with your hands facing you and your forearms in front of your chest. This time as you press the weights up, rotate your arms so that your palms face forward at the top of the rep. Pause and then lower the weights back down to the starting position. This type of press can ease strain on the shoulder joint compared to the regular dumbbell press.

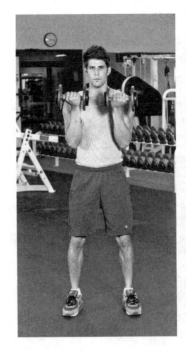
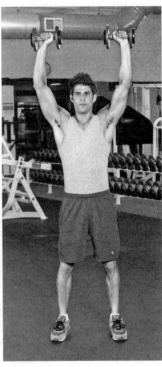

LATERAL RAISE

Stand with your feet shoulder-width apart, holding a pair of dumbbells at arm's length. Keeping a slight bend in your arms, lift your arms up until they're parallel to the ground. Pause, lower, and repeat.

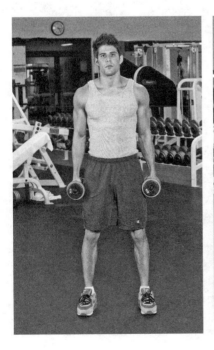
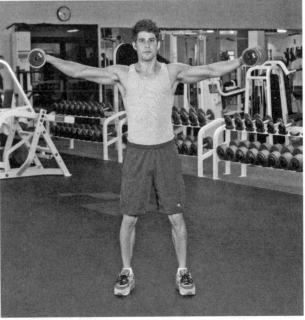

FRONT RAISE

Stand with your feet shoulder-width apart and your knees slightly bent, holding a pair of dumbbells in front of you facing your thighs. Maintaining a slight bend in your elbows, lift your right arm up in front of you until it's parallel to the ground. Pause, lower, and repeat, alternating arms.

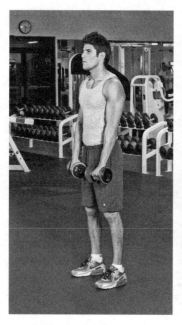
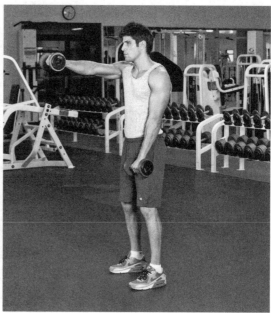

DUMBBELL SHRUG

Stand holding a pair of dumbbells at arm's length with your palms at your sides. Keeping your arms straight, raise your shoulders up toward your ears as high as possible. Pause, lower, and repeat.

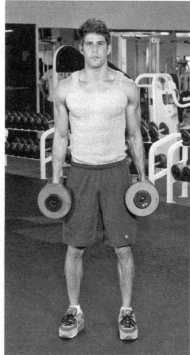
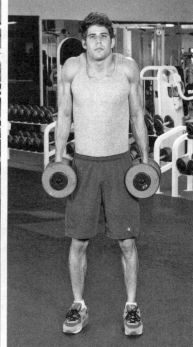

DUMBBELL UPRIGHT ROW

Stand holding a pair of dumbbells at arm's length with your palms facing your thighs. Begin by pulling the dumbbells up toward your chest, leading with your elbows. When your upper arms are parallel to the floor, pause for a second before lowering them back down to the starting position.

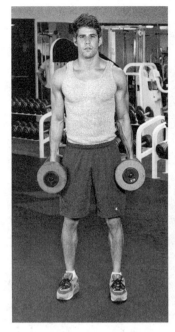 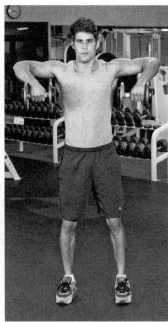

DUMBBELL SCARECROW

Grab a pair of light dumbbells and hold them at arm's length with your palms facing your thighs. Raise your upper arms so they're perpendicular to your torso and parallel to the floor. Bend your elbows 90 degrees, so that your forearms hang straight down toward the floor. Keeping your elbows, wrists, and upper arms in fixed positions, rotate the weights up and back as far as you can—you want your shoulders to act like hinges, your forearms like swinging gates. Pause, then return the forearms to the down position and repeat.

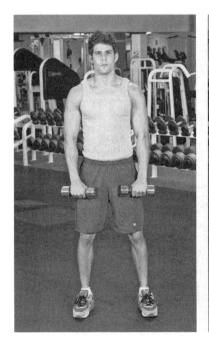 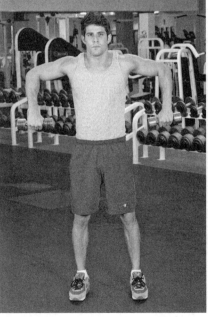 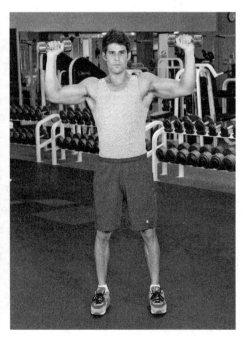

BARBELL UPRIGHT ROW

Stand holding a barbell with a pronated, shoulder-width grip in front of your thighs. Begin by pulling the barbell up toward your chest, leading with your elbows. When your upper arms are parallel to the floor, pause for a second before lowering them back down to the starting position.

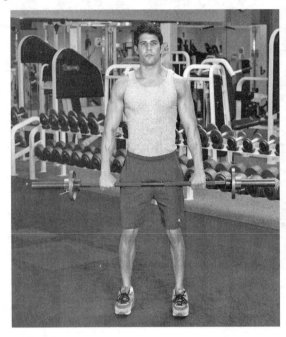 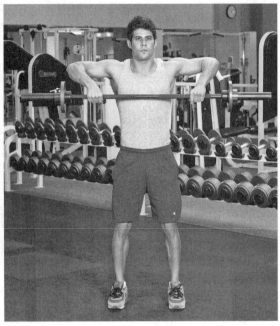

BARBELL SHRUG

Stand holding a barbell with a pronated, shoulder-width grip in front of your thighs. Keeping your arms straight, raise your shoulders up toward your ears as high as possible. Pause, lower, and repeat.

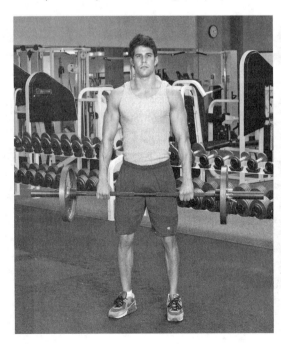 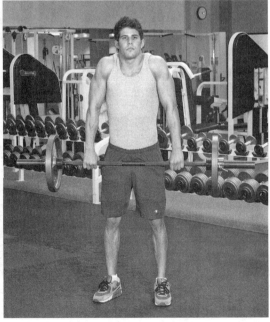

MILITARY PRESS

Grab a barbell with a shoulder-width, overhand grip. Stand holding the barbell at shoulder level, your feet shoulder-width apart and knees slightly bent. Push the weight straight overhead, leaning your head back slightly but keeping your torso upright. Pause, then slowly lower the bar back to the starting position.

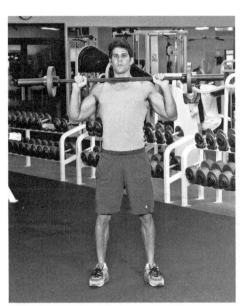
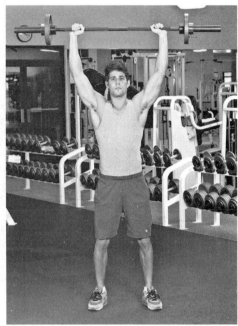

DUMBBELL ROTATIONAL PRESS

Stand as if about to perform a set of regular dumbbell shoulder presses. Begin by pressing the weights overhead as you simultaneously rotate as far as you can to one side. Pause, then lower the weights and return to the starting position. Repeat on the other side.

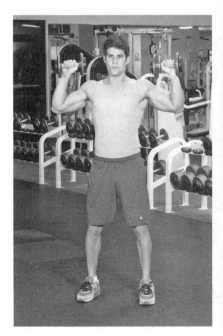
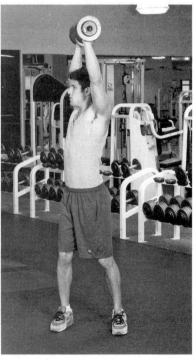

DUMBBELL OVERHEAD SHRUG

(MUSCLES TRAINED: UPPER TRAPEZIUS)

Stand and press a pair of dumbbells over your head. With your knees bent and abs held tight, raise your shoulders up toward your ears as high as possible. Once you've gone as high as you can, pause, then lower the weights back down to the starting position.

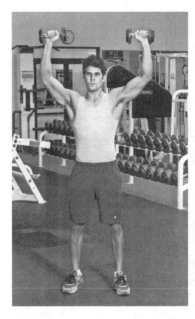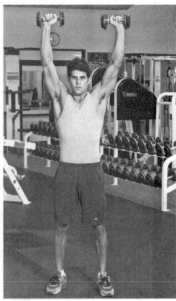

DUMBBELL HANG CLEAN

(MUSCLES TRAINED: UPPER TRAPEZIUS, SHOULDERS, BICEPS)

Grab a pair of dumbbells with an overhand, shoulder-width grip and hold them in front of your thighs while standing with your knees slightly bent. Your lower back should be in its natural alignment (in other words, slightly arched). Shrug your shoulders as you pull the weights up as hard as you can. You should rise up on your toes as you do this. When the dumbbells reach chest level, bend your knees again, rotate your forearms from the elbows, and bend your wrists so they go underneath the dumbbells as you "catch" them on the front of your shoulders. Then quickly flip the weights back down to the starting position and repeat.

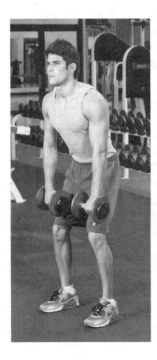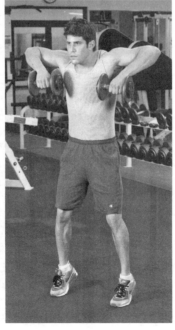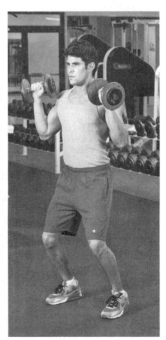

DUMBBELL CUBAN PRESS

(MUSCLES TRAINED: SHOULDERS, TRICEPS, EXTERNAL ROTATORS)

Stand holding a pair of light dumbbells just above your shoulders with your palms facing forward. Keeping your upper arms still, begin by allowing your forearms to rotate downward until almost perpendicular to the floor. Pause, reverse directions and rotate your arms back to the starting position, then press the weights overhead. Pause again, lower, and repeat.

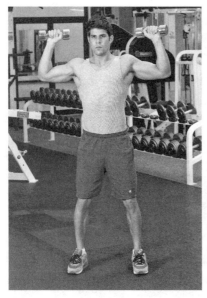
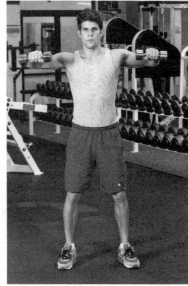
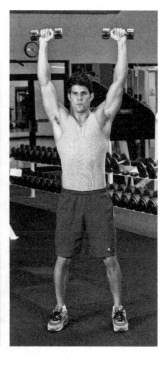

BARBELL HANG CLEAN

(MUSCLES TRAINED: UPPER TRAPEZIUS, SHOULDERS, BICEPS)

Grab a barbell with an overhand, shoulder-width grip and hold it in front of your thighs while standing with your knees slightly bent. Your lower back should be in its natural alignment (in other words, slightly arched). Shrug your shoulders as you pull the bar up as hard as you can. You should rise up on your toes as you do this. When the bar reaches chest level, bend your knees again, rotate your forearms from the elbows, and bend your wrists so they go underneath the bar as you "catch" it on the front of your shoulders. Then quickly flip the bar back down to the starting position and repeat.

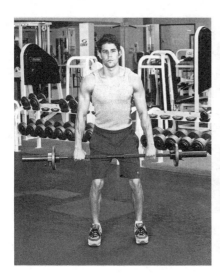
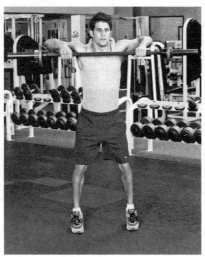
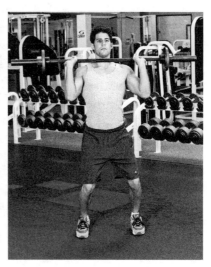

BARBELL FRONT RAISE

(MUSCLES TRAINED: SHOULDERS)

Stand holding a barbell with an overhand, shoulder-width grip in front of your thighs. Keeping your arms straight, begin by raising the bar out in front of you until it's approximately shoulder height, parallel to the ground. Pause, lower, and repeat.

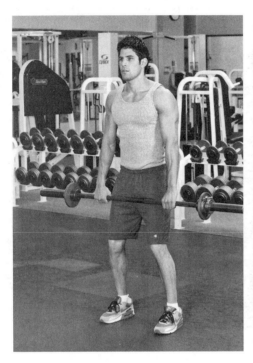 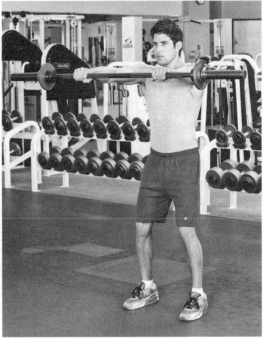

BARBELL OVERHEAD SHRUG

(MUSCLES TRAINED: UPPER TRAPEZIUS)

Stand and press a barbell over your head. With your knees bent and abs held tight, raise your shoulders up toward your ears as high as possible. Once you've gone as high as you can, pause, then lower the weight back down to the starting position.

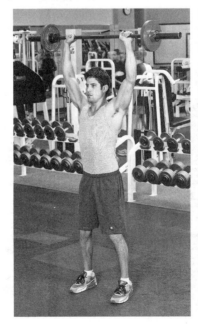 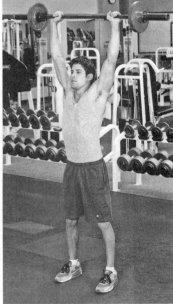

BRADFORD PRESS

(MUSCLES TRAINED: SHOULDERS, UPPER TRAPEZIUS, TRICEPS)

Begin holding a barbell just above your upper chest with your knees bent and back straight. Press the weight up until it just clears the top of your head and then immediately lower it behind you toward the base of your neck. Once there, press it back over to the front and repeat.

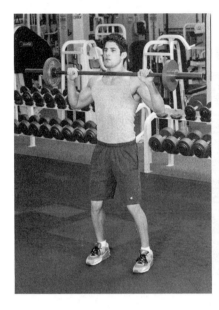
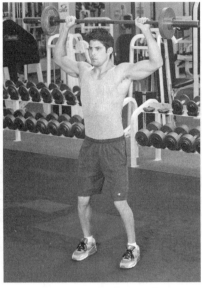
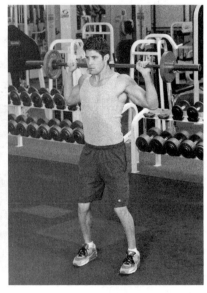

OVERHEAD DUMBBELL TRICEPS EXTENSION

(MUSCLES TRAINED: TRICEPS)

Grasp a dumbbell with a hand-over-hand grip and lift it up over your head. Keeping your elbows as close together as possible, lower the dumbbell behind your head until it almost touches the base of your neck. Pause for a second and then lift it back up by straightening your arms. This can also be done with one arm at a time with the nonworking arm being used to help keep the working arm in place.

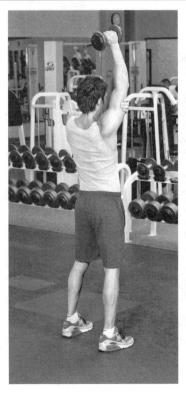
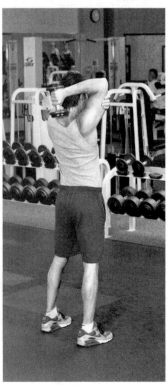

LYING DUMBBELL TRICEPS EXTENSION

(MUSCLES TRAINED: TRICEPS)

Grab a pair of dumbbells and lie back on an exercise bench, positioning your outstretched arms directly above your shoulders. Keeping your upper arms straight, bend at the elbow and lower the weights down toward the crown of your head. Pause an inch off your head and press back up to the starting position. This exercise can also be done by alternating raising and lowering the dumbbells, or with an E-Z curl bar.

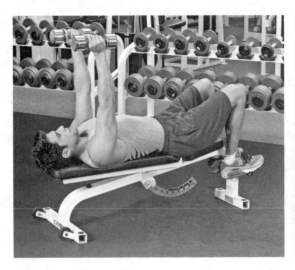
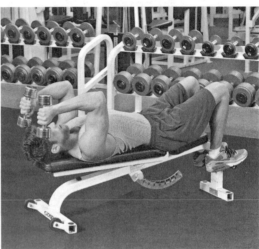

E-Z BAR OVERHEAD TRICEPS EXTENSION

(MUSCLES TRAINED: TRICEPS)

Grasp an E-Z bar and press it overhead. Keeping your upper arms as close to your head as possible, lower the bar until it almost touches the base of your neck. Press back up until your arms are completely straight.

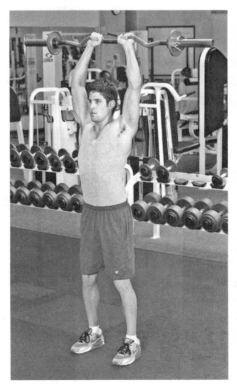
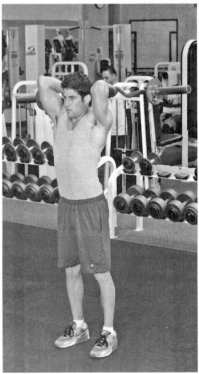

CLOSE-GRIP BENCH PRESS

(MUSCLES TRAINED: TRICEPS, CHEST)

Lie back on a bench press and take a close grip (hands 12 to 16 inches apart) on the bar. Begin by lowering the weight down toward your chest. Pause when the bar is almost in contact with your chest and then press back up to the starting position.

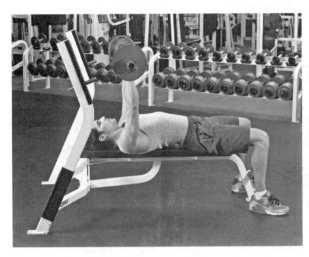
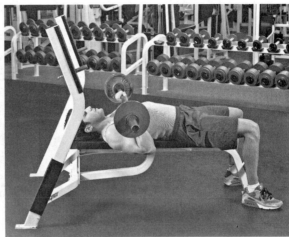

STANDING DUMBBELL CURL

(MUSCLES TRAINED: BICEPS, FOREARMS)

Stand holding a pair of dumbbells with your palms facing forward. Keeping your upper arms still, curl the dumbbells until your palms are almost in contact with your shoulders. Pause, lower, and repeat. Using a neutral grip with the dumbbells facing each other (known as a Hammer Curl) will bring the brachioradialis more into play. Either of these exercises can also be done by alternating arms.

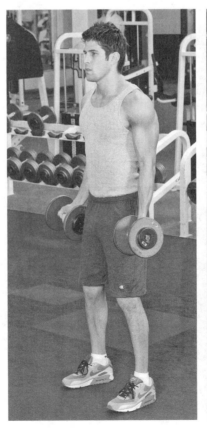
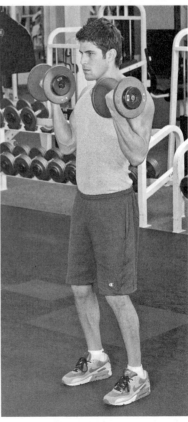

STANDING BARBELL CURL

Stand holding a barbell with a supinated, slightly wider than shoulder-width grip. Keeping your upper arms still, curl the bar until your palms are almost in contact with your shoulders. Pause, lower, and repeat.

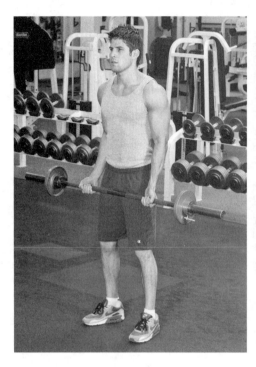
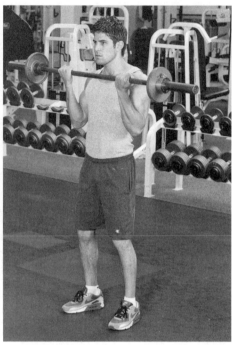

STANDING CONCENTRATION CURL

Stand holding a dumbbell in one hand. Bend your knees and lean forward at the waist, resting the back of your working arm on the inside of your thigh on that same side. With your other arm braced against your other leg, keep your back flat as you curl the weight up toward your shoulder. Pause at the top, lower, and repeat.

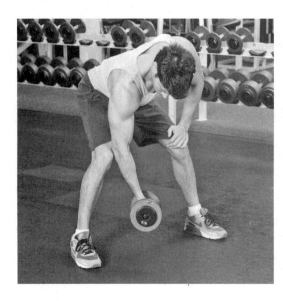
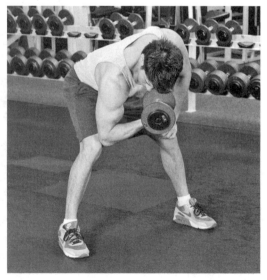

E-Z BAR REVERSE GRIP CURL

(MUSCLES TRAINED: BICEPS, BRACHIORADIALIS, FOREARMS)

Grab an E-Z bar with a pronated, medium grip with your palms facing your thighs. Keeping your back straight and knees bent, curl the weight until the backs of your hands are as close to your shoulders as possible. Pause, lower, and repeat.

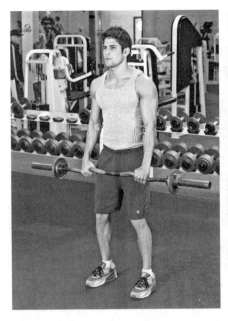
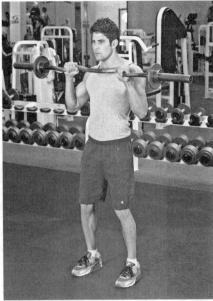

STANDING BARBELL WRIST CURL

(MUSCLES TRAINED: WRIST FLEXORS)

Stand holding a barbell behind your back with your palms facing behind you. Begin by allowing the barbell to roll down into your fingertips and then reverse directions and pull it back up as high as it can go without bending your arms. Pause, lower, and repeat.

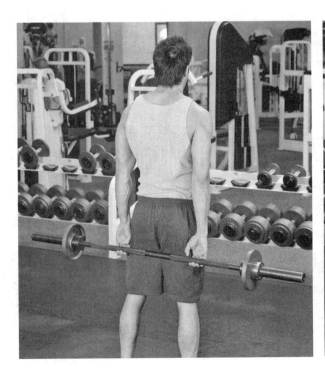
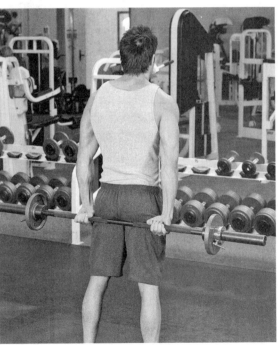

ZOTTMAN CURL

(MUSCLES TRAINED: BICEPS, BRACHIORADIALIS)

Stand holding a pair of dumbbells with a supinated grip just outside your thighs. Begin by curling the weights up toward your shoulders. At the top of the movement, rotate your wrists so that your palms face down (pronated grip) and lower the dumbbells back down to the starting position. At the bottom, go back to a supinated grip again and continue.

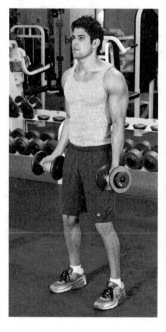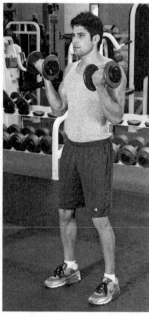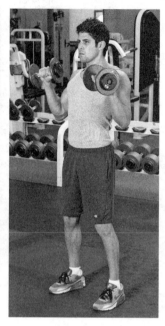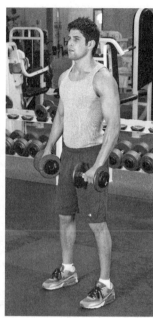

BARBELL CURL PLUS

(MUSCLES TRAINED: BICEPS, FOREARMS, SHOULDERS)

Adopt the same position as you would when doing the Standing Barbell Curl. This time, instead of finishing the exercise when your palms are in front of your wrists, continue the motion by bringing your elbows up and slightly forward. This little addition will further intensify the contraction of the biceps since they also contribute to flexing the shoulders (bringing your arms forward).

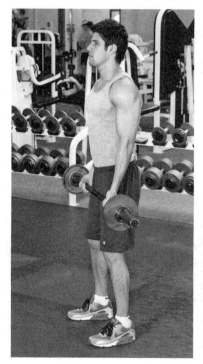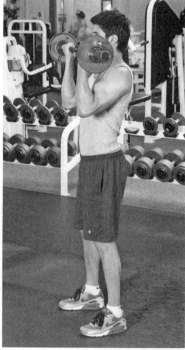

LOWER BODY

BEGINNER/INTERMEDIATE	ADVANCED
Dumbbell Squat	Dumbbell Side Lunge
Dumbbell Sumo Squat	Dumbbell Power Clean
Dumbbell Reverse Lunge	Jump Squat
Dumbbell Split Squat	Barbell Side Lunge
Dumbbell Front Lunge	Deadlift
Dumbbell Front Squat	Suitcase Deadlift
Dumbbell Romanian Deadlift	Barbell Romanian Deadlift
Dumbbell Unilateral Calf Raise	Good Morning
Barbell Reverse Lunge	Barbell Power Clean
Barbell Front Lunge	

DUMBBELL SQUAT

(MUSCLES TRAINED: QUADRICEPS, GLUTES, HAMSTRINGS)

Grab a pair of dumbbells and hold them at arm's length at your sides. Set your feet shoulder-width apart, knees slightly bent, back straight, eyes focused straight ahead. Slowly lower your body as if you were sitting back into a chair, keeping your back in its natural alignment and lower legs nearly perpendicular to the floor. When your upper thighs are parallel to the floor, pause, then return to the starting position.

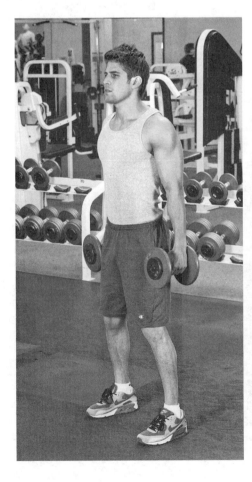
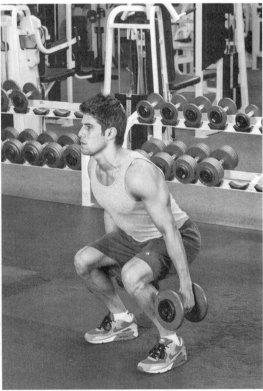

DUMBBELL SUMO SQUAT

(MUSCLES TRAINED: QUADRICEPS, ADDUCTORS, GLUTES, HAMSTRINGS)

Hold a heavy dumbbell by its sides between your legs with a wide stance and your toes turned out approximately 45 degrees. Holding a natural arch in your back, keep your shoulder blades together as you sit back into a squat. Once your thighs are parallel to the floor, keep your torso as upright as possible as you push back up to the starting position.

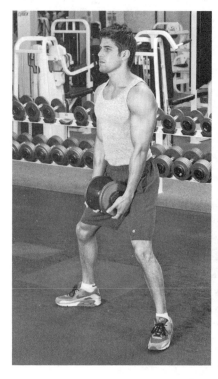
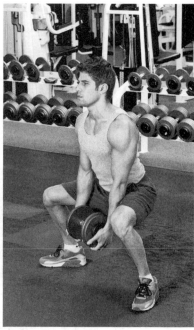

DUMBBELL REVERSE LUNGE

(MUSCLES TRAINED: GLUTES, HAMSTRINGS, QUADRICEPS)

Grab a pair of dumbbells and hold them at your sides. Stand with your feet hip-width apart. Step backward with your nondominant leg (your left if you're right-handed) and lower your body until your front knee is bent 90 degrees and your rear knee nearly touches the floor. Your front lower leg should be perpendicular to the floor and your torso should remain upright. Push yourself back up to the starting position as quickly as you can and repeat with your dominant leg.

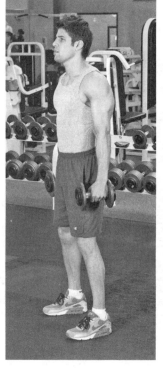
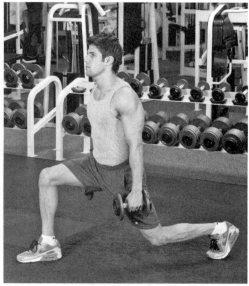

DUMBBELL SPLIT SQUAT

(MUSCLES TRAINED: QUADRICEPS, GLUTES, HAMSTRINGS)

Grab a pair of dumbbells and hold them at your sides. Stand in a staggered stance with your feet 2½ to 3 feet apart, your left foot in front of your right. Lower your body until your front knee is bent 90 degrees and your rear knee nearly touches the floor. Your front lower leg should be perpendicular to the floor and your torso should remain upright. Push yourself back up to the starting position as quickly as you can. Finish all of your repetitions, then repeat the exercise with your right foot in front of your left.

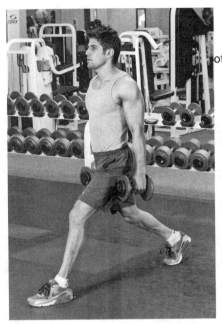
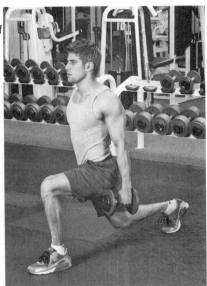

DUMBBELL FRONT LUNGE

(MUSCLES TRAINED: QUADRICEPS, GLUTES, HAMSTRINGS)

Grab a pair of dumbbells and hold them at your sides. Stand with your feet hip-width apart. Step forward with your non-dominant leg (your left if you're right-handed) and lower your body until your front knee is bent 90 degrees and your rear knee nearly touches the floor. Your front lower leg should be perpendicular to the floor and your torso should remain upright. Push yourself back up to the starting position as quickly as you can, and repeat with your dominant leg. That's one repetition.

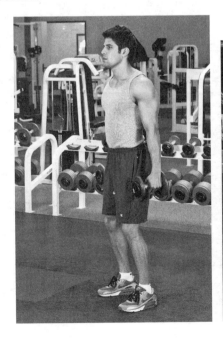
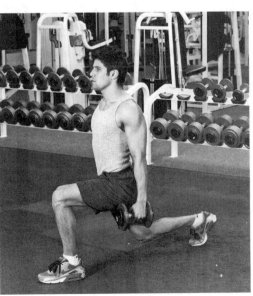

DUMBBELL FRONT SQUAT

(MUSCLES TRAINED: QUADRICEPS, GLUTES, HAMSTRINGS)

Lift a pair of dumbbells so they sit end to end on top of your shoulders. Holding them in place with your upper arms parallel to the floor, squat down until your thighs are parallel to the floor. Pause for a second, then press back up to the starting position.

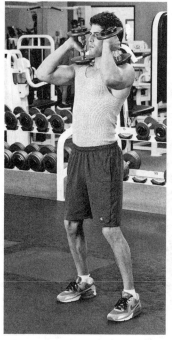
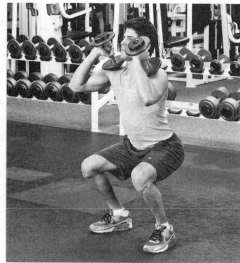

DUMBBELL ROMANIAN DEADLIFT

(MUSCLES TRAINED: HAMSTRINGS, GLUTES)

Grab a pair of dumbbells and stand holding them at arm's length in front of your thighs. Keep your feet shoulder-width apart, your knees slightly bent, and your eyes focused straight ahead. Slowly bend at the hips as you lower the dumbbells just below your knees. Don't change the angle of your knees. Keep your head and chest up and your lower back flat or slightly arched. Lift your torso back to the starting position, keeping the dumbbells as close to your body as possible.

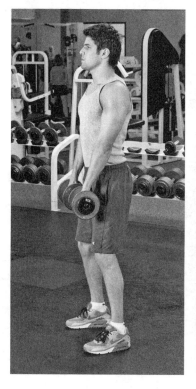
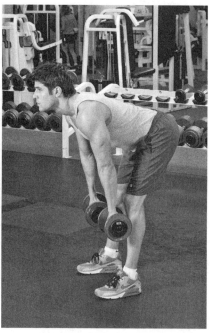

DUMBBELL UNILATERAL CALF RAISE

(MUSCLES TRAINED: CALVES)

Grab a dumbbell in one hand and place the ball of your foot on that same side on a calf block or step. Hold on to something for balance with your opposite hand as you begin with the heel of your working leg below the level of the surface you're standing on. Next, press up as high as you can onto the ball of your foot and hold for a second at the top. Pause, lower, and repeat.

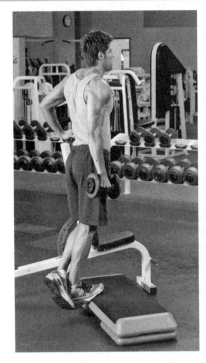
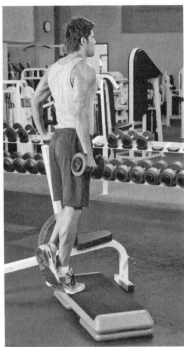

BARBELL REVERSE LUNGE

(MUSCLES TRAINED: GLUTES, HAMSTRINGS, QUADRICEPS)

Stand holding a barbell across your upper trapezius, your feet hip-width apart. Step backward with your non-dominant leg (your right if you're left-handed) and lower your body until your front knee is bent 90 degrees and your rear knee nearly touches the floor. Your front lower leg should be perpendicular to the floor and your torso should remain upright. Push yourself back up to the starting position as quickly as you can and repeat with your dominant leg.

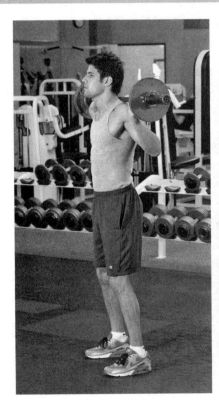
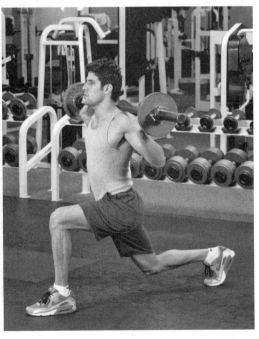

BARBELL FRONT LUNGE

(MUSCLES TRAINED: QUADRICEPS, GLUTES, HAMSTRINGS)

Stand holding a barbell across your upper trapezius, your feet hip-width apart. Step forward with your nondominant leg (your left if you're right-handed) and lower your body until your front knee is bent 90 degrees and your rear knee nearly touches the floor. Your front lower leg should be perpendicular to the floor and your torso should remain upright. Push yourself back up to the starting position quickly as you can, and repeat with your dominant leg.

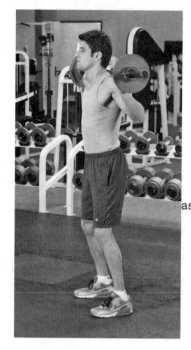
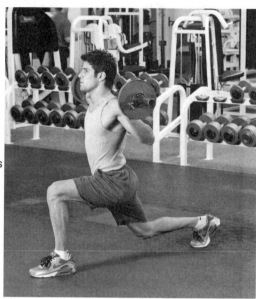

DUMBBELL SIDE LUNGE

(MUSCLES TRAINED: QUADRICEPS, ADDUCTORS, GLUTES, HAMSTRINGS)

Stand holding a pair of dumbbells at arm's length at your side. Step out sideways and squat into that hip as you keep your other leg perfectly straight. In the bottom position, your working leg should be parallel to the floor and you should have a normal arch in your spine, with your arms hanging on either side of your lead knee. As soon as you get to the bottom, push yourself back up to the starting position.

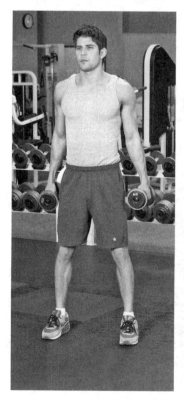
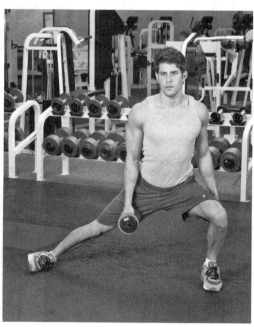

DUMBBELL POWER CLEAN

(MUSCLES TRAINED: GLUTES, HAMSTRINGS, QUADRICEPS, UPPER BACK, BICEPS)

Grab a pair of dumbbells with a pronated, shoulder-width grip and squat over them on the floor. Using your hips to start the movement, press your feet into the floor as you drive upward, extending your hips and torso in the process. As the weights approach your waist, quickly rise up onto the balls of your feet as you pull them up toward your chest. Then quickly drop underneath the weight and catch the dumbbells on top of your shoulders in a squat position. Stand up, flip the weights down, squat down, and repeat.

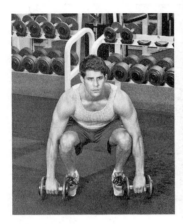
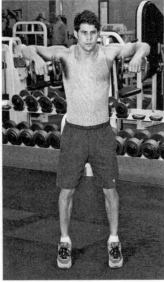
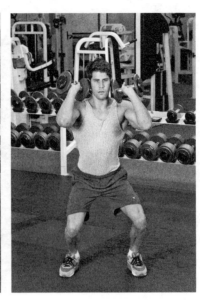

JUMP SQUAT

(MUSCLES TRAINED: QUADRICEPS, GLUTES, HAMSTRINGS, CALVES)

Stand with your feet hip-width apart, holding a light barbell across your upper trapezius. Quickly descend until your thighs are bent about 45 degrees (a half-squat position) and then immediately fire up using your thighs and calves to jump off the floor. Land as softly as possible and immediately descend into your next repetition.

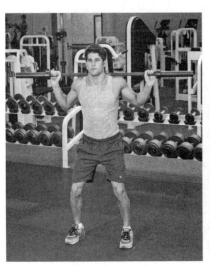
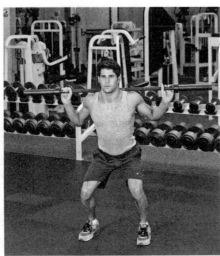
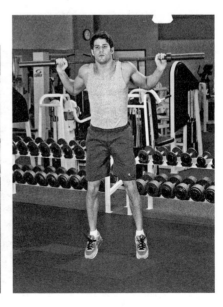

BARBELL SIDE LUNGE

(MUSCLES TRAINED: QUADRICEPS, ADDUCTORS, GLUTES, HAMSTRINGS)

Stand with your feet hip-width, holding a light barbell across your upper trapezius. Step out sideways and squat into that hip as you keep your other leg perfectly straight. In the bottom position your working leg should be parallel to the floor and you should have a normal arch in your spine. As soon as you get to the bottom, push yourself back up to the starting position and repeat.

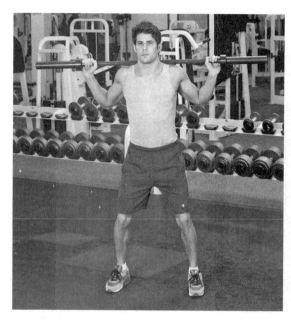 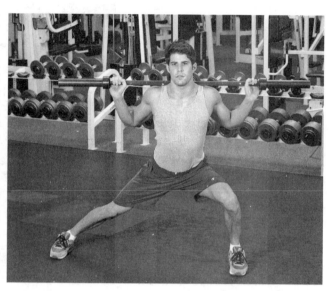

DEADLIFT

(MUSCLES TRAINED: GLUTES, HAMSTRINGS, QUADRICEPS, UPPER BACK)

Set a barbell on the floor and stand facing it. Squat down and grab it overhand with your hands just outside your legs. With your back flat and head up, stand up with the barbell, pulling your shoulder blades back. Slowly lower the bar to the starting position.

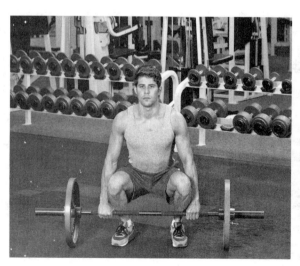 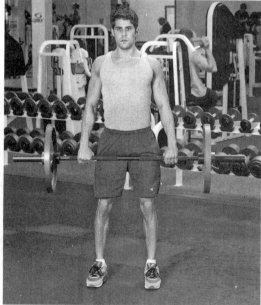

SUITCASE DEADLIFT

Stand holding an unweighted barbell at its midpoint alongside you at arm's length. Begin by sitting back into your hips as you keep your torso as erect as possible, doing your best not to favor the side holding the weight. (In other words, do the lift as if you have the bar in both hands.) Once your thighs are parallel to the ground, pause for a second before pressing your feet into the floor and bringing the bar back to the starting position.

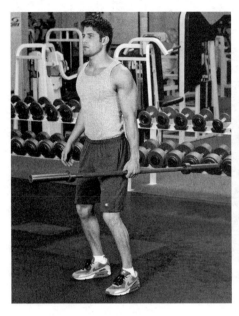
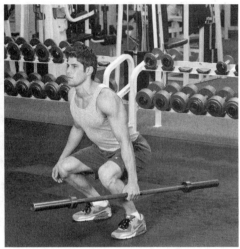

BARBELL ROMANIAN DEADLIFT

(MUSCLES TRAINED: GLUTES, HAMSTRINGS)

Stand with your feet hip-width apart and your knees slightly bent. Grab a barbell with an overhand, shoulder-width grip and hold the bar down at arm's length in front of you. Keeping your lower back arched slightly, slowly bend at the waist as far as you can without losing the arch. (The bar will probably be just below your knees.) Don't change the angle of your knees and keep the bar as close to your body as possible throughout the entire move. Pause, then lift your torso back to the starting position.

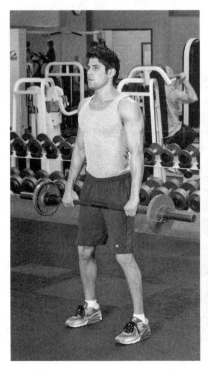
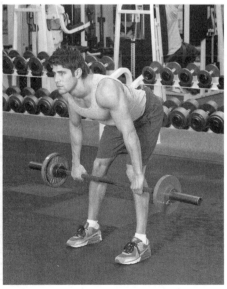

GOOD MORNING

Grab a barbell with an overhand grip and place it so that it rests comfortably across your upper back. Slowly bend forward at the hips as you lower your chest as far as you can go while maintaining the natural arch in your lower back or until your upper body is parallel to the floor. Keep your head up and maintain the same angle of your knees. Lift your upper body back to the starting position.

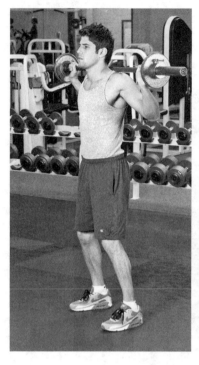
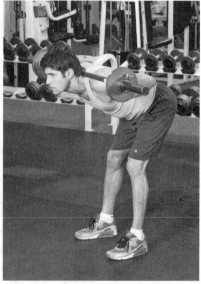

BARBELL POWER CLEAN

(MUSCLES TRAINED: GLUTES, HAMSTRINGS, QUADRICEPS, UPPER BACK, BICEPS)

Squat down over a loaded barbell and grab it with a pronated, shoulder-width grip. Using your hips to start the movement, press your feet into the floor as you drive upward, extending your hips and torso in the process. As the bar approaches your waist, quickly rise up onto the balls of your feet as you pull it up toward your chest. Then quickly drop underneath the bar and catch it on top of your shoulders in a squat position. Stand up, flip the weight down, squat down, and repeat.

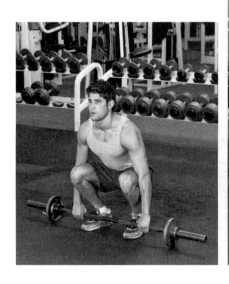
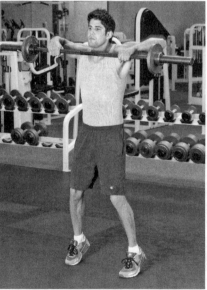
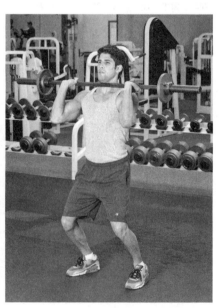

INTEGRATED LIFTS

BEGINNER/ INTERMEDIATE	ADVANCED
Split Squat and Press	Overhead Squat
Floor-to-Ceiling One-Arm Row	Overhead Lunge
Lateral Raise with Rotation	Bent-Over Row with Back Extension
Thruster	

SPLIT SQUAT AND PRESS

(MUSCLES TRAINED: QUADRICEPS, GLUTES, HAMSTRINGS, SHOULDERS, TRICEPS, CORE)

Stand in a split squat position holding a barbell or a pair of dumbbells just above shoulder height. Begin by descending into a split squat as you simultaneously press the weight overhead. In the bottom position both your knees should be bent approximately 90 degrees with your back knee almost touching the floor and the weight up above your head. Pause for a second, then return to the starting position.

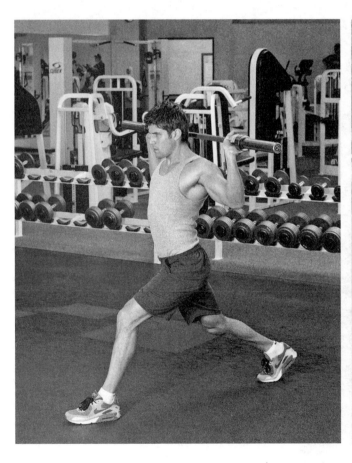 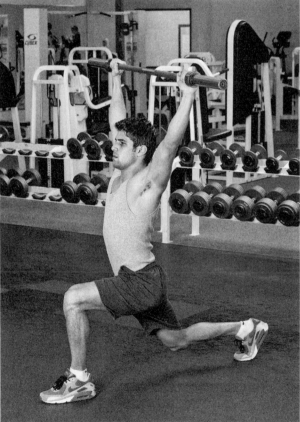

FLOOR-TO-CEILING ONE-ARM ROW

(MUSCLES TRAINED: UPPER BACK, BICEPS, GLUTES, HAMSTRINGS, CORE)

Stand in a slight lunge position with one foot in front of the other and only the ball of your back foot touching the floor. Holding a dumbbell at arm's length pointing toward the floor, begin by pulling the dumbbell up as you simultaneously extend your legs. At the top of the movement your working arm's elbow will be up above the level of your shoulder and your legs will be completely straight. Pause, lower, and repeat.

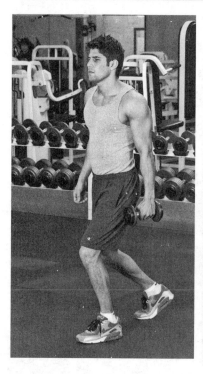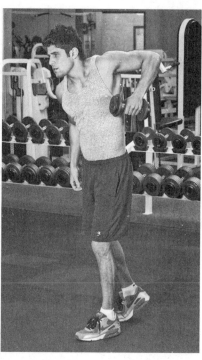

LATERAL RAISE WITH ROTATION

(MUSCLES TRAINED: SHOULDERS, CORE)

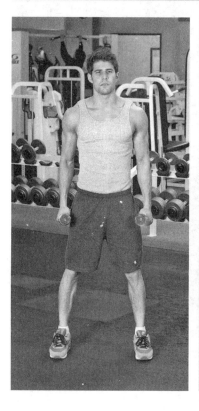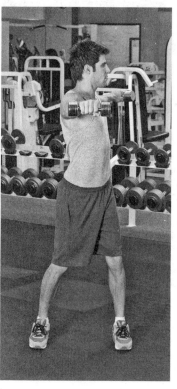

Stand with your feet shoulder-width apart and hold a pair of dumbbells at arm's length. Keeping a slight bend in your arms, begin by lifting your arms up until they're parallel to the ground. Hold there and then rotate as far as you can in one direction without allowing your arms to drop. Pause for a second and then repeat to the other side.

THRUSTER

Stand with your feet shoulder-width apart and hold a pair of dumbbells just above your shoulders. Begin by descending into a squat, then once your thighs are parallel to the floor, reverse directions and stand back up as you simultaneously press the weights up overhead. Pause for a second, lower the weights back down, and repeat.

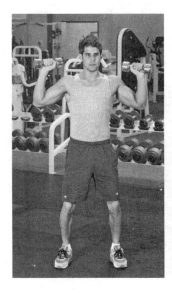 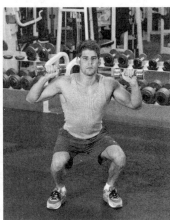 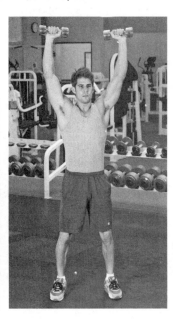

OVERHEAD SQUAT

Stand holding a light barbell overhead with a grip that's twice shoulder-width. Begin by descending into a squat, making sure that the barbell stays out of your peripheral vision and doesn't drift forward as you do. When your thighs are parallel to the floor, pause for a second before pressing back up to the starting position.

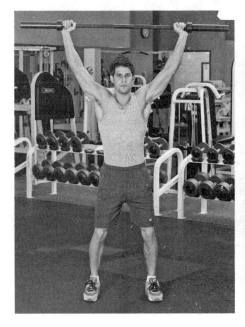 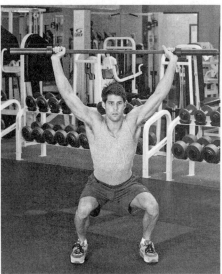

OVERHEAD LUNGE

(MUSCLES TRAINED: QUADRICEPS, GLUTES, HAMSTRINGS, UPPER BACK)

Begin the same way as you would the Overhead Squat, only this time take a lunge step forward as you keep the bar held overhead. In the bottom position, both knees should be bent approximately 90 degrees with your arms completely straight. As soon as you reach the bottom, push back and up to the starting position.

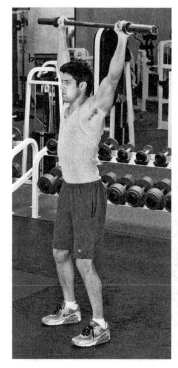
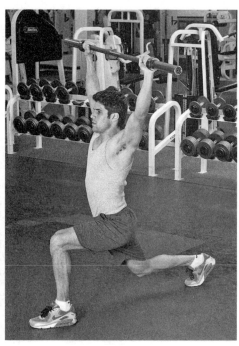

BENT-OVER ROW WITH BACK EXTENSION

(MUSCLES TRAINED: HAMSTRINGS, GLUTES, UPPER BACK, BICEPS)

Stand holding a barbell with a pronated, shoulder-width grip. Keeping your knees slightly bent, bend over at the waist until your torso is almost parallel to the floor and your arms are lined up underneath your shoulders. Once there, maintain an arch in your lower back as you row the weight up to your chest. Hold the weight there as you use your lower back muscles to extend back up to a standing position. Lower your arms back down and repeat.

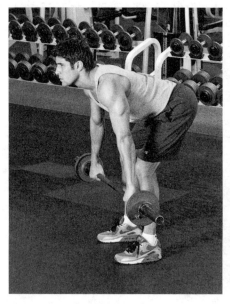
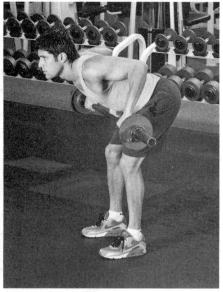

THREE WAYS TO WEIGH IN

Although we can't predict what type of dumbbells your gym or club may have, they come in three specific styles.

Fixed-weight dumbbells: This type of dumbbell is what most gyms and clubs stock up on. Made from materials ranging from cheap cast iron to highly expensive polished chrome, fixed-weight dumbbells can be either a solid piece of metal or a series of weight plates. Either way, they're typically stamped with whatever weight they are so you know exactly what you're grabbing off the rack—and that's it. You can't change their weight—what you see is what you get—which is why many gyms will stock a range from as little as 1 pound a piece to as heavy as 200 pounds each.

Plate-loaded adjustable dumbbells: Although not as common in gyms, this type of dumbbell is generally a small, 12- to 15-inch bar that holds standard or Olympic weight plates in the same way as a barbell, allowing you the benefit of adding or removing weight plates on either end. Holding the plates on each end are a pair of collars that clamp, spin, or pinch the bar (depending on the type of collars your gym has).

Selectorized adjustable dumbbells: Another not-so-common style of dumbbell (although we've seen them in a few places), selectorized adjustable dumbbells rely on a series of thin, interconnecting plates that all rest inside a base. You can change how many plates are lifted from the base—which lets you adjust the weight of each dumbbell to your tastes—by sliding a lever, pushing a button, or turning a knob (depending on the manufacturer). Doing so connects the right amount to the handle, so when you lift the dumbbell straight up from its base, you have the exact amount you need while the remaining plates stay unused inside the base.

CHAPTER NINE

BASIC CABLE

Discover the Power of the Gym's Most Versatile Machine

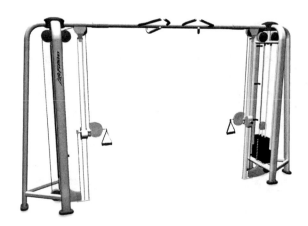

IF FREE WEIGHTS ARE THE MEAT and potatoes of your workout, think of a cable station as the dessert. It's a fun-looking piece of equipment that most folks can't wait to try out, and like free weights, it offers you tremendous versatility in terms of the number of different exercises you can perform with it. And if it's adjustable to a variety of different angles—as most commercial models found in gyms are—so much the better. True, it is still technically a machine, so your movement is at least partially controlled, but the large ranges of motion it allows for still make it a very functional piece of equipment with a great deal of carryover to three-dimensional sport and leisure activities, like swinging a golf club.

The two main types of cable stations most gyms have are the traditional cable crossover station and the single adjustable cable column. The only major difference between the two is that the cable crossover allows you to do bilateral (both limbs working simultaneously) exercises like chest flys and standing cable crossovers. In fact, to watch some of your fellow gym goers use them, you'd think that's all they were good for. Despite their enormous popularity though, these two exercises merely scratch the surface of what can be accomplished with a cable station. The fact that they have both high and low settings and can be adjusted to various levels in between make the number of exercises you're capable of doing on either variety practically endless.

Besides versatility, another big benefit of using cables is the tension factor. This doesn't mean that by sticking with

cables you'll be less apt to piss off all the big, burly types in the free weight area, leading to a more harmonious gym environment. What we mean here is that unlike free weights, cables keep your muscles under constant tension throughout the entire range of motion. Ever notice how when you use free weights, exercises like biceps curls and especially flys suddenly become easier at certain points in the lift? That's because the amount of force your muscles have to exert to overcome the resistance changes due to the affects of gravity. A fly, for instance, is pretty tough when the dumbbells are out away from your body, near parallel to the floor, but gets increasingly easier as you bring the weights up over your chest.

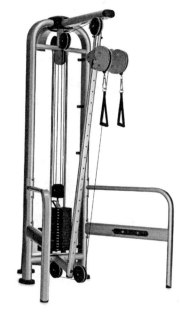

Not so with cables! The constant tension they provide means that you'll be more effectively overloading your muscles throughout the entire range of motion. Not that they're perfect, mind you. It's pretty difficult to work certain muscle groups thoroughly like your legs and chest using cables exclusively. You can, however, use them to perform some good complementary exercises to use as "finishers" once you've already fatigued these areas with more compound lifts. Plus, they're great for upper back, shoulder, and arm training—and don't even get us started on core work. As you're about to see, there are about a dozen different ways to work your core on an adjustable cable station—and probably even more if you put your mind to it. It all depends on just how creative you want to get.

GET A HANDLE ON IT

One thing you'll invariably notice about working with any type of cable station is the number of handles and attachments that can be used with it. Most gyms have these displayed either on a wall right next to the unit or in a large bin nearby. At first glance, some of these contraptions may look like they're right out of a medieval torture chamber. As you get used to them, though, you'll find they're quite necessary and when used properly can really add some nice variety to your workouts. So without any further ado, let's meet these little guys and find out exactly what they do.

1. **Closed stirrup handle:** This is most often made of metal, but can also be made of nylon with a plastic handle. It is used for all forms of chest work, unilateral rowing exercises, arm work, and shoulder work, and also for core exercises. Easily the most common handle used with a cable unit.

2. **Open stirrup handle:** Made of metal, this U-shaped handle has one open side. The only difference between these and the closed stirrup handles is that the handle is able to roll, making certain exercises like arm curls and various triceps exercises much more comfortable on the wrists.

3. **Rope attachment:** This long, V-shaped rope handle is most commonly used for triceps exercises, but is also great for face pulls, both of which are featured in the exercises in this chapter.

4. **V bar:** Its unique shape is designed to ease tension on the wrists when doing triceps exercises.

5. **E-Z bar:** Like the V bar, it's also used for easing wrist strain on triceps, biceps, and shoulder exercises.

6. **Ankle cuffs:** These little buggers allow you to perform a number of challenging lower-body isolation exercises aimed at strengthening often underused muscle groups like the glutes, as well as the inner and outer thighs.

7. **Straight bar (short):** This short bar is used for various types of arm and shoulder exercises. But it's less popular because of the unforgiving wrist position it forces.

8. **Lat bar:** This long bar can be used for both lat pulldowns and rows if the specified lat pulldown/low row machine is already being used. Since it's a longer bar, you can also use it for wider grip biceps curls, triceps extensions, and upright rows.

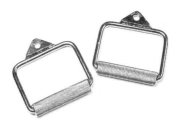
Closed stirrup handle

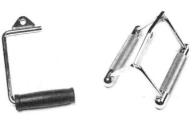
Open stirrup handle   **V bar**

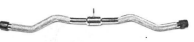
E-Z bar

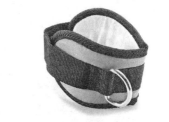
Ankle cuffs

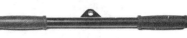
Straight bar

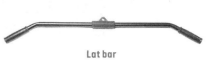
Lat bar

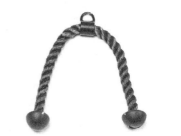
Rope attachment

CORE

<table>
<tr><th>BEGINNER/
INTERMEDIATE</th><th>ADVANCED</th></tr>
<tr><td>Standing Cable
Crunch</td><td>Woodchopper:
High to Low</td></tr>
<tr><td>Kneeling Cable
Crunch</td><td>Woodchopper:
Low to High</td></tr>
<tr><td>Reverse Cable
Crunch</td><td>Cable Rotation</td></tr>
<tr><td></td><td>Overhead Reach</td></tr>
</table>

STANDING CABLE CRUNCH

(MUSCLES TRAINED: ABDOMINALS)

Attach a rope handle to a high pulley and stand with your back to the pulley with your neck between the ropes. Holding the handle to your chest, bend forward at the waist, rounding your back, and aim your chest toward your pelvis. Hold the contracted position for a second, then raise the weight back up and repeat.

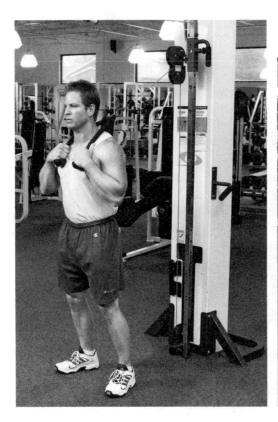
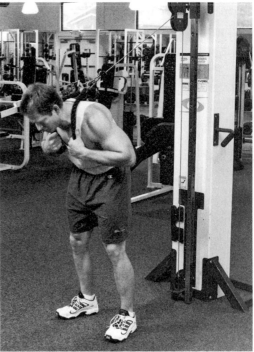

KNEELING CABLE CRUNCH

(MUSCLES TRAINED: ABDOMINALS)

Attach the rope handle to a high pulley and kneel down facing the machine with your buttocks near your heels but not resting on them. Holding the ropes at the sides of your head, crunch your rib cage toward your pelvis without moving any other part of your body. Pause when your elbows touch your knees, then slowly return the weight to the starting position. You can also crunch down bringing one elbow to the opposite knee to involve the obliques more.

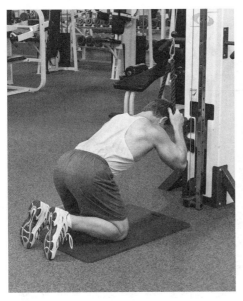 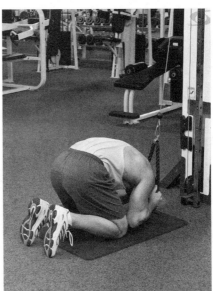

REVERSE CABLE CRUNCH

(MUSCLES TRAINED: ABDOMINALS)

Lie down on the floor in front of a low pulley and loop the ankle straps around your ankles. Keeping your knees bent about 90 degrees, use your abs to roll your hips back toward your chest. At the top of the movement your thighs should be close to your chest with your tailbone off the ground. Pause there for a second, lower, and repeat.

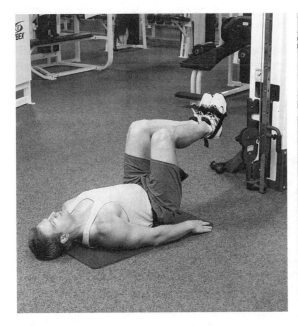 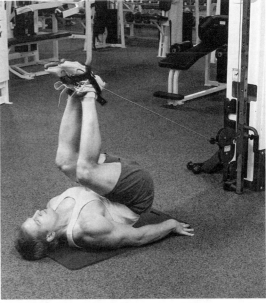

WOODCHOPPER: HIGH TO LOW

(MUSCLES TRAINED: ABDOMINALS, OBLIQUES)

Attach a rope handle to a high cable pulley, grab it with both hands, and stand with your right side facing the cable station and your feet shoulder-width apart. Hold the rope over your inside shoulder, as if it were an ax you were about to swing. Pull the rope down and across your torso by bending and twisting at your waist so that it ends up on the far side of your outside calf. Pause at the bottom, then slowly straighten back to the starting position. Finish the repetitions on this side, then switch sides to complete the set.

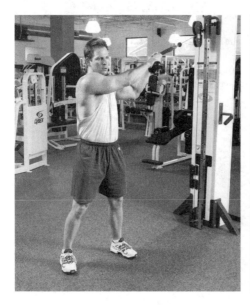 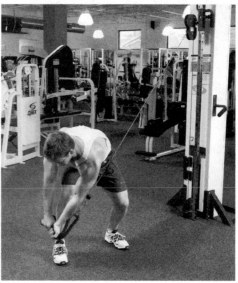

WOODCHOPPER: LOW TO HIGH

(MUSCLES TRAINED: ABDOMINALS, OBLIQUES)

Attach a rope handle to a low cable pulley, grab it with both hands, and stand with your right side facing the cable station and your feet shoulder-width apart. Bend over and hold the handle with both hands just outside your right calf muscle. Your shoulders will be rotated toward the cable machine. Straighten your arms and maintain this position throughout the entire movement. Pull the handle up and across your torso as you straighten your body and twist your shoulders to the left. Your right arm ends up in front of your face, and the handle is at the same height as your ear. Pause, then slowly return to the starting position. Finish the repetitions on this side, then switch sides to complete the set.

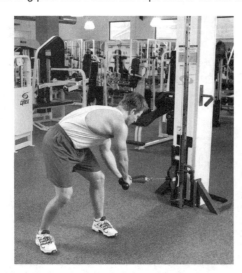 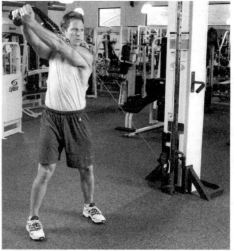

CABLE ROTATION

Stand aside an adjustable cable station with the pulley set at about chest height. Reach across your body and grab the handle with the hand furthest away from the weight stack and then wrap the other hand over it. Keeping your knees bent and arms straight but not locked, use your core muscles to work the weight around in a wide, arcing motion. When your arms are in a perpendicular line to the weight stack and the cable is in contact with your shoulder, pause for a second, then return the weight to the starting position.

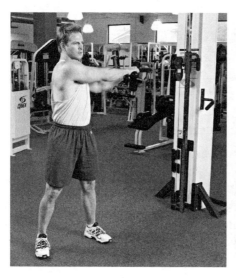
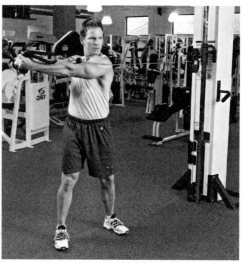

OVERHEAD REACH

Attach a rope handle to a high cable pulley and grasp it at both ends as you raise your arms overhead. Stand with a slightly staggered stance as you use your core muscles to go from a slightly extended spine to a slightly rounded back position. To do this, use your abdominals to pull your chest toward your pelvis. Pause for a second, then return the weight to the starting position.

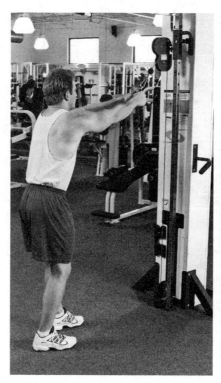
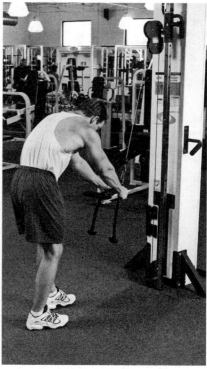

CHEST AND UPPER BACK

	BEGINNER/INTERMEDIATE	ADVANCED
CHEST	Unilateral High Cable Fly Unilateral Low Cable Fly Cable Crossover: High to Low Cable Crossover: Low to High	Bent-Over Cable Crossover
BACK	Double Pulldown Seated Row Standing Unilateral High Row Standing Unilateral Low Row Standing Pullover Bent-Over Rear Lateral Raise Standing Rear Lateral Raise	Face Pull Bent-Over Row

UNILATERAL HIGH CABLE FLY

(MUSCLES TRAINED: CHEST, FRONT DELTOIDS)

Stand aside a cable station with a stirrup handle attached to a high pulley. With your knees slightly bent, reach up and grasp the handle as you use your chest to bring your arm down in an arcing motion in front of your body. Once you've reached the point where your arm is across the midline of your body, pause for a second, and then return the weight to the starting position.

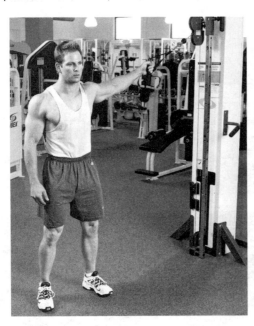
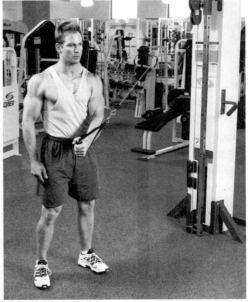

UNILATERAL LOW CABLE FLY
(MUSCLES TRAINED: CHEST, FRONT DELTOIDS)

Stand aside a cable station with a stirrup handle attached to a low pulley. With your knee slightly bent, reach down and grasp the pulley handle as you use your chest to bring the weight up in an arcing motion across your body. Once you reach the point where your arm is across the midline of your body, pause for a second, and then return the weight to the starting position.

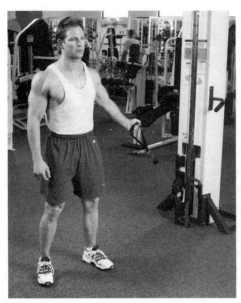
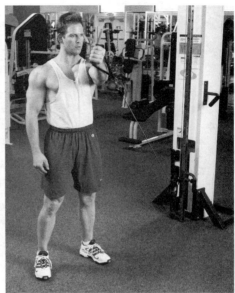

CABLE CROSSOVER: HIGH TO LOW
(MUSCLES TRAINED: CHEST, FRONT DELTOIDS)

Stand inside a cable crossover with the stirrup handles attached to the high pulleys. With your knees slightly bent, use your chest to bring your arms down until they cross in front of your body. Pause for a second and then return the weights to the starting position.

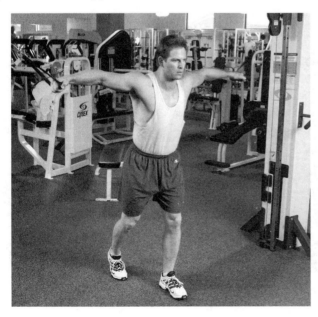
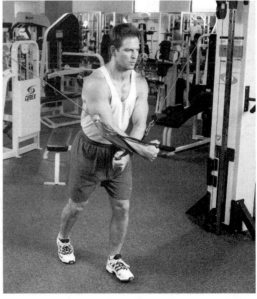

CABLE CROSSOVER: LOW TO HIGH

(MUSCLES TRAINED: CHEST, FRONT DELTOIDS)

Stand inside a cable crossover with the stirrup handles attached to the low pulleys. With your knees slightly bent, use your chest to bring your arms up so they cross in front of your body. Pause for a second and then return the weights to the starting position.

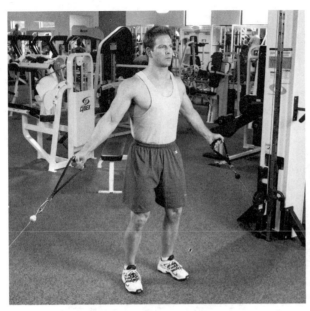 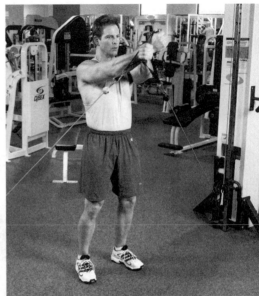

BENT-OVER CABLE CROSSOVER

(MUSCLES TRAINED: CHEST, FRONT DELTOIDS)

Stand inside a cable crossover with the stirrup handles attached to the high pulleys. Begin by bringing the weights down across the front of your body. Once there, bend forward at the waist until your torso is parallel to the ground and allow your arms to drift up past your torso in a wide arc. When your elbows are slightly past your torso, reverse directions and bring your arms down across the front of your body.

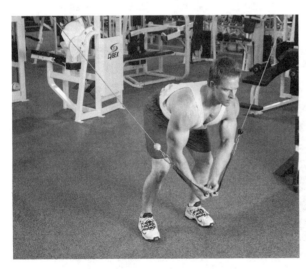 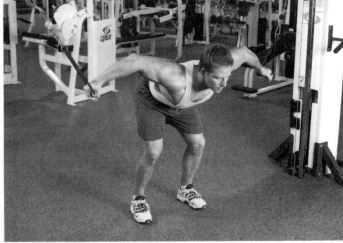

DOUBLE PULLDOWN

(MUSCLES TRAINED: UPPER BACK, BICEPS)

Stand inside a cable crossover with the stirrup handles attached to the high pulleys. Kneel down and keep your torso as erect as possible as you pull your arms down and in toward your body. When your elbows are just slightly behind your back, pause and return the weight to the starting position.

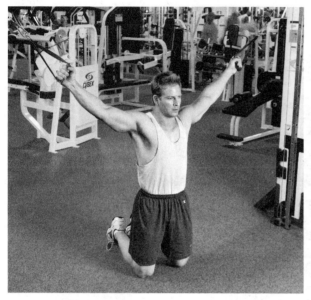 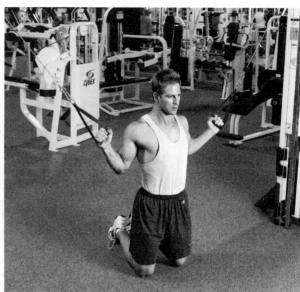

SEATED ROW

(MUSCLES TRAINED: UPPER BACK, BICEPS)

Attach a long, straight bar to the cable and position yourself in the machine. Grab the bar with an overhand grip that's just beyond shoulder-width. Sit up straight and pull your shoulders back. Pull the bar to your abdomen. Pause and then slowly return to the starting position.

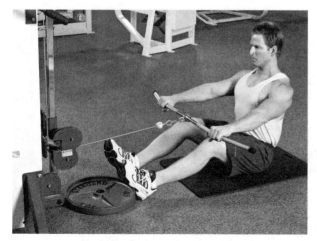 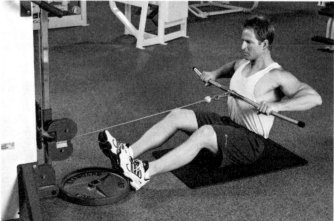

STANDING UNILATERAL HIGH ROW

(MUSCLES TRAINED: UPPER BACK, BICEPS)

Stand inside a cable station facing the weight stack with a stirrup handle attached to a high pulley. Reach up and grab the handle as you adopt a staggered stance with your opposite leg one full stride behind the other (left leg if you have the handle in your right hand). With your lead knee slightly bent and torso held straight, draw your elbow back until it passes your torso. Pause and then return the weight to the starting position. Keeping your elbow in close to your body will involve the lats more, while performing the exercise with your elbow out away from your body will recruit the scapular retractors more.

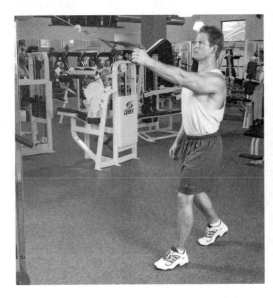 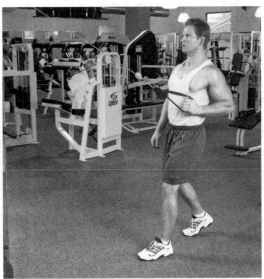

STANDING UNILATERAL LOW ROW

(MUSCLES TRAINED: UPPER BACK, BICEPS)

Stand inside a cable station facing the weight stack with a stirrup handle attached to a low pulley. Reach down and grab the handle as you adopt a staggered stance, with the leg on the side of your working arm one full stride behind the other. Draw your elbow back until it passes your torso. Pause and then return the weight to the starting position. Keeping your elbow in close to your body will involve the lats more, while performing the exercise with your elbow out away from your body will recruit the scapular retractors more.

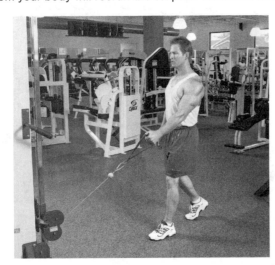 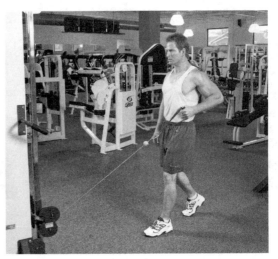

STANDING PULLOVER

Stand facing a cable station with a bar attached to the high pulley. Grasp the bar with an overhand grip as you bend your knees and lean forward approximately 45 degrees. Keeping your torso still and arms straight but not locked, bring the bar down until it makes contact with your thighs. Pause and then return the weight to the starting position.

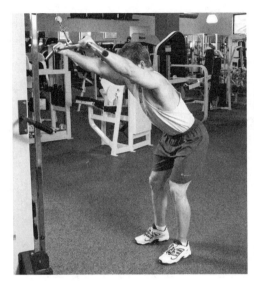 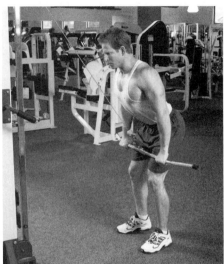

BENT-OVER REAR LATERAL RAISE

Stand inside a cable crossover with the handles attached to the low pulleys. Bend over at the waist and grab both handles across your body (in other words, your right hand grabs the left handle and vice versa). Keeping your knees bent, back straight, and arms slightly bent, work your arms up in a wide arc until your elbows slightly pass your torso. Pause, lower, and repeat.

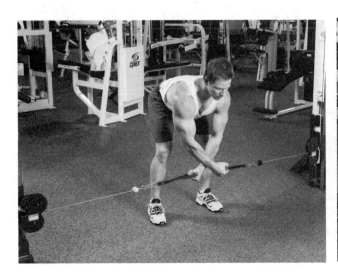 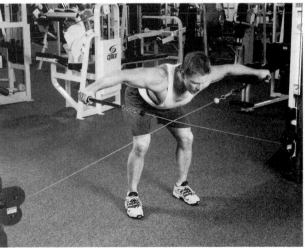

STANDING REAR LATERAL RAISE

(MUSCLES TRAINED: UPPER BACK, SHOULDERS)

Stand inside a cable crossover with the handles attached to the high pulleys. Grasp the handles with a crossover grip (in other words, your right hand grabs the left handle and vice versa). With your hands crossed in front of your face, keep your knees bent, back straight, and arms straight but not locked, and work your arms down in a wide arcing motion until your elbows slightly pass your torso. Pause for a second and then return the weight to the starting position.

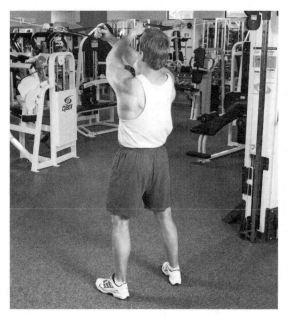 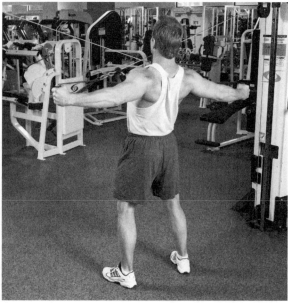

FACE PULL

(MUSCLES TRAINED: UPPER BACK, TRAPEZIUS, BICEPS)

Stand facing a cable station with the rope handle attached to the high pulley. Keep your knees bent and back straight as you grasp the handles and pull them back with your elbows held high until they slightly pass your torso. Pause for a second and then return the weight to the starting position.

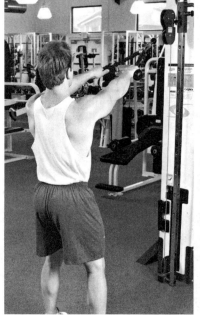 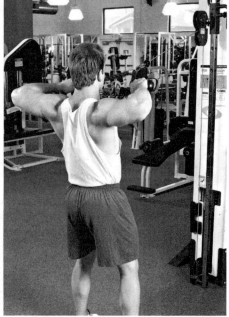

BENT-OVER ROW

Stand in front of a cable station with a straight bar attached to the low pulley. Bend over at the waist with your knees bent and back straight as you grasp the bar with a pronated, shoulder-width grip and pull the bar up until it touches your torso. Pause, lower, and repeat. Using a pronated grip with your elbows out away from your body will target the scapular retractors more, while a supinated grip with your elbows held in close will lead to greater lat and biceps involvement.

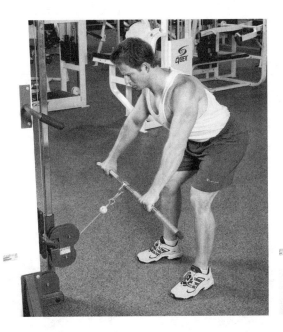
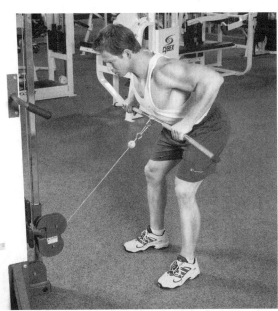

SHOULDERS AND ARMS

	BEGINNER/INTERMEDIATE	ADVANCED
SHOULDERS	Upright Row	Cable Muscle-Up
	Cable Shrug	Dumbbell Cable Press
	Lateral Raise	Unilateral Shoulder Press
	Front Raise	
	Lateral External Rotation	
	Lateral Internal Rotation	
	Unilateral Scarecrow	
	Sword Draw	
TRICEPS	Cable Kickback	Crossover Pushdown
	Triceps Pushdown	Bent-Over Triceps Extension
BICEPS	Cable Curl	Lean Away Concentration Curl
	Reverse Curl	Cable Curl Plus
	Crucifix Curl	
FOREARMS	Standing Wrist Curl	

UPRIGHT ROW

(MUSCLES TRAINED: UPPER TRAPEZIUS, SHOULDERS, BICEPS)

Attach an E-Z curl bar to the low pulley of a cable station. Stand facing the weight stack and grab the bar with a shoulder-width, overhand grip. Hold the bar at arm's length in front of your thighs. Pull the bar up until your upper arms are parallel to the floor. Pause, lower, and repeat.

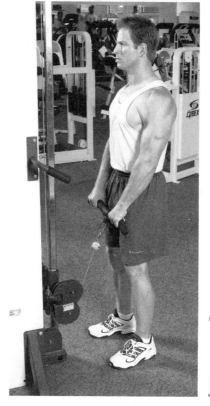
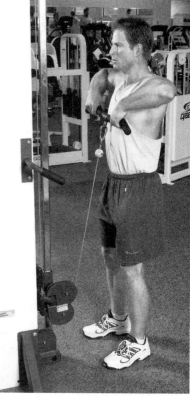

CABLE SHRUG

(MUSCLES TRAINED: UPPER TRAPEZIUS)

Attach a straight bar to a low pulley and hold with a pronated, shoulder-width grip. With your knees slightly bent and back flat, keep your arms straight as you bring your shoulders up as close to your ears as possible. Pause, lower, and repeat.

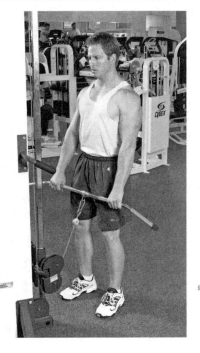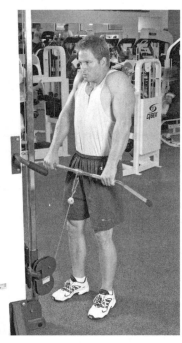

LATERAL RAISE

(MUSCLES TRAINED: MEDIAL DELTOIDS)

Stand inside a cable station with the stirrup handles attached to the low pulleys. Your knees should be slightly bent. Grabbing the handles with a crossover grip (in other words, your right hand grabs the left handle and vice versa), begin with your hands in front of your body. Next, keeping your elbows slightly bent, bring your arms up in a wide arcing motion until they're parallel to the ground. Try to lead more with your elbows than your wrists as you do this. Pause, lower, and repeat.

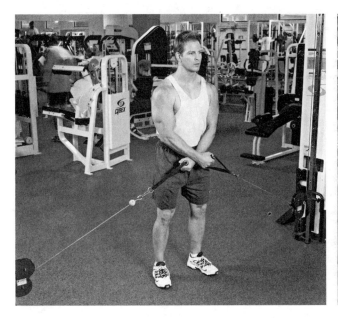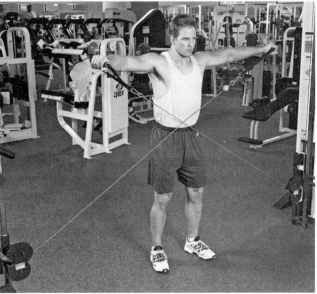

FRONT RAISE

(MUSCLES TRAINED: FRONT DELTOIDS)

Stand in front of a cable station with a straight bar attached to the low pulley. Bend down and grab the bar with a pronated, shoulder-width grip. With your knees bent and back straight, keep a slight bend in your elbows as you lift the weight out in front of you in a wide, arcing motion until your arms are parallel to the floor. Avoid leaning your torso back at any point during the movement. Pause, lower, and repeat.

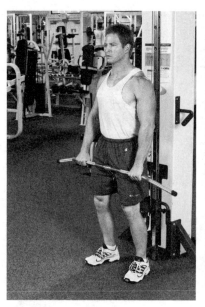 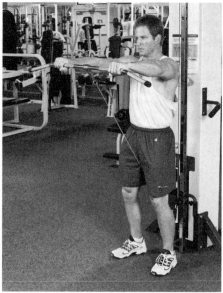

LATERAL EXTERNAL ROTATION

(MUSCLES TRAINED: EXTERNAL ROTATORS)

Stand aside an adjustable cable column with the pulley set to about hip height. Next, reach across your body and grab the handle with the arm that's furthest away from the weight stack. With a rolled-up towel placed between your working arm and the hip on that side, keep your elbow bent 90 degrees as you work the weight out in a short, arcing motion. Avoid lifting your elbow away from the towel or extending your wrist to do so. Stop when you've gone out as far as you can, or when your forearm is perpendicular to your torso. Pause for a second and then return the weight to the starting position.

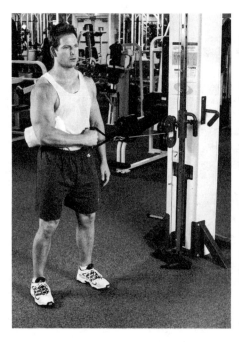 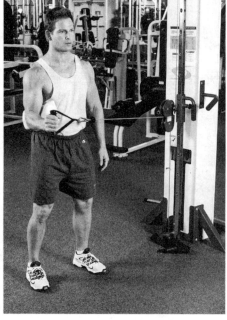

LATERAL INTERNAL ROTATION

Stand aside an adjustable cable column with the pulley set to about hip height. Next, grab the handle with the arm that's closest to the weight stack. With a rolled-up towel placed between your working arm and the hip on that side, keep your elbow bent 90 degrees as you work the weight toward your torso in a short, arcing motion. Avoid lifting your elbow away from the towel or curling your wrist to do so. Stop when you've gone out as far as you can or when your forearm is touching your abdomen. Pause for a second and then return the weight to the starting position.

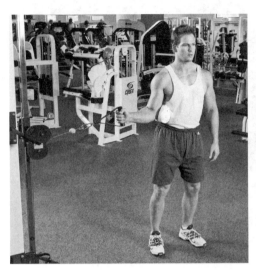 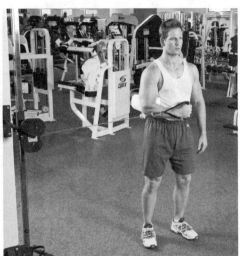

UNILATERAL SCARECROW

Stand in front of a cable station with a stirrup handle attached to the low pulley. Bend down and grab the handle, bringing it up to a position where your arm is bent approximately 90 degrees in front of your body—similar to the way it looks at the top of a unilateral row. With your knees bent and back flat, keep your upper arm still as you pivot on your elbow and work your forearm up in an arcing motion. Go up as high as you can, or until your forearm is perpendicular to the ground. Pause, lower, and repeat.

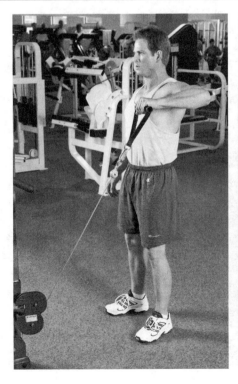 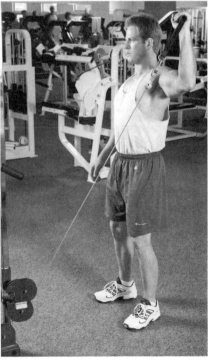

SWORD DRAW

(MUSCLES TRAINED: SHOULDERS, EXTERNAL ROTATORS)

Stand aside a cable station with the stirrup handle attached to the low pulley. Next, reach across your body and grab the handle with the arm furthest away from the weight stack. With your knees bent and your back straight, work the weight up and back in an arc-like manner until your hand is just about in line with your head. Pause, lower, and repeat.

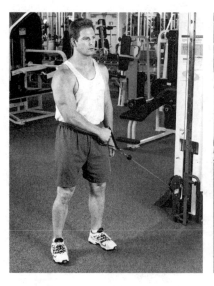

CABLE MUSCLE-UP

(MUSCLES TRAINED: UPPER TRAPEZIUS, SHOULDERS, BICEPS, TRICEPS)

Stand facing a cable station with an E-Z bar or straight bar handle attached to the pulley. Begin by performing a cable upright row by drawing your elbows up toward the ceiling. Once you get the bar just above your collarbone, rotate your forearms underneath the bar and then press it overhead by extending your arms. Pause, lower, and repeat.

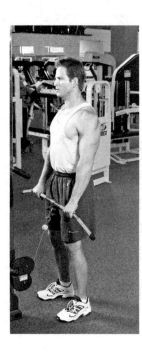
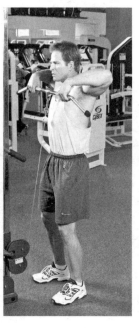
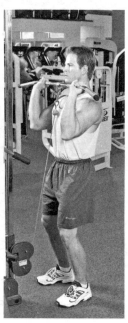
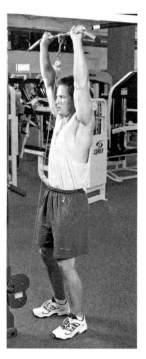

DUMBBELL CABLE PRESS

(MUSCLES TRAINED: SHOULDERS, TRICEPS)

Stand inside a cable crossover with a pair of ankle straps attached to your wrists and a pair of dumbbells at your feet. Next, attach the cable weight to the ankle straps and grab the dumbbells as you get into position to do a set of shoulder presses. Begin by pressing the weights up over your head. Pause at the top, then lower and repeat. These will give you a much different feel than regular free weight shoulder presses since you'll have to overcome both vertical resistance (from the dumbbells) and horizontal resistance (from the cables), forcing your shoulders to work harder. Because they're so tough we recommend you only use one-half to three-quarters as much weight as you normally would for dumbbell shoulder presses and a light weight on the cables.

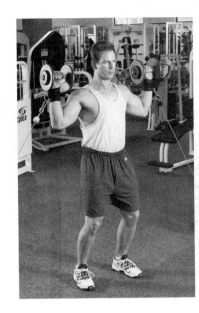 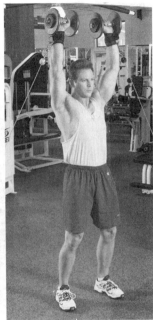

UNILATERAL SHOULDER PRESS

(MUSCLES TRAINED: SHOULDERS, TRICEPS)

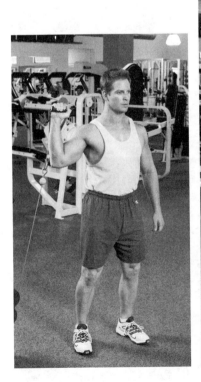 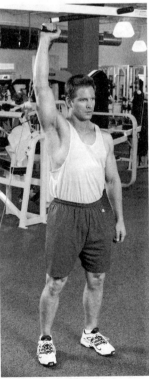

Stand aside a cable station with a stirrup handle attached to the low pulley. Begin by bending down and grabbing the handle and positioning the weight just above your shoulder, with your knees bent and back straight. Begin by pressing the weight up over your head until your arm is straight. Pause, lower, and repeat.

CABLE KICKBACK

(MUSCLES TRAINED: TRICEPS)

Stand in front of a cable station with a stirrup or rope handle attached to the low pulley. Next, bend over at the waist with one leg positioned a full stride behind the other. Grab the handle with the same hand as the leg that's extended behind you while resting your other hand on your front thigh. With your knees bent and back straight, keep your working elbow tucked in close to your side as you extend your arm until straight. Pause for a second and then return the weight to the starting position.

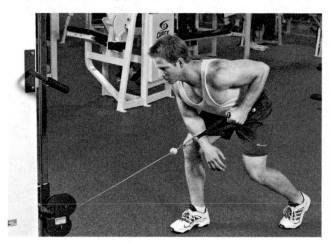 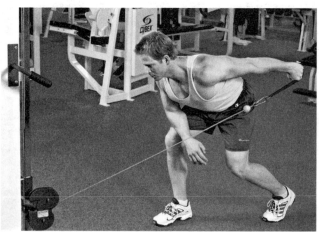

TRICEPS PUSHDOWN

(MUSCLES TRAINED: TRICEPS)

Stand in front of a cable station with a V bar, E-Z bar, or rope handle attached to the high pulley. Keeping your knees bent and your back straight, grab the handles and, with your upper arms positioned close to your torso, extend your arms from your chest down toward the floor until straight. Pause for a second and then return the weight back to the starting position.

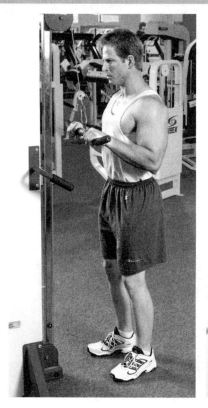 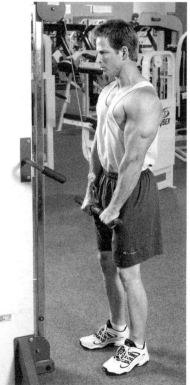

CROSSOVER PUSHDOWN

(MUSCLES TRAINED: TRICEPS)

Stand inside a cable crossover with stirrup handles attached to the high pulleys. Grab the handles with a crossover grip (your right hand grabs the left handle and vice versa) and, starting with your arms crossed in front of your chest, extend them down and out toward the floor. When your arms are straight, pause and then return the weights to the starting position.

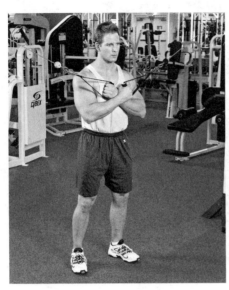 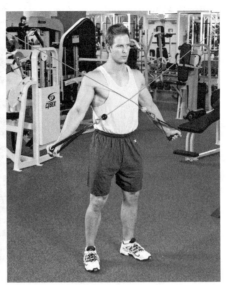

BENT-OVER TRICEPS EXTENSION

(MUSCLES TRAINED: TRICEPS)

Stand with your back to a cable station with a V bar, E-Z bar, or rope handle attached to the high pulley. Grab the handle and bend over at the waist with one leg a full stride in front of the other. With your torso almost parallel to the floor and upper arms held close to your head, extend your arms out until completely straight. Pause for a second and then return the weight to the starting position.

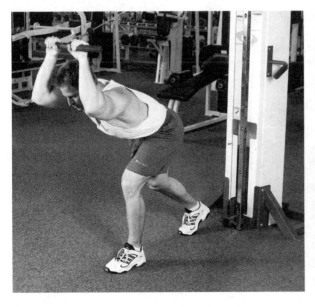 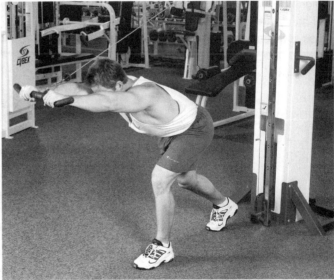

CABLE CURL

(MUSCLES TRAINED: BICEPS)

Stand in front of a cable station with a straight bar or E-Z bar attached to the low pulley. Bend down and grab the weight with a supinated grip and, standing with your knees bent and back straight, curl the weight up until your palms are in front of your shoulders. Pause, lower, and repeat.

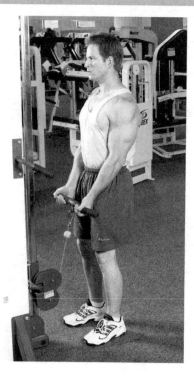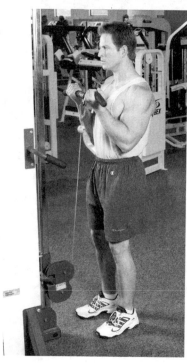

REVERSE CURL

(MUSCLES TRAINED: BICEPS, BRACHIORADIALIS)

Stand in front of a cable station with a straight bar or E-Z bar attached to the low pulley. Grab the bar with a pronated grip and, standing with your knees bent and your back straight, curl the weight up until the backs of your hands are in front of your shoulders. Pause, lower, and repeat.

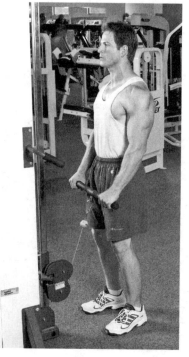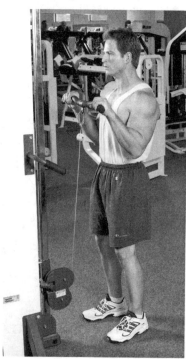

CRUCIFIX CURL

Stand inside a cable crossover with stirrup handles attached to the high pulleys. With your knees bent and your back straight, grab the handles with a supinated grip and your arms held out to the sides, parallel to the floor. Keeping your upper arms still, curl the weights in until your hands are next to your head. Pause for a second and then return the weight to the starting position.

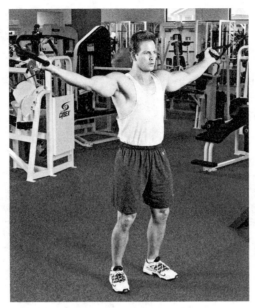
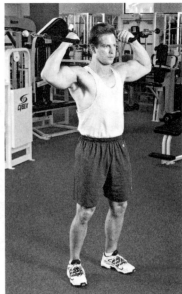

LEAN AWAY CONCENTRATION CURL

Stand inside a cable station with a stirrup handle attached to the low pulley. Grab the handle and lunge away from the pulley, with your torso almost parallel to the floor and one leg one-and-a-half to two strides behind the other. Keeping your upper arm perfectly still and reaching back toward the low pulley, curl the weight until it's just in front of your shoulder. Pause for a second and then return the weight to the starting position.

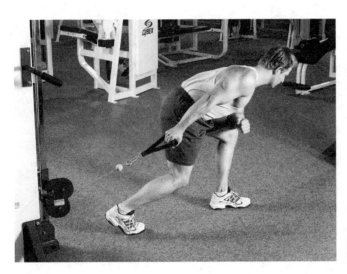
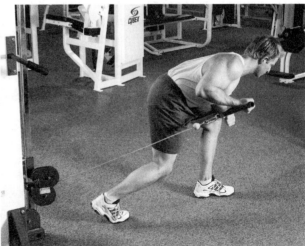

CABLE CURL PLUS

(MUSCLES TRAINED: BICEPS, SHOULDERS)

Stand in front of a cable station with a straight bar or E-Z bar attached to the low pulley. Bend down and grab the weight with a supinated grip and, standing with your knees bent and your back straight, curl the weight up until your palms are in front of your shoulders. Once there, draw your elbows up and forward as you give your biceps an extra squeeze. Pause, lower, and repeat.

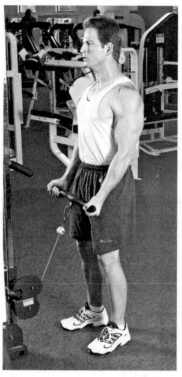 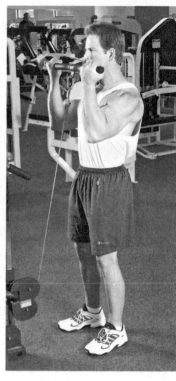

STANDING WRIST CURL

(MUSCLES TRAINED: FOREARMS)

Stand facing away from a cable station with a straight bar attached to the low pulley. Bend down and grab the handle, then stand up and hold it at arm's length behind your back. Allow the bar to roll down into your fingertips and then curl it back up toward your forearms. Pause, lower, and repeat.

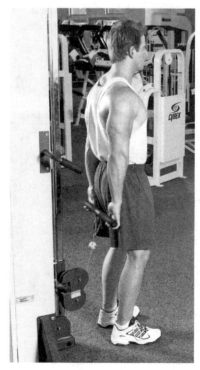 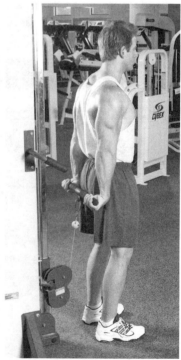

LOWER BODY

SPLIT SQUAT

(MUSCLES TRAINED: QUADRICEPS, HAMSTRINGS, GLUTES)

Stand in front of a cable station with a stirrup handle attached to the low pulley. Adopt a split squat stance with one foot 2½ to 3 feet in front of the other and only the ball of your back foot in contact with the ground. Holding the cable in the same hand as your back leg, begin by bending both knees and descending straight down. In the bottom position both knees should be bent approximately 90 degrees and your back knee should almost touch the floor. Pause for a second and then press back up to the starting position.

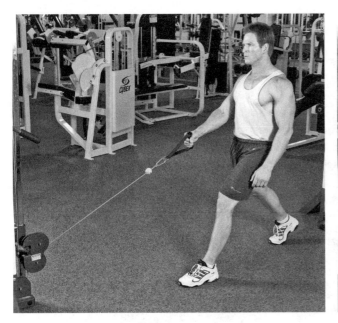
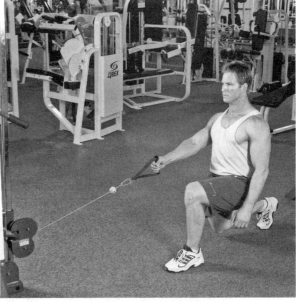

FORWARD LUNGE

(MUSCLES TRAINED: QUADRICEPS, HAMSTRINGS, GLUTES)

Stand in front of a cable station with a stirrup handle attached to the low pulley. Grab the handle, and while standing a full stride away from the pulley, begin by taking a big lunge step forward with the opposite leg of the hand holding the weight. In the bottom position both knees should be bent approximately 90 degrees and your back knee should almost touch the floor. Pause for a second and then press back up to the starting position. This differs from the split squat in that the dynamic nature of the lunge step forward directs even more stress to the quadriceps.

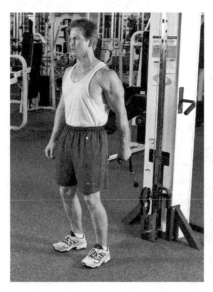 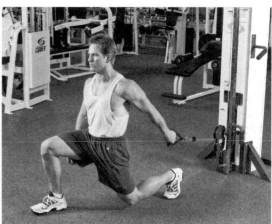

REVERSE LUNGE

(MUSCLES TRAINED: QUADRICEPS, HAMSTRINGS, GLUTES)

Stand in front of a cable station with a stirrup handle attached to the low pulley. Grab the weight and while standing close to the pulley, take a lunge stride straight back, landing only on the ball of your back foot. In the bottom position both knees should be bent approximately 90 degrees and your back knee should almost touch the floor. Pause for a second and then press back up to the starting position. This differs from the front lunge in that the step backward puts more stress on the glutes of the front leg when you push back up.

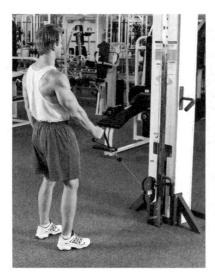 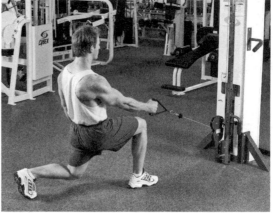

STANDING ABDUCTION

Stand next to a cable station wearing an ankle strap on your outside leg. Bend down and attach the weight, then stand up and, with your back straight and support knee slightly bent, lift your outer leg out as far away from your body as possible without changing the position of your torso. Pause, lower, and repeat.

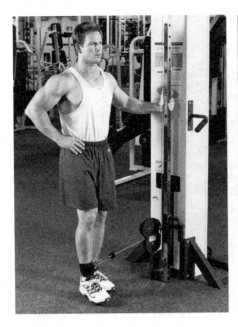 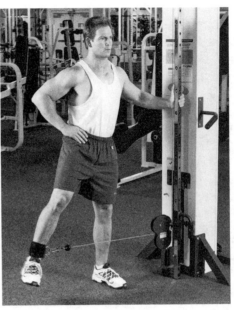

STANDING ADDUCTION

Stand next to a cable station wearing an ankle strap on your inside leg. Bend down and attach the weight, then stand up and, with your back straight and support knee slightly bent, draw your working leg across the front of your body as far as you can without changing the position of your torso. Pause, lower, and repeat.

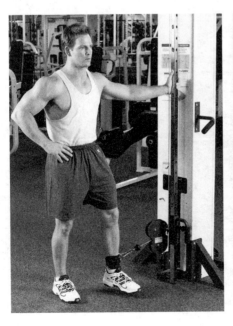 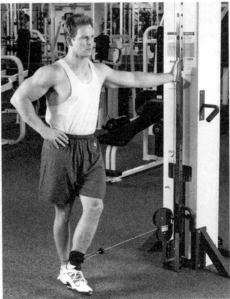

STANDING HIP EXTENSION

(MUSCLES TRAINED: GLUTES)

Stand facing a cable station wearing an ankle strap attached to one leg. Attach the weight to the strap and begin by leaning forward at the waist slightly as you support yourself against the handles of the cable station. Keeping your working leg straight and support leg slightly bent, extend your leg back until it forms a diagonal line with your torso. Pause, lower, and repeat.

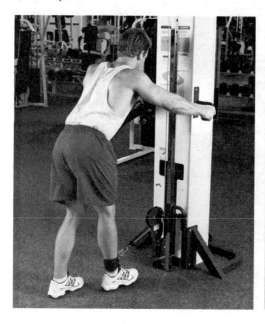 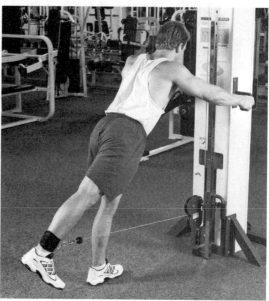

UNILATERAL STANDING CALF RAISE

(MUSCLES TRAINED: GASTROCNEMIUS, SOLEUS)

Stand facing a cable station with a stirrup handle attached to the low pulley and a calf block or thick weight plate positioned right in front of it. Bend down and grab the handle as you step up with the leg of the same side on the block, with only the ball of your foot in contact with it. Starting with your heel below the level of the block, keep your back and arm straight as you raise up as high on the ball of your foot as possible. Pause, lower, and repeat.

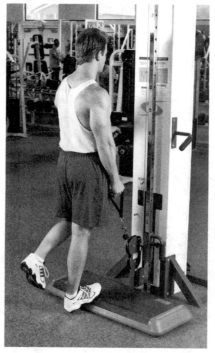 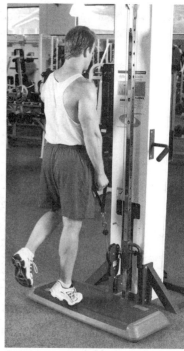

OFFSET SQUAT

Stand facing a cable station with a stirrup handle attached to the low pulley. Bend down and grab the handle with one hand as you lift that same foot off the floor and balance on your other leg. Keeping your arm extended out in front of you, begin by squatting down as low as possible, holding your nonworking leg up toward your butt. When your working leg is parallel to the floor, push back up to the starting position and repeat without putting your foot down until the end of the set.

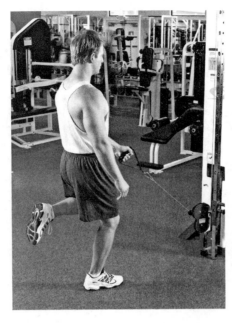
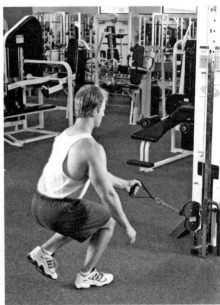

LEG CURL AND HIP EXTENSION

(MUSCLES TRAINED: HAMSTRINGS, GLUTES)

Stand facing a cable station wearing an ankle strap attached to one leg. Attach the weight to the strap and begin by leaning forward at the waist slightly as you support yourself against the handles of the cable station. Keeping your working leg straight and support leg slightly bent, curl your foot up toward your butt. Once your shin is parallel to the floor, use your glutes to push straight back until your leg is almost straight. Pause for a second before returning the weight to the starting position.

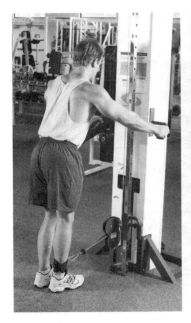
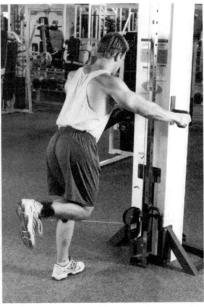
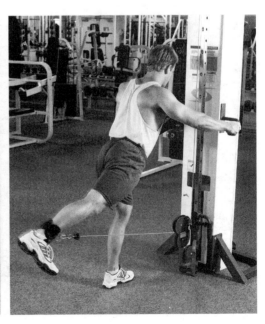

PULL THROUGH

Stand with your back to a cable station, with a rope handle attached to the low pulley. Reach down between your legs and grab the pulley as you walk out a step away from the weight stack. Once there, with your feet slightly wider than shoulder-width apart, bend over and reach back between your legs while keeping your back flat and arms straight. From there, push your feet into the ground and stand up, pulling the weight forward until it lines up right around the tops of your quads.

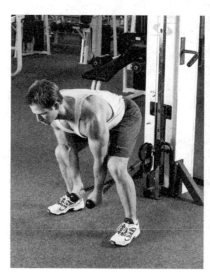

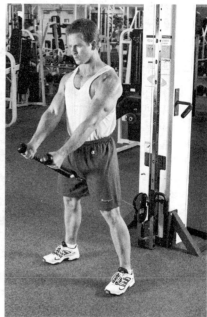

STEP OUT SIDE LUNGE

Stand next to a cable station with a stirrup handle attached to a low pulley. Grab the weight with the hand closest to the pulley as you step out sideways into a lunge position. In the bottom position your outside leg will be parallel to the floor with your trailing leg perfectly straight and both feet pointing forward. You'll also be leaning slightly forward at the waist with a flat back. Once there, immediately push back up to the starting position.

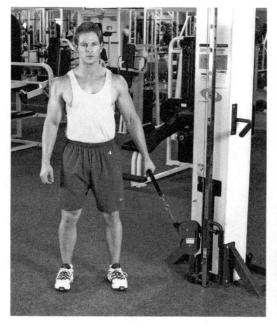

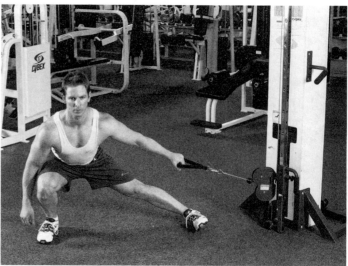

CHAPTER TEN

APPROACH THE BENCH

Laying the Foundation for Big Gains

IF YOU THOUGHT YOUR LIST OF available exercise options was pretty long with just a couple of free weights and a cable station, get ready to be blown away! Adding a bench to the mix exponentially increases the number of exercises you can do. And we're not just talking about lots of different chest exercises here, although that is one of the more obvious advantages of using a bench. We're also talking about all sorts of challenging upper- and lower-body lifts you can incorporate into your program with a standard flat bench. If the bench is adjustable to a variety of angles, as many are, that much more can be accomplished with it.

Adjustable benches can usually be found over by the dumbbell rack in most gyms, although they often have wheels so they can be easily transported where needed. You can use these for a variety of barbell and dumbbell exercises as well as set them up for use inside of cable stations and squats racks (more on these in the next chapter). Most adjust from flat to both incline and decline positions.

Because of their tremendous versatility, these babies can become pretty hot commodities during peak hours of operation, so keep that in mind when planning your workout. If you are lucky enough to snag one when the gym is packed, be sure to share with your fellow gym rats—no one likes an equipment hog. (See Chapter Nineteen on gym etiquette.)

Somewhat less versatile but equally valuable are the nonadjustable benches, which provide the support for various types of pressing movements. These include the flat, incline, and decline bench presses, as well as the smaller, upright shoulder press bench. You'll usually find these clustered together somewhere in the free weight area, and depending on the size of your gym, you'll often find them in pairs. Because bench pressing is so popular many gyms find it necessary to have multiple pressing stations open to its members. This also enables people of similar strength levels to train together. Nothing disrupts the flow of a workout more than having to load and unload multiple plates between sets because two guys, or a guy and a girl of vastly different strength levels, both want to use the gym's only bench press at the same time.

ISN'T THAT SPECIAL

While both the preset and adjustable benches get all the attention, there are a couple of other specialized benches that you'll probably find lying about that can also prove quite useful. For core training, a Roman chair, also called a hyperextension bench, is a good tool to have. This rather odd-looking contraption enables you to lock your legs in place as you flex, extend, and/or rotate your torso. Positioning yourself facedown and extending upward works your lower back, while facing up and flexing your torso hits the abdominals and hip flexors more. You can even lie on your side and flex your torso laterally to target the obliques or rotate a bit to bring just about all of your core musculature into play. Look for them near the abdominal training equipment.

The other type of bench that gets a decent amount of usage is the preacher curl bench. Getting its name for being shaped like a preacher's pulpit, this triangular-shaped bench allows you to target your biceps by effectively taking both your shoulders and lower back out of the exercise. By locking you into position, the preacher curl bench makes it pretty much impossible to cheat by thrusting your hips or shoulders forward, as is often the case during standing barbell curls. (Sadly, this phenome-

non occurs all too often in weight rooms nationwide.) You'll usually find these types of benches mixed in amongst the arm equipment and almost always facing a mirror.

Now that you know where to find them and how they're best used, let us show you just how much you can get done by incorporating a bench into your program.

CORE

BEGINNER/ INTERMEDIATE	ADVANCED
Incline Reverse Crunch	Elevated Side Bridge
V-Leg Raise	Back Extension
	Roman Chair Situp

INCLINE REVERSE CRUNCH

(MUSCLES TRAINED: ABDOMINALS, HIP FLEXORS)

Lift the top end of an adjustable flat bench up so that it's in a slight incline position. Lie on the bench with your hips lower than your head and grab the end of it for support. Bend your hips and knees 90 degrees. Pull your hips upward and crunch them inward, as if you were emptying a bucket of water that was resting on your pelvis. Keep your hips and knees at 90-degree angles. Pause, lower, and repeat.

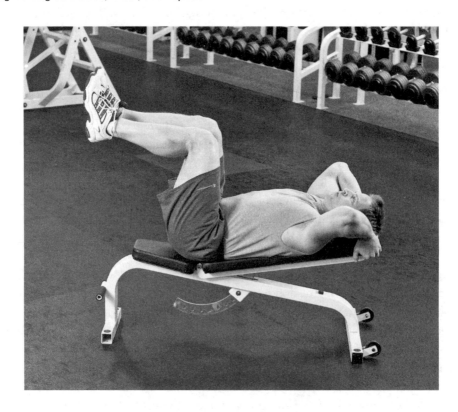

V-LEG RAISE

Sit crossways on a flat bench with your legs slightly bent and your hands just outside your hips. Lean back, and without changing the amount of bend in your knees, use your abs and hip flexors to bring your torso and legs as close together as possible. Hold the highest point for a second, lower, and return back to the starting position.

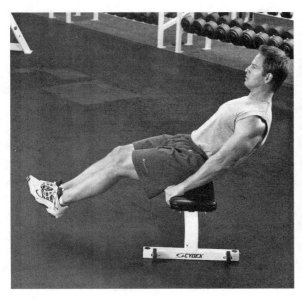
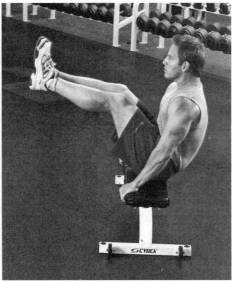

ELEVATED SIDE BRIDGE

Position one forearm at the end of an exercise bench with your legs outstretched in front of it stacked one on top of the other. Keeping your body in line with the bench, begin with your hips below the level of the bench. Lift your hips up until your body forms a diagonal line from your head to your feet. Pause, lower, and repeat.

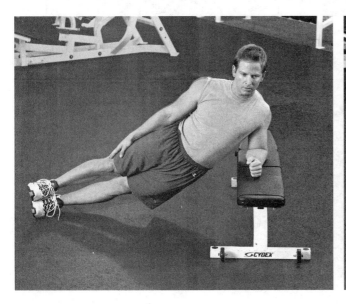
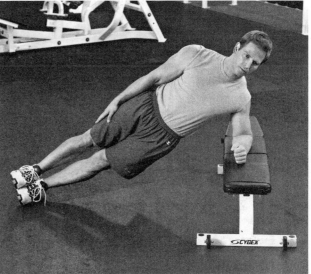

BACK EXTENSION

Position yourself in a Roman chair so that your lower legs are underneath the supports and your hips are on top of the front pad with your entire torso hanging off. Starting with your torso below parallel, use your spinal erectors to slowly raise yourself up until your torso is slightly higher than your hips. Pause, lower, and repeat.

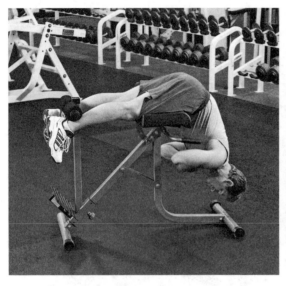
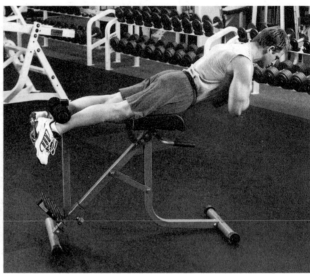

ROMAN CHAIR SITUP

Position yourself in a Roman chair opposite the way you would to perform a set of back extensions: Shins under the supports and glutes on the front pad. With your arms folded across your chest, begin with your body in a straight line and slowly curl your upper body up toward your hips. Pause at the highest point, lower, and repeat.

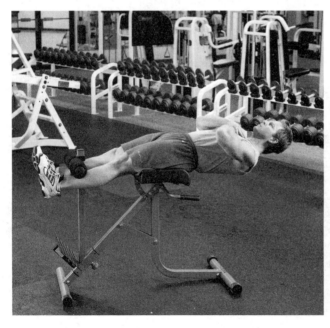
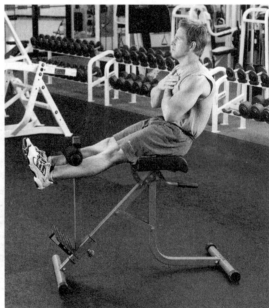

CHEST AND UPPER BACK

	BEGINNER/INTERMEDIATE	ADVANCED
CHEST	Dumbbell Flat Bench Press	Unilateral Bench Press
	Flat Fly	Triple-Angled Press
	Dumbbell Incline Bench Press	Telle Fly
	Incline Fly	Reverse-Grip Bench Press
	Dumbbell Decline Bench Press	Close-Grip Bench Press
	Decline Fly	Dumbbell Cable Press (all three angles)
	Barbell Flat Bench Press	
	Barbell Incline Bench Press	
	Barbell Decline Bench Press	
	Cable Fly (all three angles)	
BACK	One-Arm Row	Prone Row with Abduction
	Dumbbell Pullover	Barbell One-Arm Row
	E-Z Bar Pullover	Lying Cable Reverse Fly
	Dumbbell Prone Row	
	Reverse Fly (various grips)	

DUMBBELL FLAT BENCH PRESS
(MUSCLES TRAINED: CHEST, SHOULDERS, TRICEPS)

Lie on a flat bench holding a pair of dumbbells above your chest, with your back in a normal arch. Lower the dumbbells toward the sides of your chest (stop when your elbows are at torso level or just a little lower), pause, and then push them back up the starting position.

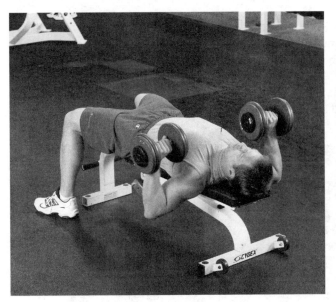
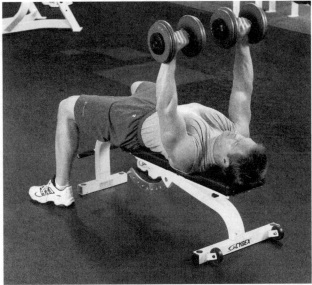

FLAT FLY

Lie on a flat bench holding a pair of dumbbells above your chest, with your feet flat on the floor. Keeping a slight bend in your elbows, work the weights down in a wide, arcing motion until your upper arms are parallel to the floor and your hands are in line with your ears. Pause for second and then raise the weights back up to the starting position.

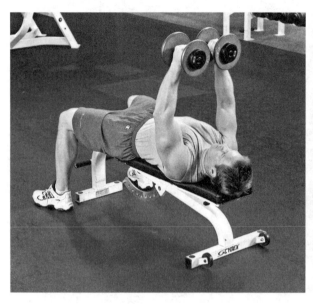 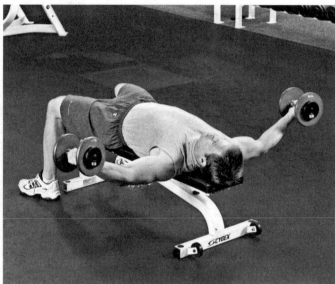

DUMBBELL INCLINE BENCH PRESS

(MUSCLES TRAINED: UPPER CHEST, SHOULDERS, TRICEPS)

Grab a pair of dumbbells and lie on your back on an incline bench with your feet flat on the floor. Lift the dumbbells so they're above your chin, and hold them with your palms turned out (thumbs facing each other). Slowly lower the weights to your upper chest, pause, and then push them back up above your chin.

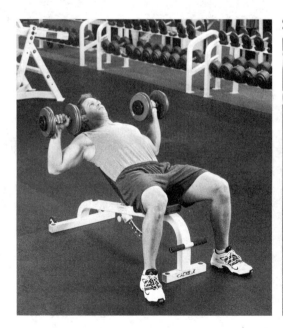 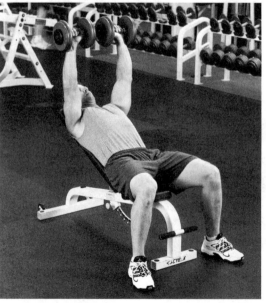

INCLINE FLY

Lie down on an incline bench holding a pair of dumbbells above your chest, with your feet flat on the floor. Keeping a slight bend in your elbows, work the weights down in a wide, arcing motion until your upper arms are parallel to the floor and your hands are in line with your ears. Pause for a second, then raise the weights back up to the starting position.

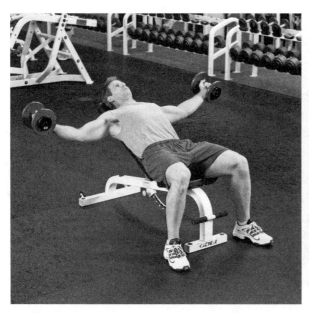 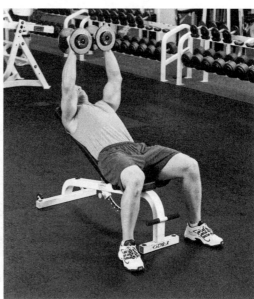

DUMBBELL DECLINE BENCH PRESS

Lie back on a decline bench holding a pair of dumbbells in your hands, with your legs locked underneath the supports. As you lie back, position the weights just above your shoulders and then press them up over your chest until your arms are completely straight. Pause, lower, and repeat.

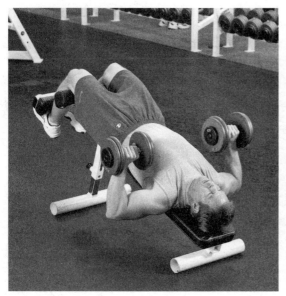 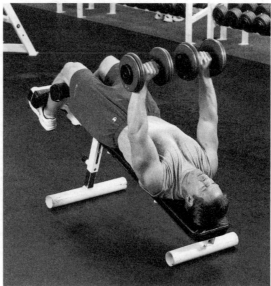

DECLINE FLY

Lie back on a decline bench holding a pair of dumbbells, with your legs hooked underneath the supports. Begin by positioning the weights just above your shoulders and working them down in a wide arc until your upper arms are parallel to the floor and your hands are in line with your jaw. Pause for a second, then raise the weights back up to the starting position.

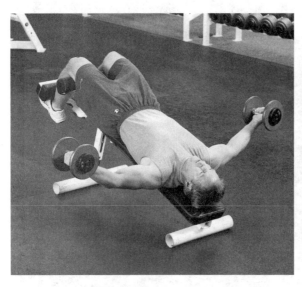 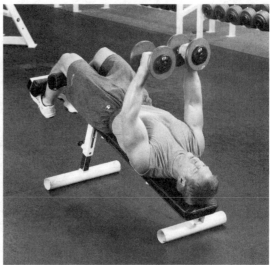

BARBELL FLAT BENCH PRESS

Grab a bar with your hands just wider than shoulder-width, your back in a normal arch, and feet flat on the floor. Lift the bar off the uprights and hold it over your chest. Lower the bar to the midline of your chest, pause, then push it back to the starting position.

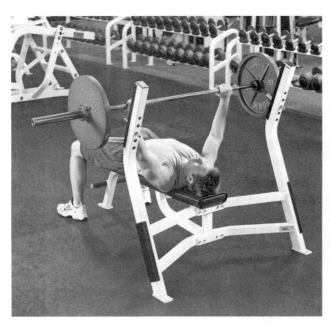 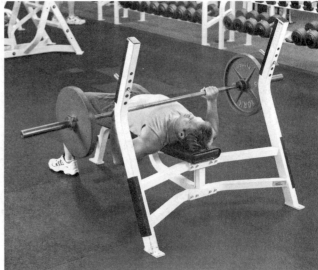

BARBELL INCLINE BENCH PRESS

(MUSCLES TRAINED: UPPER CHEST, SHOULDERS, TRICEPS)

Lie on your back on an incline bench with your feet flat on the floor and grab the bar with an overhand grip that's just wider than shoulder width. Lift the bar off the supports so it's lined up over your chin. Slowly lower the weight to your upper chest, pause, then push it back up above your chin.

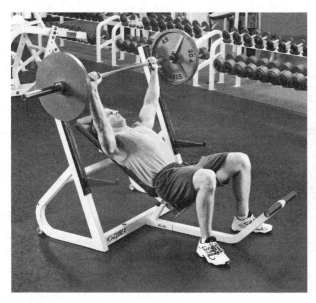 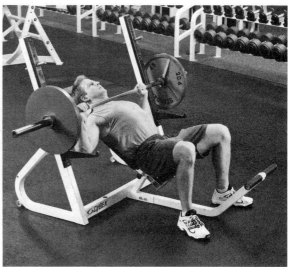

BARBELL DECLINE BENCH PRESS

(MUSCLES TRAINED: LOWER CHEST, SHOULDERS, TRICEPS)

Lie on a decline bench with your feet underneath the supports and grab a bar with a grip that's just wider than shoulder width. Lift the bar off the supports so it's lined up over your lower chest. Slowly lower the weight down to your lower chest, pause, and press it back up.

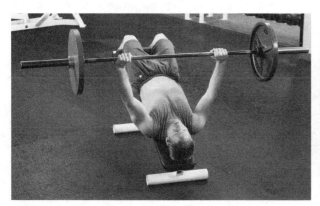 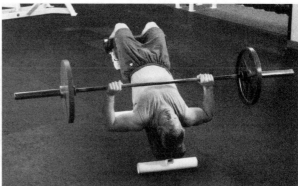

CABLE FLY (ALL THREE ANGLES)

(MUSCLES TRAINED: CHEST, SHOULDERS)

These can be done from any of the three angles (flat, incline, or decline). Whichever angle you choose, the basic premise remains the same: Place an adjustable bench inside the cable crossover station set to the angle of your choice, with the stirrup handles attached to the low pulleys. Begin by grabbing the handles and lying back on the bench. Raise the handles up over your middle, upper, or lower chest depending on which angle you choose and, keeping your elbows slightly bent, work the weights down in a wide, arcing motion. When your upper arms are parallel to the floor, reverse directions and bring the handles back up to the starting position.

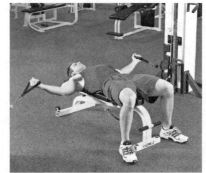
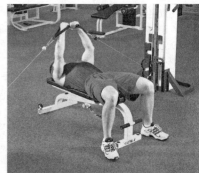
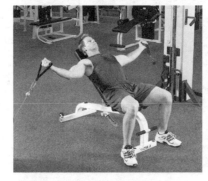
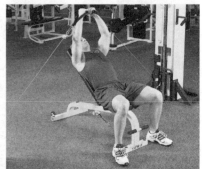
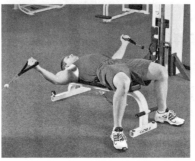
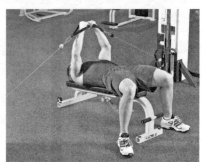

UNILATERAL BENCH PRESS

(MUSCLES TRAINED: CHEST, SHOULDERS, TRICEPS)

This more challenging version of the traditional dumbbell bench press can be done at any angle and is great for correcting strength imbalances if one side of your chest is stronger than the other—just do either more sets or more reps for the weaker side. Simply grab a single dumbbell and lie back on the bench; let your free arm help secure you by grabbing its side. From there, just perform the exercise as you normally would.

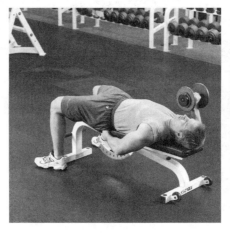
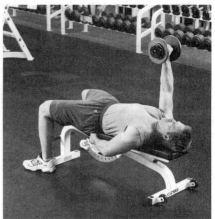

TRIPLE-ANGLED PRESS

(MUSCLES TRAINED: CHEST, SHOULDERS, TRICEPS)

This superintense version of the dumbbell press is best saved for experienced lifters. Begin by selecting your weight and performing 6 to 8 reps of incline dumbbell presses. Once you're done, quickly put the weights down and lower the angle of the bench to a flat press. Crank out another 6 or so reps. Finally, put the weights down and quickly drop the angle of the bench to decline and go for broke. You'll find that even though you're exhausting your muscles at each angle, you'll still be able to use the same weight by simply dropping the angle of the bench.

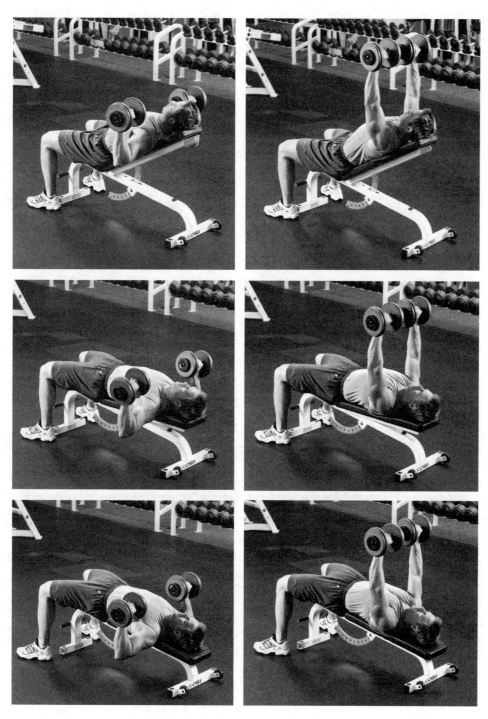

TELLE FLY

(MUSCLES TRAINED: CHEST, SHOULDERS, TRICEPS)

Named for innovative trainer Jerry Telle, this advanced technique allows you to use a more challenging weight than you normally would when doing flys. Position the weights over your shoulders and work the weights down in a wide, arcing motion. When your upper arms are parallel to the floor, bend your elbows and bring the weights in toward your chest as you press them back up to the starting position.

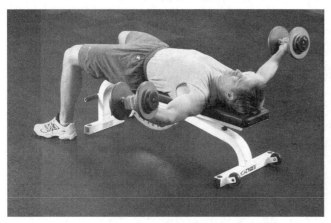
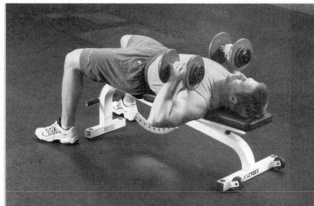

REVERSE-GRIP BENCH PRESS

(MUSCLES TRAINED: CHEST, SHOULDERS, TRICEPS)

This advanced version of the bench press really targets the front deltoids. Simply lie down and grab a bar with a supinated, shoulder-width grip. Lower the bar down toward the midline of the chest, pause, and then press it back up to the starting position.

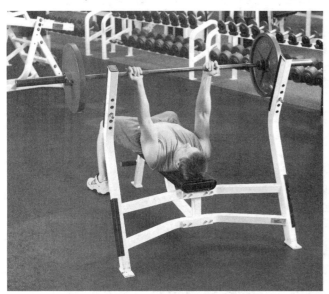
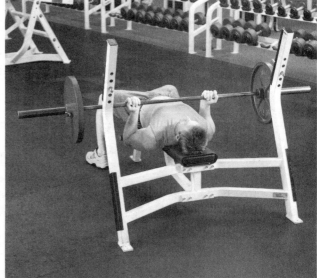

CLOSE-GRIP BENCH PRESS

(MUSCLES TRAINED: TRICEPS, CHEST, SHOULDERS)

Lie on your back on a flat bench with your feet on the floor. Grab a bar with an overhand grip, your hands a bit narrower than shoulder-width apart. Lift it off the uprights and hold it over your lower chest at arm's length. Slowly lower the bar until it touches or is close to your chest. Pause, then push the bar straight up until your arms are straight and the bar is above your lower chest again. Keep your butt on the bench and avoid arching your back beyond its natural position.

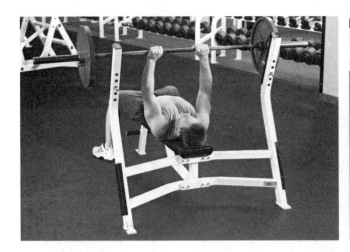
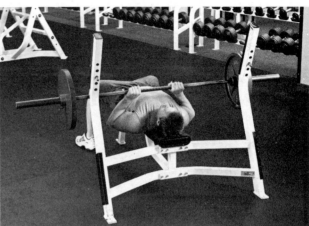

DUMBBELL CABLE PRESS (ALL THREE ANGLES)

(MUSCLES TRAINED: CHEST, SHOULDERS, TRICEPS)

Like the Cable Fly, this exercise can also be done from all three angles by placing an adjustable bench inside the cable crossover station. Hook the stirrup handles up to the low pulleys and lie back on the bench. Position the weights directly above your shoulders and press them up until your arms are completely straight. Pause, lower, and repeat.

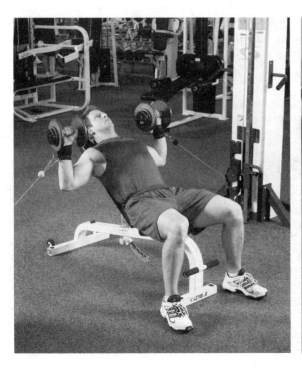
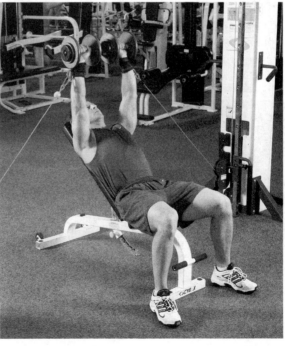

ONE-ARM ROW
(MUSCLES TRAINED: UPPER BACK, BICEPS)

Grab a dumbbell in your left hand and place your right hand and right knee on a flat bench. Keep your back flat and your upper body parallel to the floor. Let your left arm hang straight down from your shoulder with your palm facing your torso. Raise your left upper arm up until it's just past parallel to the floor, with your elbow above the level of your torso. Pause, lower, and repeat. Keeping your elbow in close to your body and your palm in a neutral position will target the lats more, while turning your palm to face your feet and rowing with your elbow out will hit the scapular retractors to a greater degree.

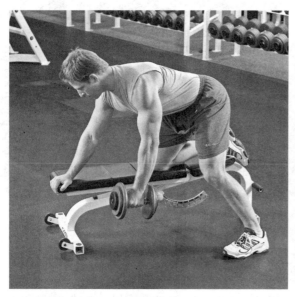 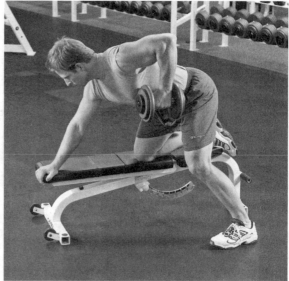

DUMBBELL PULLOVER
(MUSCLES TRAINED: LATS, CHEST, TRICEPS)

Lie on an exercise bench holding a dumbbell with a hand-over-hand grip. With your feet flat on the floor and a normal arch in your back, begin with the weight directly above your upper chest and lower it with your arms slightly bent until your upper arms are in line with your head. Pause for a second, then, without changing the amount of bend in your arms, bring the weight back to the starting position.

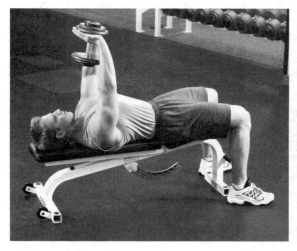 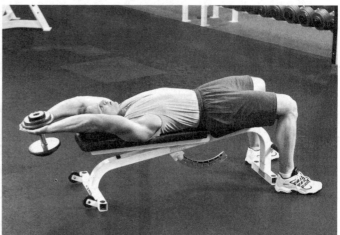

E-Z BAR PULLOVER

(MUSCLES TRAINED: LATS, CHEST, TRICEPS)

The Dumbbell Pullover can also be done with an E-Z bar to allow for greater comfort in the wrists and shoulders and range of motion. Simply grab an E-Z bar and perform the exercise the same way as described for the Dumbbell Pullover.

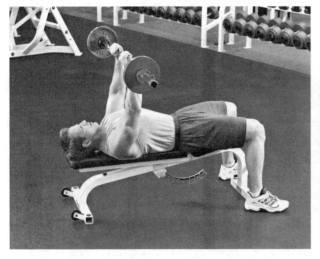 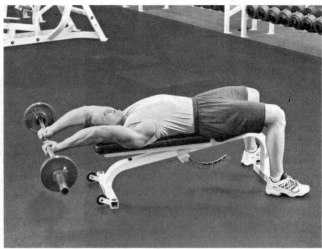

DUMBBELL PRONE ROW

(MUSCLES TRAINED: UPPER BACK, BICEPS)

Set an incline bench to a 45-degree angle. Grab a pair of dumbbells and lie chest-down against the pad. Let your arms hang straight down from your shoulders and turn your palms so that your thumbs are facing each other. Lift your upper arms as high as you can by bending your elbows and squeezing your shoulder blades together. Your upper arms should be almost perpendicular to your body at the top of the move. Your lower arms should point toward the floor. Pause, lower, and repeat. Keeping your elbows in close to your body and your palms facing each other will target the lats more, while turning your palms to face your feet and rowing with your elbows out will hit the scapular retractors to a greater degree.

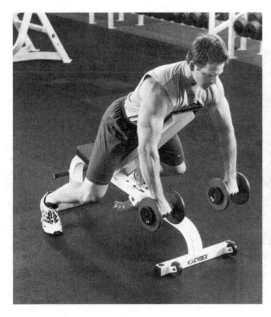 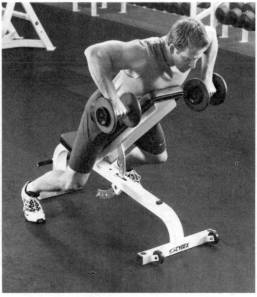

REVERSE FLY (VARIOUS HAND POSITIONS)

(MUSCLES TRAINED: UPPER BACK, REAR DELTOIDS)

Lie chest-down on an exercise bench set to a 45-degree angle holding a pair of light dumbbells at arm's length beneath your shoulders. With a slight bend in your elbows, begin by working the weights up in a wide arc until your upper arms are parallel to the floor. Pause, lower, and repeat. Doing the exercise with a neutral grip (palms facing each other) will hit the entire upper back, while a pronated grip (thumb sides facing each other) will hit the rear deltoids more and a supinated grip (pinky sides facing each other) will put more stress on the external rotators.

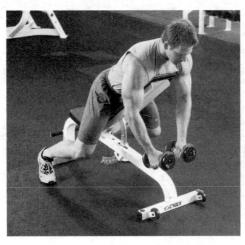 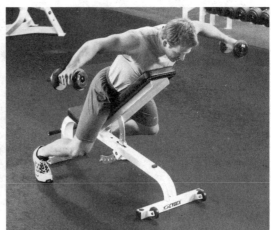

PRONE ROW WITH ABDUCTION

(MUSCLES TRAINED: UPPER BACK, BICEPS)

Begin as you would a regular prone dumbbell row: lying on a bench set to a 45-degree angle holding a pair of dumbbells at arm's length beneath your shoulders. Using a neutral grip with your elbows close to your body, row the weight up until your elbows pass your torso. Once there, swing your elbows out wide to the sides before slowly lowering the weight back to the starting position. Like the Telle Fly, this advanced version of the row challenges you more on the negative (lowering) portion of the repetition where you're naturally stronger by allowing you to use a heavier weight than normal in the elbow-out position.

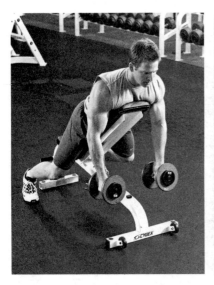 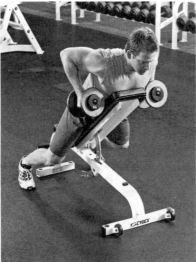 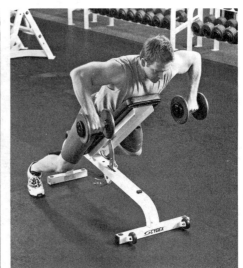

BARBELL ONE-ARM ROW

This tougher version of the traditional dumbbell one-arm row will be a real challenge for your shoulders and forearms to properly stabilize the weight. Grab a barbell in your left hand and place your right hand and right knee on a flat bench. Keep your back flat and your upper body parallel to the floor. Let your left arm hang straight down from your shoulder with your palm facing your torso. Raise your left upper arm up until it's just past parallel to the floor, with your elbow above the level of your torso. Try to keep the entire barbell parallel to the floor throughout the lift. Pause, lower, and repeat.

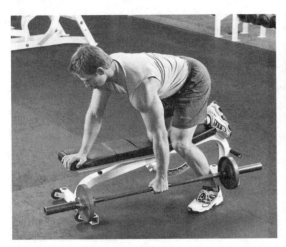
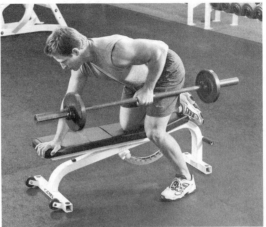

LYING CABLE REVERSE FLY

Place a flat bench inside a cable crossover with the stirrup handles attached to the upper pulleys. Grab the handles with a crossover grip (your right hand grabs the left handle and vice versa) and lie down on the bench. With your feet flat on the floor and elbows slightly bent, work the weights down in a wide, arcing motion until your upper arms just pass your torso. Pause there for a second, lower, and repeat.

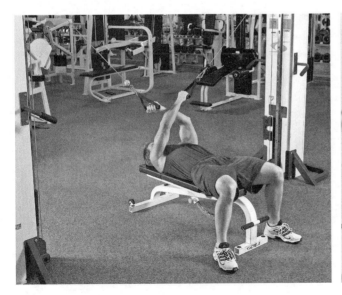
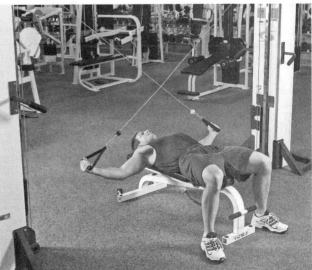

SHOULDERS AND ARMS

	BEGINNER/INTERMEDIATE	ADVANCED
SHOULDERS	Seated Dumbbell Press	Dumbbell Prone Scarecrow
	Seated Barbell Press	Side Lying Dumbbell External Rotation
	Incline Dumbbell Front Raise	Angled Dumbbell Shrug
	Dumbbell Lying Triceps Extension (all three angles)	Unilateral Triceps Extension with a Lean
	Lying Cross-Body Unilateral Extension	JM Press
	Seated Overhead Dumbbell Extension (Bi- and Unilateral)	
	Dumbbell Kickback	
	Overhead E-Z Bar Extension	
	Lying E-Z Bar Extension	
	Lying Cable Extension	
	Seated Overhead Cable Extension	
BICEPS	Seated Dumbbell Biceps Curl	Seated Biceps Curl with Isometric Hold
	Seated Dumbbell Reverse Curl	Seated Zottman Curl
	Incline Dumbbell Biceps Curl	Prone Dumbbell Curl
	Incline Reverse Dumbbell Curl	Rope Pull-Apart Curl
	Seated Dumbbell Hammer Curl	Prone Barbell Curl
	Incline Dumbbell Hammer Curl	Prone Reverse Barbell Curl
	Concentration Curl	
	Dumbbell Preacher Curl	
	Barbell Preacher Curl	
	Lying Cable Curl	
	Dumbbell Wrist Curl	
	Dumbbell Reverse Wrist Curl	
	Barbell Wrist Curl	
	Barbell Reverse Wrist Curl	

SEATED DUMBBELL PRESS

(MUSCLES TRAINED: SHOULDERS, TRICEPS)

Sit on an exercise bench or specialized shoulder press bench holding a pair of dumbbells. Lift the dumbbells up just above your shoulders and, with your feet flat on the floor, press the weights up until your arms are straight. Pause, lower, and repeat. You can also do this exercise with a neutral grip to ease strain on your shoulder joints.

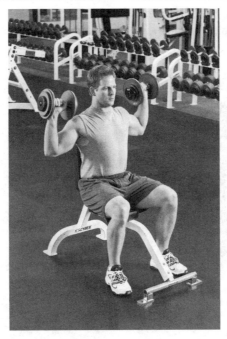
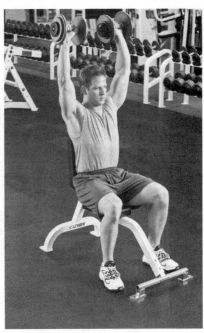

SEATED BARBELL PRESS

(MUSCLES TRAINED: SHOULDERS, TRICEPS)

Sit on a specialized shoulder press station and grab the bar with a grip that's slightly wider than shoulder width. With your back against the pad and feet flat on the floor, lift the weights off the supports and lower it in front of your face, just below your chin. Pause there for a second before pressing the weights up until your arms are straight. Lower in front of your face again and repeat. You can also do this exercise by lowering the bar behind you, just above the base of your neck, but this is best left to experienced lifters with no history of shoulder problems.

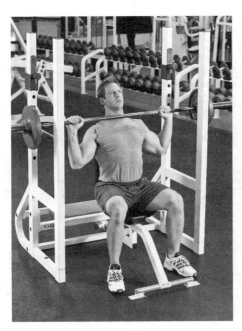
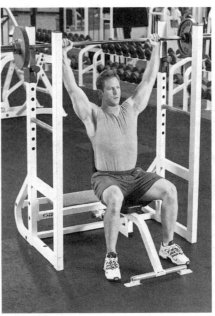

INCLINE DUMBBELL FRONT RAISE

(MUSCLES TRAINED: FRONT DELTOIDS, TRAPEZIUS)

Lie chest-down on an incline bench set to a 45-degree angle holding a pair of light dumbbells at arm's length beneath your shoulders. Keeping your arms straight but not locked, lift your arms up in front of you until they're parallel to the floor. Pause, lower, and repeat.

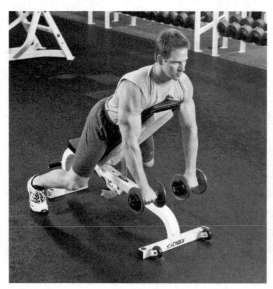 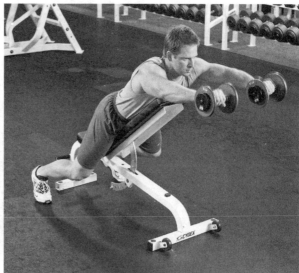

DUMBBELL PRONE SCARECROW

(MUSCLES TRAINED: EXTERNAL ROTATORS, SHOULDERS)

Set an incline bench to 45 degrees. Holding a pair of light dumbbells, lie chest-down on the bench. Raise your upper arms so they're perpendicular to your torso and parallel to the floor. Bend your elbows 90 degrees so your forearms hang straight down toward the floor. Keeping your elbows, wrists, and upper arms in fixed positions, rotate the weights up and back as far as you can—you want your shoulders to act like hinges, your arms like swinging gates. Pause, lower, and repeat.

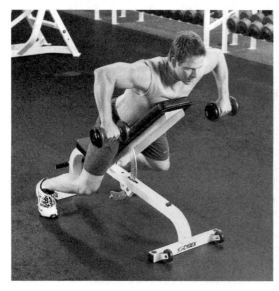 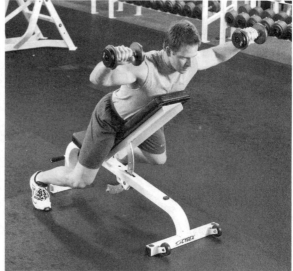

SIDE LYING DUMBBELL EXTERNAL ROTATION

(MUSCLES TRAINED: EXTERNAL ROTATORS)

Lie sideways on an exercise bench holding a dumbbell in the hand of your top arm. Place a rolled up towel between your top hip and elbow and rest your upper arm on it, bent at a 90-degree angle. Start with your forearm across your abs and work the weight up in a wide, arcing motion until your forearm is as close to perpendicular to the floor as possible. Be sure not to lift your elbow off the towel or break your wrist back in attempting to raise the weight higher. Pause in the top position, lower, and repeat.

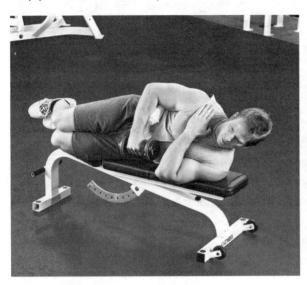 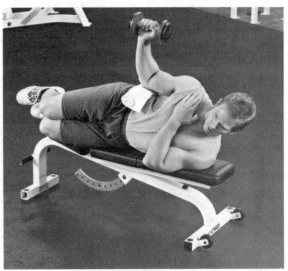

ANGLED DUMBBELL SHRUG

(MUSCLES TRAINED: UPPER TRAPEZIUS, UPPER BACK)

Lie chest-down on an exercise bench set to a 75-degree angle, holding a pair of dumbbells at arm's length beneath your shoulders. Keeping your arms straight, shrug your shoulders up and back as you lift the weights as high as possible. When you've reached your highest point, pause, lower, and repeat.

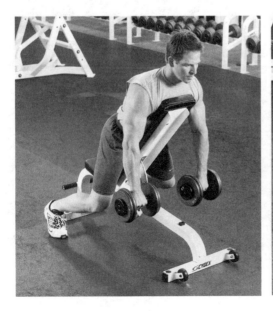 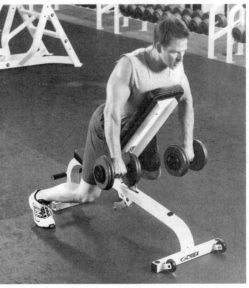

DUMBBELL LYING TRICEPS EXTENSION (ALL THREE ANGLES)

(MUSCLES TRAINED: TRICEPS)

These can be done on any of the three angles, but the basic premise remains the same. Lie on a bench holding a pair of dumbbells extended above your chest. Keeping your upper arms still, lower the dumbbells toward your head. Once you're about an inch away from your head, press back up to the starting position.

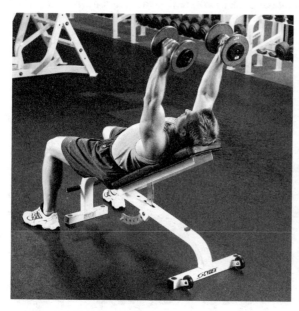 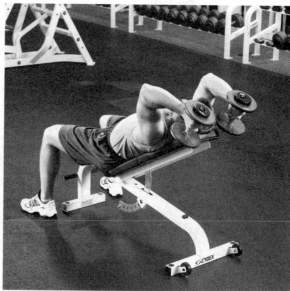

LYING CROSS-BODY UNILATERAL EXTENSION

(MUSCLES TRAINED: TRICEPS)

Lie on a flat bench holding a dumbbell in one hand extended above your chest. Using your free arm to support the working arm, lower the weight down across your body toward your opposite cheek. When you're about an inch away from your cheek, pause before pressing the weight back up to the starting position.

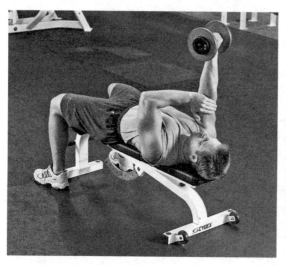 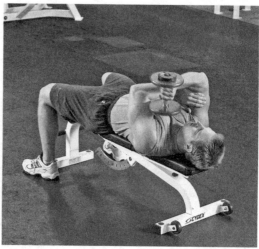

SEATED OVERHEAD DUMBBELL EXTENSION (BI- AND UNILATERAL)

(MUSCLES TRAINED: TRICEPS)

These can be done either with one arm or two. For the single-arm version, sit on the bench holding a dumbbell over your head, supporting your working arm with your free arm. Lower the dumbbell until it's just above the base of your neck. Pause there for second before pressing the weight back up to the starting position. When working with two dumbbells, lift them both over your head and keep your upper arms still as you lower the dumbbells behind your head and press them back up to the starting position.

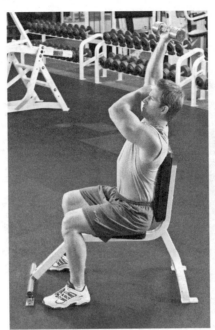 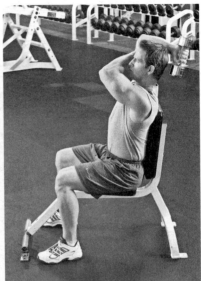

DUMBBELL KICKBACK

(MUSCLES TRAINED: TRICEPS)

Holding a dumbbell in one hand, place your other hand and same-side leg on a bench with your back straight and your other leg on the floor. Lift your working arm up and tuck it to your side as you extend the dumbbell back until your arm is straight and parallel to the floor. Pause, lower, and repeat.

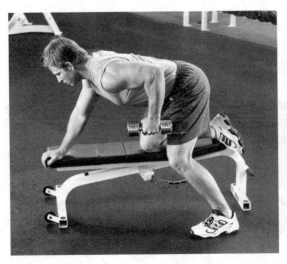 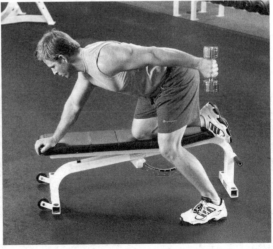

OVERHEAD E-Z BAR EXTENSION

(MUSCLES TRAINED: TRICEPS)

Sit on a bench and grab an E-Z bar with the closer of the two provided grips. Raise the bar over your head until your arms are straight. Keeping your back perfectly straight and upper arms over your head, lower the weights down behind your head. Pause just before you touch the base of your neck, then extend the weights back up to the starting position.

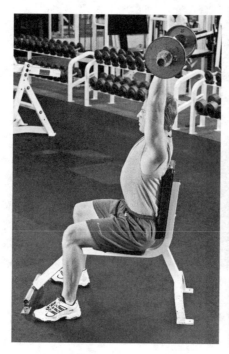 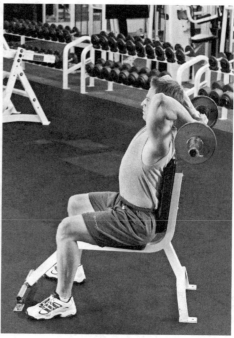

LYING E-Z BAR EXTENSION

(MUSCLES TRAINED: TRICEPS)

Lie back on an exercise bench holding an E-Z bar with the closer of the two provided grips. Extend your arms up over your chin. Keeping your upper arms still, lower the bar down to within an inch of your forehand. Pause, then push the weights back up to the starting position.

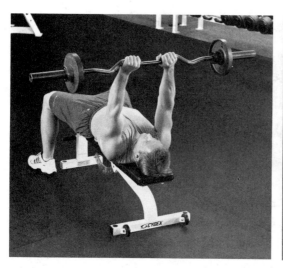 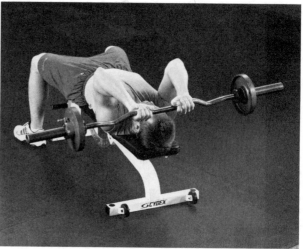

LYING CABLE EXTENSION

(MUSCLES TRAINED: TRICEPS)

Position a flat bench in front of a cable station lengthwise with either a V bar, E-Z bar, or rope handle attached to the low pulley. Grab the handle and lie back on the bench as you extend your arms up over your chin. Keeping your upper arms still, lower the handle to within an inch of your head. Pause, then push the weights back up to the starting position.

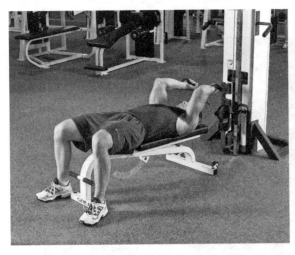 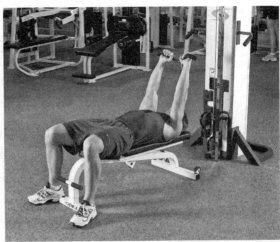

SEATED OVERHEAD CABLE EXTENSION

(MUSCLES TRAINED: TRICEPS)

Position a flat bench in front of a cable station crossways with either a V bar, E-Z bar, or rope handle attached to the low pulley. Grab the handle and sit on the bench with your back straight and feet flat on the floor. Raise the handle up above your head until your arms are straight, then, keeping your upper arms close to your head, lower the weight down toward the base of your neck. Pause, then extend the weight back up to the starting position.

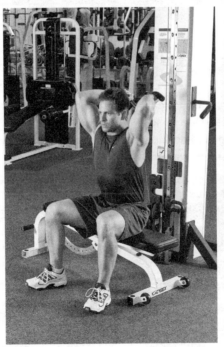 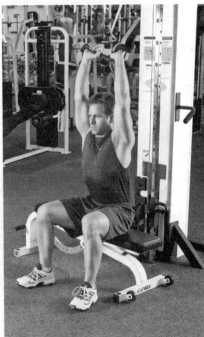

UNILATERAL TRICEPS EXTENSION WITH A LEAN

(MUSCLES TRAINED: TRICEPS)

Sit crossways on an exercise bench with a dumbbell in one hand extended above your head. Lean over to your opposite side and brace yourself with the opposite arm. Keeping your torso leaned to your nonworking side, lower the dumbbell down behind your head until it almost reaches the base of your neck. Pause, then raise the weight back up to the starting position. Leaning to one side increases the difficulty level by making it harder to straighten your arm out at the top of the repetition.

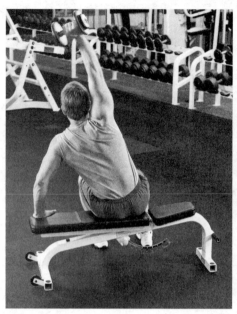
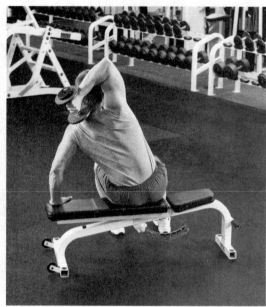

JM PRESS

(MUSCLES TRAINED: TRICEPS)

This exercise is like a Close-Grip Bench Press mixed with a Triceps Extension, but with variations on both. Start the exercise the same way you would a Close-Grip Bench Press, except make sure the bar is set in a direct line above your upper chest. Beginning from a fully extended position, lower the bar down until you reach the halfway point. At this point let the bar roll back about 1 inch, then press the bar back up.

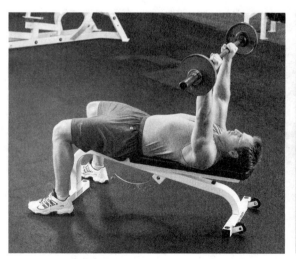
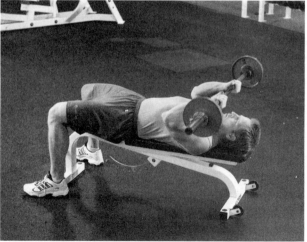

SEATED DUMBBELL BICEPS CURL

(MUSCLES TRAINED: BICEPS, FOREARMS)

Sit on an exercise bench holding a pair of dumbbells in your hands with a supinated grip. Keeping your upper arms perfectly still, curl the weights up until your palms are in front of your shoulders. Pause, lower, and repeat.

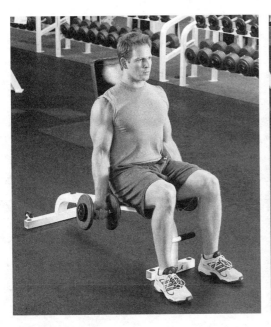 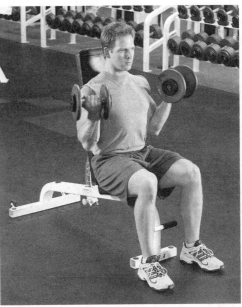

SEATED DUMBBELL REVERSE CURL

(MUSCLES TRAINED: BRACHIORADIALIS, BICEPS)

Execute this the same way as the regular Seated Dumbbell Biceps Curl with the one exception that you use a supinated grip throughout.

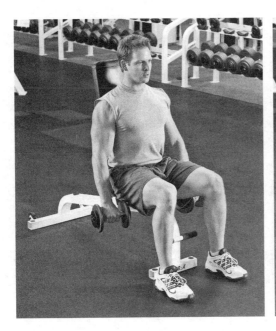 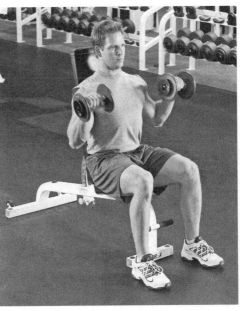

INCLINE DUMBBELL BICEPS CURL

(MUSCLES TRAINED: BICEPS, FOREARMS)

Lie back on an incline bench holding a pair of dumbbells in your hands at arm's length underneath your shoulders. Keeping your upper arms still, curl the weights up until your palms are in front of your shoulders. Pause, lower, and repeat. The angle of the bench will slightly increase the difficulty of the exercise.

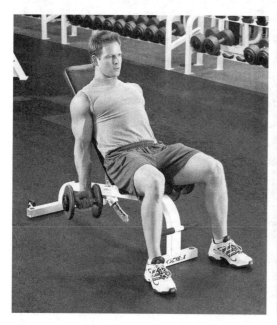 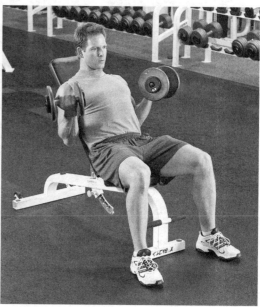

INCLINE REVERSE DUMBBELL CURL

(MUSCLES TRAINED: BRACHIORADILALIS, BICEPS)

Execute the same way as described above, except use a pronated grip throughout.

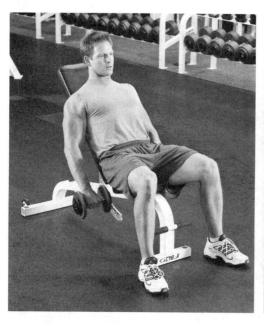 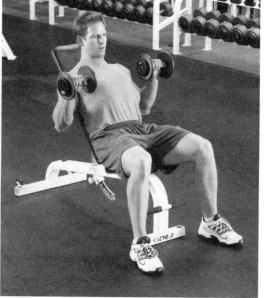

SEATED DUMBBELL HAMMER CURL

(MUSCLES TRAINED: BRACHIORADIALIS, BICEPS)

Execute the same way you would as the Seated Dumbbell Biceps Curl, except with a neutral or Hammer grip.

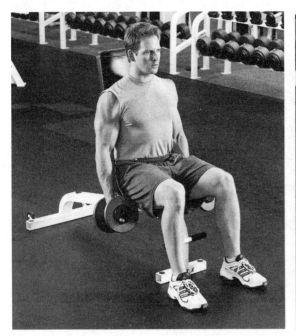 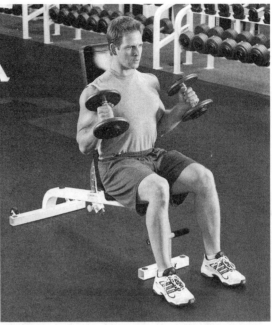

INCLINE DUMBBELL HAMMER CURL

(MUSCLES TRAINED: BRACHIORADIALIS, BICEPS)

Execute the same way you would as the Incline Dumbbell Biceps Curl, except with a neutral or Hammer grip.

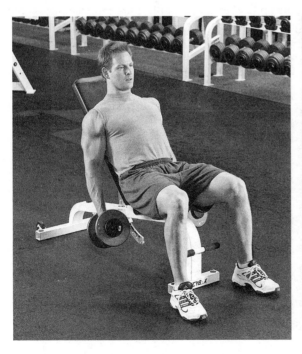 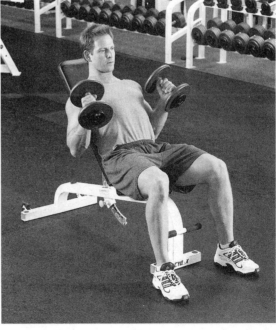

CONCENTRATION CURL

Sit at the end of an exercise bench holding a dumbbell at arm's length between your thighs. With the back of your working arm resting against your inner thigh on that same side, lean forward at the waist and brace yourself with your nonworking arm on your opposite thigh. Hold this position as you curl the weight up as high as you can toward your chest. Pause, lower, and repeat.

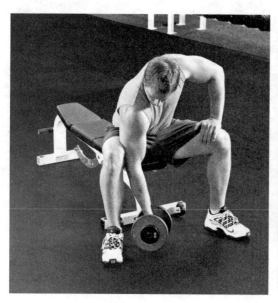 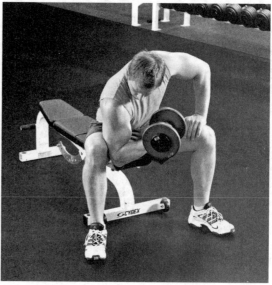

DUMBBELL PREACHER CURL

Sit on a preacher bench with it set so that the pad fits comfortably into your armpits with your arms extended and the backs of your elbows in contact with the pad. Curl both weights up to your shoulder. Start the exercise by lowering the weights down until your elbows are almost completely straight. Pause and then bring the weights back up to the starting position. Be careful not to allow your elbows to straighten out completely, as that may lead to injury.

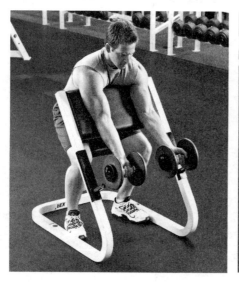 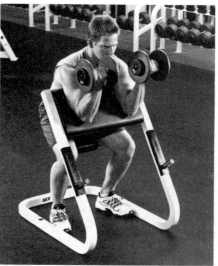

BARBELL PREACHER CURL

Sit on a preacher bench with it set so that the pad fits comfortably into your armpits with your arms extended and the backs of your elbows in contact with the pad. Begin by reaching over and grabbing the bar and bringing it up to the starting position as you sit down. Start the exercise by lowering the bar down until your elbows are almost completely straight. Pause, and then bring the weight back up to the starting position. Be careful not to allow your elbows to straighten out completely, as that may lead to injury. An E-Z bar can also ease elbow strain.

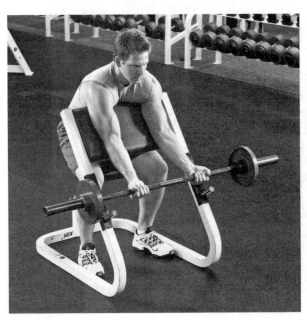
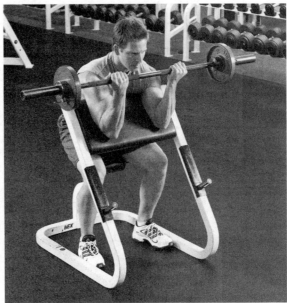

LYING CABLE CURL

(MUSCLES TRAINED: BICEPS, FOREARMS)

Sit in front of a cable station with your legs extended and a bar attached to the low pulley. Lie back until your body is completely straight. Keeping your elbows in close to your body, curl the weights out in front of you in a wide arc until the bar is in front of your shoulders. Pause, lower, and repeat.

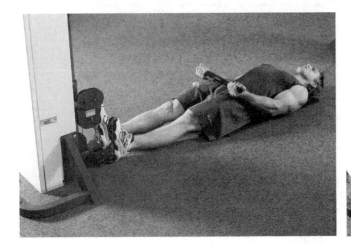
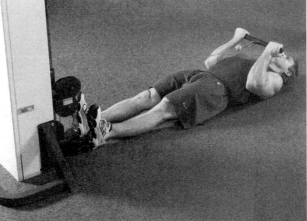

DUMBBELL WRIST CURL

(MUSCLES TRAINED: FOREARMS)

Kneel down in front of an exercise bench holding a dumbbell in each hand, with your wrists extended out over the edge. Begin by allowing the weights to roll down into your fingertips, then immediately curl the weights up so that your palms face your elbows. Pause, lower, and repeat.

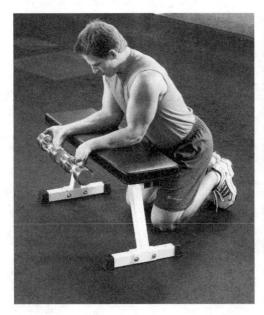
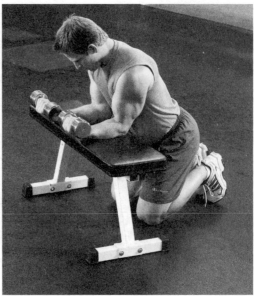

DUMBBELL REVERSE WRIST CURL

(MUSCLES TRAINED: FOREARMS)

Execute this exercise the same way you would a regular Dumbbell Wrist Curl, except using a pronated grip throughout.

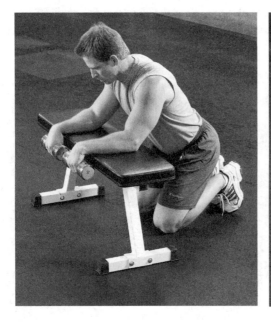
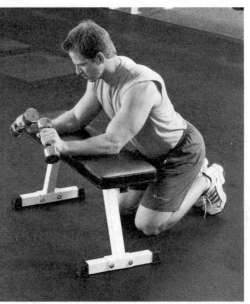

BARBELL WRIST CURL

Execute this exercise the same way you would a Dumbbell Wrist Curl.

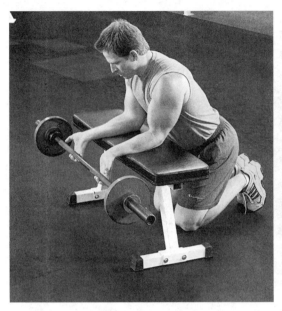 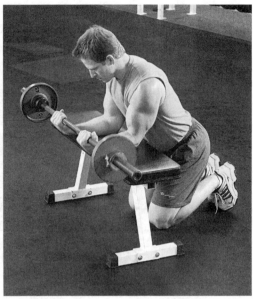

BARBELL REVERSE WRIST CURL

Execute this exercise the same way you would a Barbell Wrist Curl, except hold the bar with a pronated grip instead of a supinated grip. An E-Z bar will be more comfortable for the wrists.

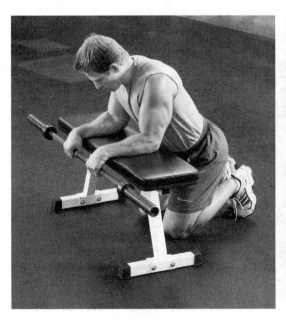 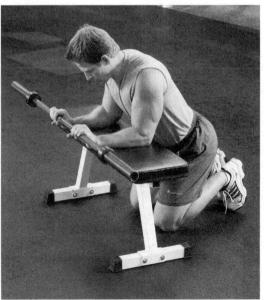

SEATED BICEPS CURL WITH ISOMETRIC HOLD

(MUSCLES TRAINED: BICEPS, FOREARMS)

Execute this exercise the same way as you would a regular Seated Dumbbell Biceps Curl, except start with one weight curled up to the halfway position with your forearm parallel to the floor. Hold that there as you then curl the other dumbbell through the full range of motion for the desire number of reps. After completing the last rep, lower the weight to the halfway position. Now curl the other arm for the same number of reps.

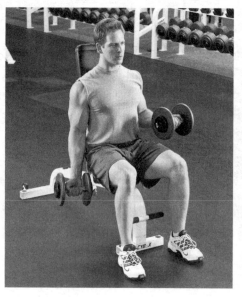 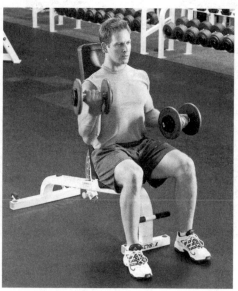

SEATED ZOTTMAN CURL

(MUSCLES TRAINED: BICEPS, BRACHIORADIALIS)

Execute this exercise the same way as you would a regular Seated Dumbbell Biceps Curl, except at the top turn your wrists so that your palms face forward, and lower the dumbbells that way. At the bottom, when your arms are almost completely straight, turn your palms back up and continue.

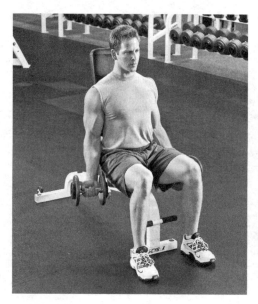 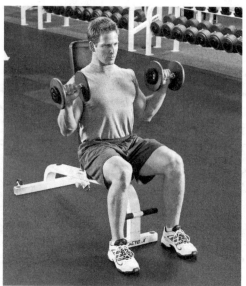

PRONE DUMBBELL CURL

(MUSCLES TRAINED: BICEPS, FOREARMS)

Lie prone on an exercise bench holding a pair of dumbbells at arm's length beneath your shoulders. Keeping your upper arms still, curl the weights up until your palms are in front of your shoulders. Pause, lower, and repeat.

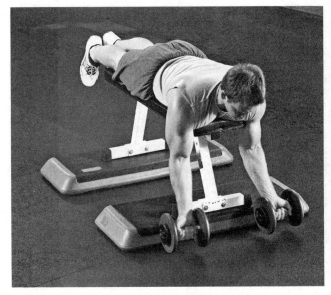
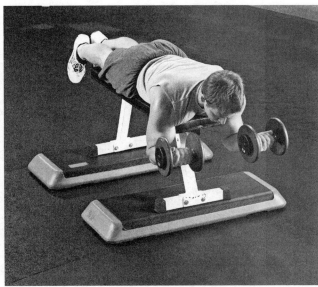

ROPE PULL-APART CURL

(MUSCLES TRAINED: BRACHIORADIALIS, BICEPS)

Stand in front of a cable station with a rope handle attached to a low pulley. Bend over and grab the weight. With your knees slightly bent and back straight, keep your upper arms still as you curl the weights up, pulling the handles apart as far as possible as you do. Pause when your hands are just outside your shoulders, then lower and repeat.

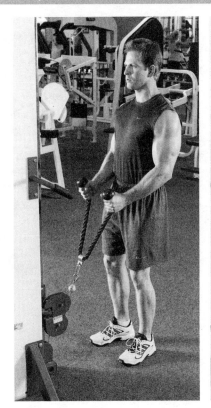
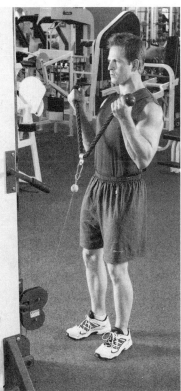

PRONE BARBELL CURL

Lie prone on an exercise bench holding a barbell at arm's length beneath your shoulders. Keeping your upper arms still, curl the weights up until your palms are in front of your shoulders. Pause, lower, and repeat.

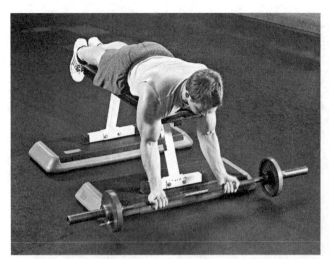 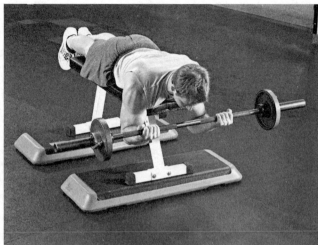

PRONE REVERSE BARBELL CURL

Perform this exercise the same way you would a regular Prone Barbell Curl, except use a pronated grip throughout. An E-Z bar would be more comfortable for the wrists.

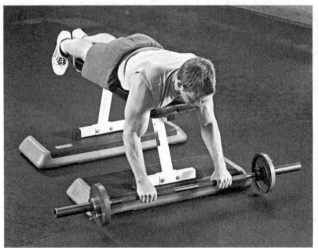 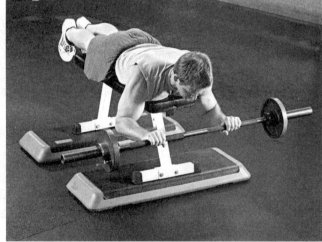

LOWER BODY

BEGINNER/ INTERMEDIATE	ADVANCED
Dumbbell Stepup	Cable Bulgarian Split Squat
Dumbbell Bulgarian Split Squat	Dumbbell Crossover Stepup
Barbell Stepup	Reverse Hyperextension
Barbell Bulgarian Split Squat	

DUMBBELL STEPUP

(MUSCLES TRAINED: QUADRICEPS, GLUTES, HAMSTRINGS)

Grab a pair of dumbbells and stand in front of a standard flat bench. Lift your foot and place it firmly on the bench, push down with your heel, and step up onto the bench. Step down with your opposite foot and then your working leg before repeating for the desired number of reps.

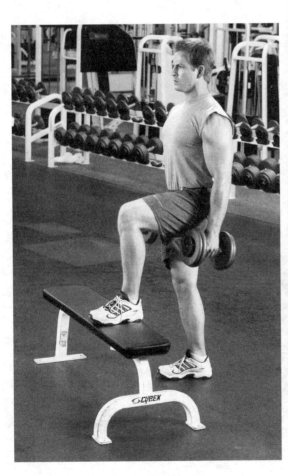
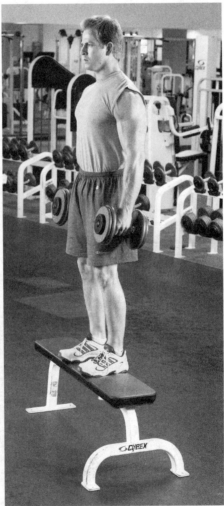

DUMBBELL BULGARIAN SPLIT SQUAT

(MUSCLES TRAINED: QUADRICEPS, GLUTES, HAMSTRINGS)

Stand facing away from an exercise bench positioned crossways a full stride behind you. Holding a pair of dumbbells at arm's length, reach one leg back and rest your instep on the bench. Balance on one leg as you keep your back straight and bend both knees as you lower yourself toward the floor. In the bottom position your back leg should be almost touching the floor, with your front leg bent at a 90-degree angle. Pause for a second, then push back up to the starting position.

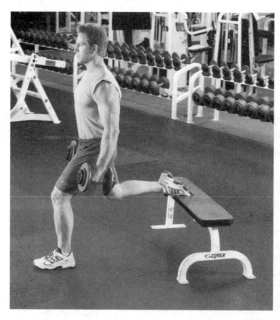 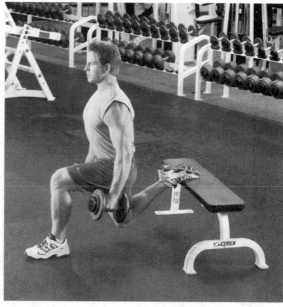

BARBELL STEPUP

(MUSCLES TRAINED: QUADRICEPS, GLUTES, HAMSTRINGS)

Execute this exercise the same way you would a Dumbbell Stepup, but with a barbell resting on your upper back.

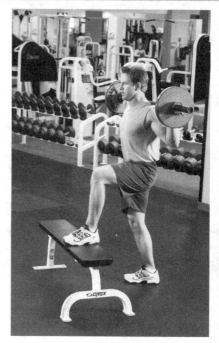 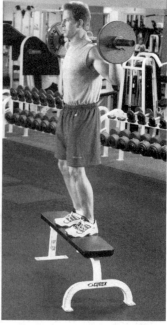

BARBELL BULGARIAN SPLIT SQUAT

(MUSCLES TRAINED: QUADRICEPS, GLUTES, HAMSTRINGS)

Execute this exercise the same way you would a Dumbbell Bulgarian Split Squat except with a barbell resting on your upper back.

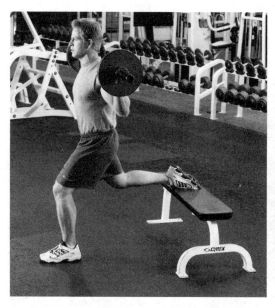 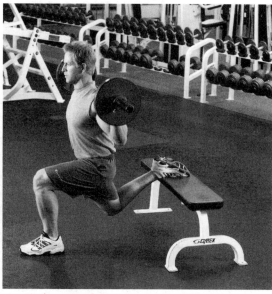

CABLE BULGARIAN SPLIT SQUAT

(MUSCLES TRAINED: QUADRICEPS, GLUTES, HAMSTRINGS)

Place a bench positioned perpendicularly in front of a cable station about 3 feet away from the pulley. With a stirrup handle attached to the low pulley, reach down and grab the handle with one hand as you position the foot of that same side on the bench behind you. Keeping your torso as upright as possible, begin by bending both knees and lowering yourself toward the floor. In the bottom position your back knee should almost be touching the floor, with your front leg bent at a 90-degree angle. Try not to allow your torso to rotate at all as you press back up to the starting position.

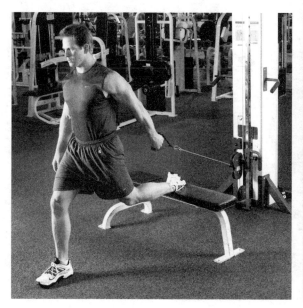 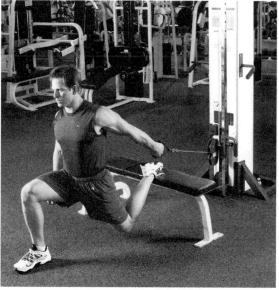

BARBELL CROSSOVER STEPUP

(MUSCLES TRAINED: QUADRICEPS, GLUTES, HAMSTRINGS)

Stand with a barbell resting across your back next to a bench positioned perpendicularly next to you. Begin by stepping up and across your body with your outside leg and planting your foot on the bench. Press up until you're standing on the bench with both legs. To get down, reverse the process by stepping down and behind you with the inside leg, followed by the leg that stepped up on the bench.

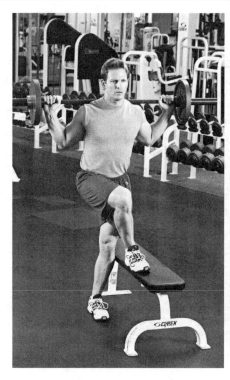
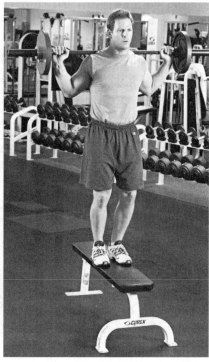

DUMBBELL CROSSOVER STEPUP

(MUSCLES TRAINED: QUADRICEPS, GLUTES, HAMSTRINGS)

Execute this exercise the same way as you would a Barbell Crossover Stepup, except hold a pair of dumbbells at your sides.

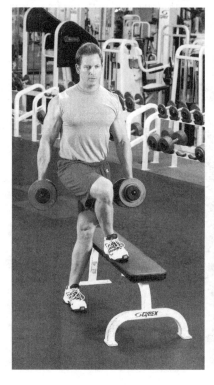
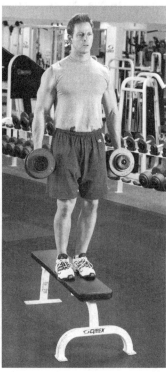

REVERSE HYPEREXTENSION

(MUSCLES TRAINED: GLUTES, HAMSTRINGS, LOWER BACK)

Lie prone on an exercise bench with your legs and hips hanging off and your legs straight. Holding on to the bench for support, lift your legs up until they're slightly past the level of the bench. Pause, lower, and repeat. You can also do the exercise with your knees bent 90 degrees for greater hamstring involvement.

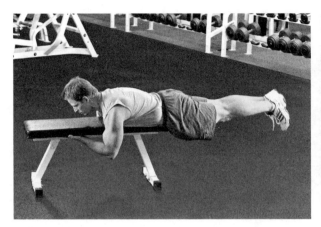 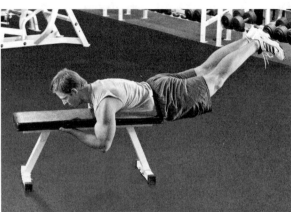

CHAPTER ELEVEN

RACK UP YOUR FREQUENT FREE WEIGHT MILES

Everything You Need to Know about Squat Racks and Power Cages

THEY'RE OFTEN FOUND IN THE DEEPEST, darkest corners of the gym: menacing-looking contraptions that look better suited to a construction site than a commercial fitness center. Throw in the fact that they're almost always inhabited by those aforementioned big guys, and it's understandable why most newbies tend to steer clear of them. Big mistake! We're here to tell you that squat racks and power cages are awesome training tools for just about anyone, and they're absolutely essential for building a strong, well-muscled physique.

So just what are these things for anyway? Fair question. Especially considering that they have a multitude of uses. Before we explain the difference between the two, the take-home point here is that these two pieces of equipment are primarily used for supporting weights that are too heavy to lift from the floor. Obviously, the exercises that squat racks and power cages facilitate are squats, but there's a lot more to it than that. You can also

use them for performing various other lower-body exercises like lunges and Romanian deadlifts, as well as upper-body lifts like bench presses, shoulder presses, heavy rowing movements, and shrugs.

It's not that you have to be some kind of hulking brute to use these pieces of equipment. Pretty much anyone can benefit from using them by working with loads that would otherwise be too difficult to position. I don't care how weak you might be, you're still going to be able to squat more off the supports in a rack or a cage than you could if you attempted to lift the weight off the floor and position it on your shoulders. The same holds true for a bench press. Trying to maneuver the weight up into position would be a heck of a lot tougher than just lying back and lifting it off the supports.

YOU *DO* KNOW SQUAT

The first and perhaps more common of these two types of apparatuses is the squat rack. This is a very open structure with a back support beam and weight supports along the sides that make it easy for you to use. One of the best features of a squat rack is that it allows you to set the bar at a variety of angles for easy racking and unracking. Plus, it also has safety supports in case you get into trouble during a lift. Bite off more than you can chew on a set of squats, for example, and you can simply set the weights down on the supports, as opposed to injuring your knees and/or back by overexerting yourself to get out of trouble.

The only downside is that because the height of the safeties is often preset, taller lifters with longer limbs may have to lower the weights farther down before being able to rest them on the supports.

Enter the power cage: This is a fully adjustable support structure that allows you to vary both the position of the weight supports as well as the safety bars, thus making any lift easier to tailor to your specific needs. This extremely sturdy, cagelike structure basically surrounds you, giving you a heightened sense of security. Regardless of what lift you're doing, the power cage affords you the peace of mind of knowing you can push yourself a little bit harder, since you essentially have a built-in spotter. The height of the weight supports and safety bars is also very easy to adjust, making it a breeze to switch from one exercise to the other.

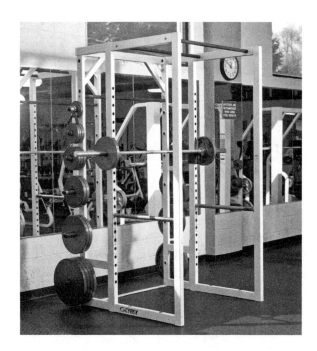

YOU CAN'T DO THAT HERE

Now that you know what they're for, but before we show you all of the different exercises you can do in them, it's important that we point out how squat racks and power cages shouldn't be used. To serious lifters, these are without question two of the most important pieces of equipment in the gym, so much so that your better gyms will often have at least two or three of them out on their floor. They are—and we cannot stress this enough—specifically for supporting weights that are otherwise too heavy to get into position. They are not for biceps curls, wrist curls, or any other exercises that could easily be performed with dumbbells, preset barbells, and cables.

This is a trap that even seasoned gym rats often fall into. Because you can easily place the bar in a convenient position from which to grab it, squat rack biceps curling has unfortunately become an all-too-common practice. So, in the interest of public safety, allow us to share with you this little pearl of wisdom that just might save you from a heated confrontation with a fellow gym member: Nothing aggravates someone looking to do squats or any other lift requiring the use of a rack or cage more than having to wait for some clown to finish doing curls. In terms of violating proper gym etiquette, this one's right up near the top of the list. (For more examples of proper gym behavior, see Chapter Nineteen.)

Now, before you go on about having every right to use the equipment because you paid your membership dues,

consider this important fact: You can do those curls just about anywhere else in the gym. The person waiting to squat can do them only in a rack or cage. Think about it for a minute: How would you like to go over and attempt to do a set of bench presses only to find someone doing crunches on the bench? Or how about trying to use the preacher curl bench and having to wait for someone else to finish a set of stepups? You'd be saying to yourself "C'mon, you could do those anywhere!" Now you know how that frustrated squatter feels. So do us all a favor and use the rack only for the types of exercise it's intended for.

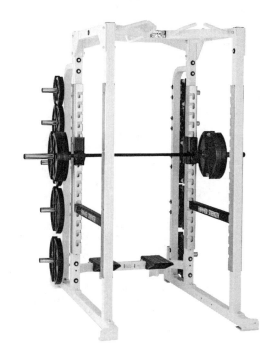

CHEST AND UPPER BACK

	BEGINNER/ INTERMEDIATE	ADVANCED
CHEST	Bench Press (various angles)	Rack Lockout
BACK	Bent-Over Row (various grips)	

BENCH PRESS (VARIOUS ANGLES)

(MUSCLES TRAINED: CHEST, SHOULDERS, TRICEPS)

Although most gyms generally have more than a few types of benches in the event they're all being used, there's no harm in taking an adjustable bench over to a rack or cage and doing your pressing there. Simply set the bench inside the rack at the appropriate angle, lie back, and lift the weight off the supports and away you go. The great part about doing these in a rack, or better yet, a cage, is that if there's no one around to spot you, you can set the safeties just above your chest so that if you get into trouble you can just set the bar down.

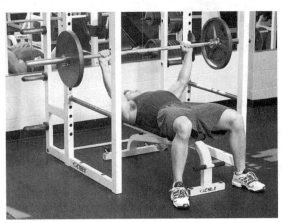 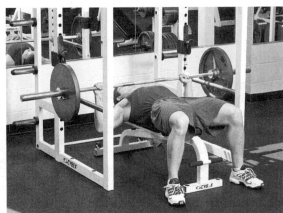

RACK LOCKOUT

(MUSCLES TRAINED: CHEST, SHOULDERS, TRICEPS)

For this, a cage really works best. This challenging exercise is designed to strengthen your triceps for the lockout position of the bench press. They can be done with any angle press, but are most commonly used for flat bench presses. Set a bench inside the power cage and position the support bars so that they're just past the midpoint of the range of motion. After unracking the bar from the supports, lower it down until it makes contact with the safety bars. Pause for a good second or two before pressing it back up until your arms are straight. Lower it again and repeat.

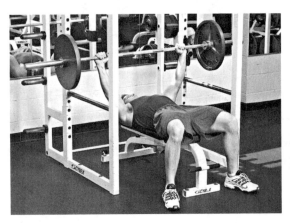 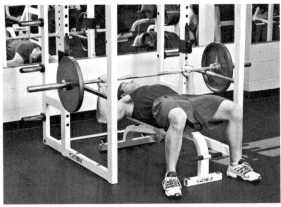

BENT-OVER ROW (VARIOUS GRIPS)

(MUSCLES TRAINED: UPPER BACK, BICEPS)

Stand facing a loaded barbell set just below waist height in the rack. Grab the bar with a pronated, shoulder-width grip and take a step back from the rack. Begin by keeping an arch in your back as you bend your knees and lean over at the waist until your torso is parallel to the floor. Once there, with your arms hanging down beneath your shoulders, use your upper back and biceps to pull the weight up to your chest. Pause, lower, and repeat. Using a pronated grip with the elbows out will target the scapular retractors more, while using a supinated grip with your elbows held in close to your body works the lats and biceps to a greater degree.

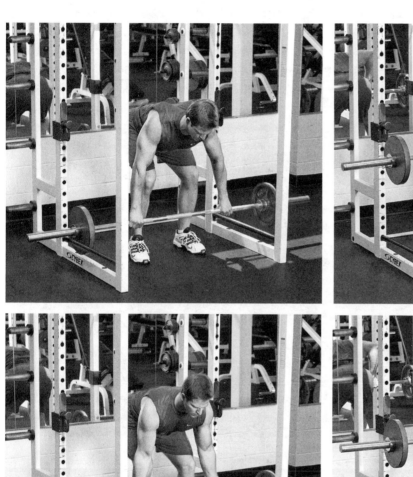
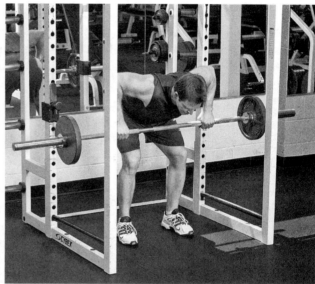
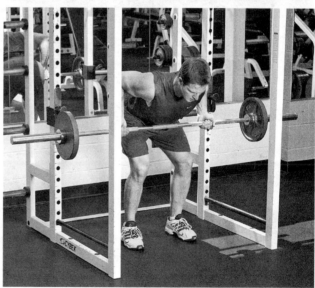

SHOULDERS AND ARMS

BEGINNER/ INTERMEDIATE	ADVANCED
Military Press	Push Press
Shrug	Hang Clean
Close-Grip Bench Press	High Pull

MILITARY PRESS

(MUSCLES TRAINED: SHOULDERS, TRICEPS)

Set a loaded barbell in a rack about chin height. Grab the bar with a shoulder-width, overhand grip and take a step back. Stand holding the barbell at shoulder level, your feet shoulder-width apart and your knees slightly bent. Push the weight straight overhead, leaning your head back slightly but keeping your torso upright. Pause, then slowly lower the bar to the starting position. More experienced lifters with no history of shoulder problems can also perform this exercise behind the neck.

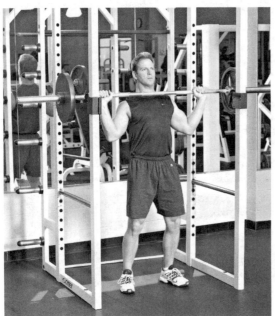 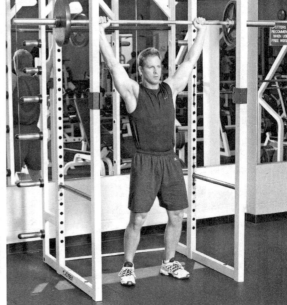

SHRUG

(MUSCLES TRAINED: UPPER TRAPEZIUS, SHOULDERS)

Set a loaded barbell in a rack just below waist height. Grab the bar with a pronated, shoulder-width grip and take a step back. Keeping your arms straight, raise your shoulders up toward your ears as high as possible. Pause, lower, and repeat.

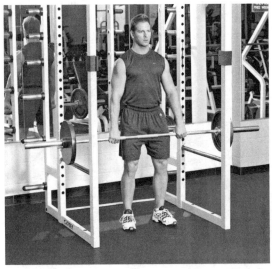 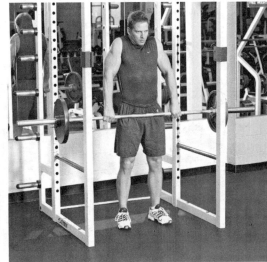

CLOSE-GRIP BENCH PRESS

(MUSCLES TRAINED: TRICEPS, CHEST)

Position a bench inside a rack or cage. Lie back on a bench press and take a close grip (narrower than shoulder width apart) on the bar. Lift the bar off the supports and slowly lower it down toward the midline of your chest. Pause when the bar is almost in contact with the chest and then press it back up to the starting position.

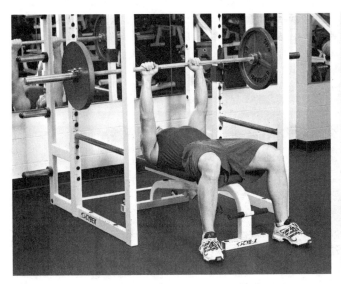 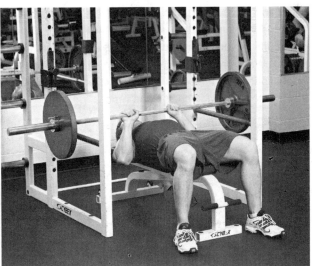

PUSH PRESS

Position a loaded barbell on the supports of a rack or cage set about level with the height of your collarbone. Using a heavier weight than you normally would for a set of Military Presses, grab the bar with a pronated, shoulder-width grip and take a step back from the rack. With the bar in front of your collarbone, just above your shoulders, quickly dip your hips and knees and then explode up to get the weight moving. Soon after you initiate this movement your arms will kick in and finish pressing the bar overhead until your arms are straight. Pause at the top before slowly lowering the bar back down and repeating. This is a great exercise for developing explosive power.

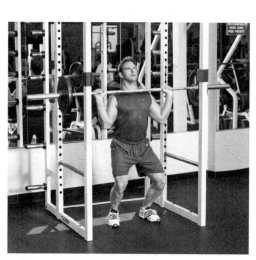 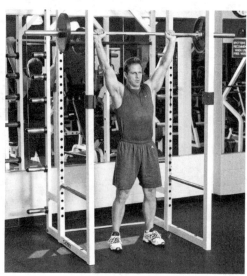

HANG CLEAN

(MUSCLES TRAINED: UPPER TRAPEZIUS, SHOULDERS, BICEPS)

Set a loaded barbell in a rack just below waist height. Grab the bar with an overhand, shoulder-width grip and take a step back. Hold it in front of your thighs while standing with your knees slightly bent. Your lower back should be in its natural alignment (in other words, slightly arched). Quickly dip into your knees and hips and then explosively change directions as you shrug your shoulders and pull the bar up as hard as you can. You should rise up on your toes as you do this. When the bar reaches chest level, bend your knees again, rotate your forearms from the elbows, and bend your wrists so they go underneath the bar as you "catch" it on the front of your shoulders. Then quickly flip the bar back down to the starting position and repeat.

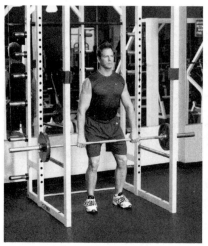 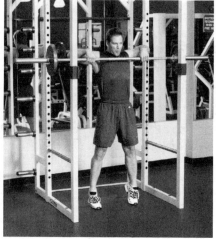 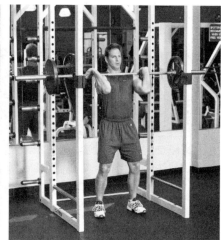

HIGH PULL

(MUSCLES TRAINED: UPPER TRAPEZIUS, SHOULDERS, BICEPS)

Set a loaded barbell in a rack, or cage just below waist level. Grab the bar with a pronated shoulder-width grip and take a step back. Then quickly dip into your hips and immediately change directions as you begin shrugging your shoulders and pulling the weight up toward your chest. Unlike a hang clean, however, you'll stop short of flipping and then catching the bar. Simply rise up on your toes and finish with the bar at about chest level. Pause for a split second and then drop back down to the starting position.

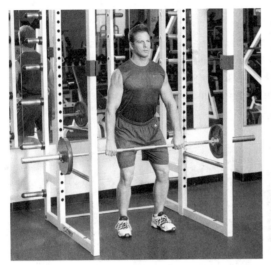 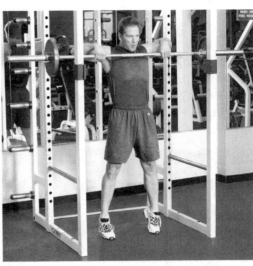

LOWER BODY

BEGINNER/ INTERMEDIATE	ADVANCED
Squat	Front Squat
Sumo Squat	Bulgarian Split Squat
Split Squat	
Romanian Deadlift	Hack Squat
Lunge (various angles)	Good Morning

SQUAT

(MUSCLES TRAINED: QUADRICEPS, HAMSTRINGS, GLUTES)

Set a loaded barbell on the supports of a rack or cage just below shoulder height. Step underneath the bar, rest it across your upper trapezius, and grab it just outside your shoulders. Lift the bar off the supports and take a step back as you set your feet shoulder-width apart. Keep your knees slightly bent, your back straight, and eyes focused straight ahead. Slowly lower your body as if you were sitting back into a chair, keeping your back in its natural alignment. When your upper thighs are parallel to the floor, pause, then return to the starting position.

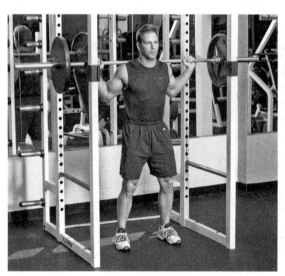 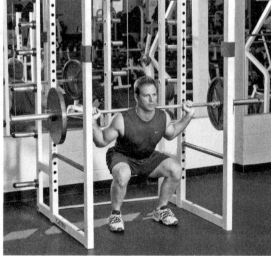

SUMO SQUAT

(MUSCLES TRAINED: QUADRICEPS, ADDUCTORS, HAMSTRINGS, GLUTES)

Set up the same way you would for the Squat, except when you walk the weight back, take a slightly wider stance and turn your toes out to the sides (using a clock reference, think of your toes pointed to ten o'clock and two o'clock.). Then simply descend to a parallel position, making sure that your knees line up over your toes throughout the movement. Pause when you hit parallel and then press back up to the starting position.

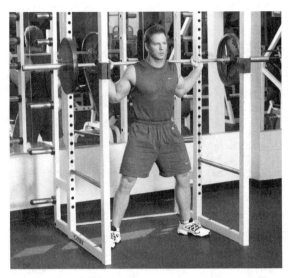 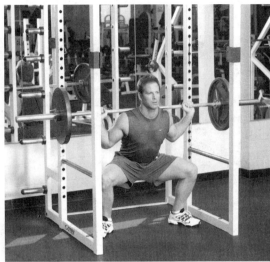

SPLIT SQUAT

(MUSCLES TRAINED: QUADRICEPS, HAMSTRINGS, GLUTES)

Set a loaded barbell on the supports of a rack or cage just below shoulder height. Step underneath the bar and rest it across your upper trapezius and grab it just outside your shoulders. Lift the bar off the supports and take a step back, positioning your feet so that one is a full 2 to 3 feet in front of the other. With only the ball of your back foot in contact with the ground, keep your back straight and bend both knees until your back knee almost touches the floor and your front leg forms a 90-degree angle. Pause for a second, then press back up to the starting position.

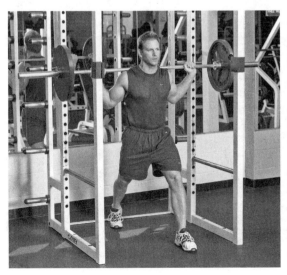 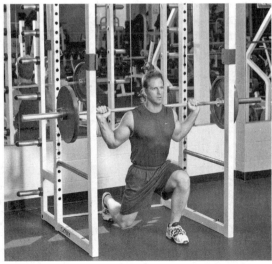

ROMANIAN DEADLIFT

(MUSCLES TRAINED: HAMSTRINGS, GLUTES, LOWER BACK)

Set a loaded barbell on the supports of a rack or cage set just below waist level. Grab the bar with an overhand grip that's just beyond shoulder width and take a step back. Stand holding the bar at arm's length and resting on the front of your thighs. Your feet are shoulder-width apart and your knees slightly bent. Your eyes are focused straight ahead. Slowly bend at the hips as you lower the bar just below your knees. Don't change the angle of your knees. Keep your head and chest up and your lower back slightly arched. Pause there and then lift your torso back to the starting position, keeping the bar as close to your body as possible.

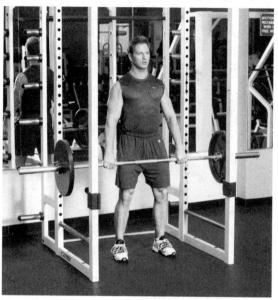 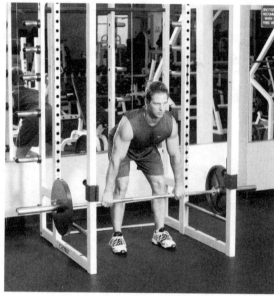

LUNGE (VARIOUS ANGLES)

(MUSCLES TRAINED: QUADRICEPS, HAMSTRINGS, GLUTES)

You can perform any type of lunge with a challenging weight by simply setting it on the supports of a rack or cage and stepping underneath it to load the barbell onto your upper back.

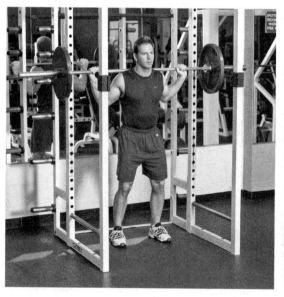 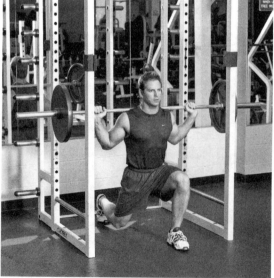

FRONT SQUAT

(MUSCLES TRAINED: QUADRICEPS, HAMSTRINGS, GLUTES)

Set a loaded barbell on the supports of a rack or cage just below shoulder height. Next, grab the bar with a shoulder-width grip and step under it, this time resting the weight across the front of your shoulders instead of your upper back. To do this, you'll need good wrist and shoulder flexibility, as you'll bring your elbows underneath the bar and forward so that the backs of your arms are parallel to the floor. Once you've got the bar supported, step back and set your feet shoulder-width apart, eyes focused straight ahead. Keep a natural arch in your back until your thighs are parallel to the floor. Pause for a second, then press back up to the starting position.

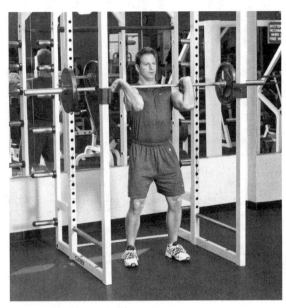 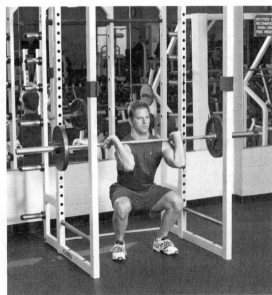

BULGARIAN SPLIT SQUAT

(MUSCLES TRAINED: QUADRICEPS, GLUTES, HAMSTRINGS)

Position a bench at the back of a squat rack or cage a full stride behind you. Set a loaded barbell on the supports of a rack or cage just below shoulder height. Step underneath the bar, rest it across your upper trapezius, and grab it just outside your shoulders. Lift the bar off the supports and take a step back as you set your feet shoulder-width apart. Keep one leg in place as you reach the other back and rest your instep on the bench. Keeping your back as straight as possible, bend both knees as you descend until your back knee almost touches the floor and your front knee forms a 90-degree angle. Pause for a second and then press back up to the starting position.

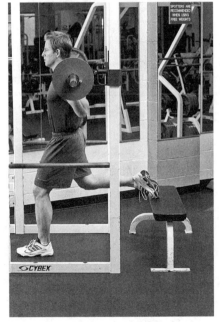 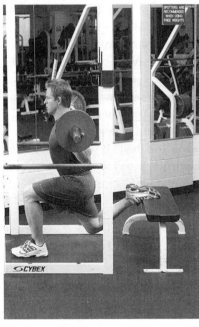

HACK SQUAT

Position a set of 25-pound plates on the floor a foot behind the supports of a rack or cage. Step around a barbell set just below waist level so that it's behind you. Grab the bar with a pronated, shoulder-width grip and lift the weight off the supports. Slowly step back and place your heels on the plates with the balls of your feet in contact with the floor. Keep your torso as erect as possible until you descend to the parallel position. Pause for a second before pressing back up to the starting position.

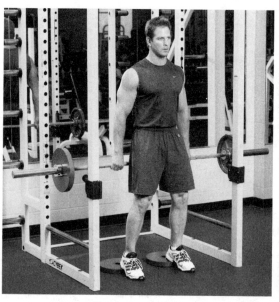 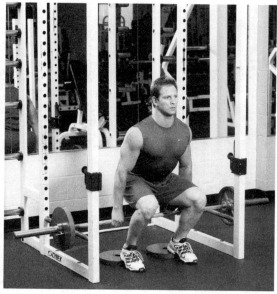

GOOD MORNING

(MUSCLES TRAINED: GLUTES, HAMSTRINGS, LOWER BACK)

Set a loaded barbell on the supports of a rack or cage just below shoulder height. Step under the bar and rest the barbell comfortably on your upper back. Slowly bend forward at the hips as you lower your chest as far as you can go while maintaining the natural arch in your lower back or until your upper body is parallel to the floor. Keep your head up and maintain the same angle of your knees. Lift your upper body back to the starting position.

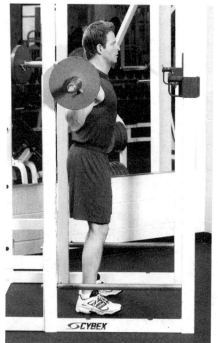 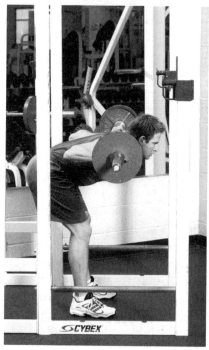

I'LL MAKE AN EXCEPTION ...

The following exercises are also considered acceptable alternatives for either a squat rack or a power cage. You still shouldn't do them there if someone else is waiting to squat, but even if you do, they'll probably earn you fewer dirty looks than biceps curls.

BEGINNER/INTERMEDIATE	ADVANCED
Reverse Pushup (supinated grip)	Reverse Pushup (pronated grip)
Chinup	Fixed-Bar Triceps Extension
	Pullup

REVERSE PUSHUP (SUPINATED GRIP)
(MUSCLES TRAINED: UPPER BACK, BICEPS)

Secure a bar 3 to 4 feet above the floor in a squat rack or cage. Lie under the bar and grab it with a shoulder-width, supinated grip. Hang at arm's length from the bar with your body in a straight line from your ankles to your shoulders. Keep your body rigid and pull your chest to the bar. Pause and then lower yourself back to the starting position. You can make this exercise more challenging by placing your feet on a bench instead of the floor.

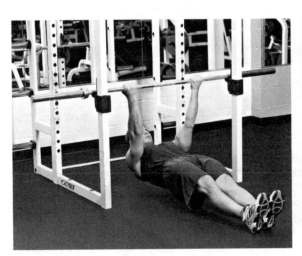 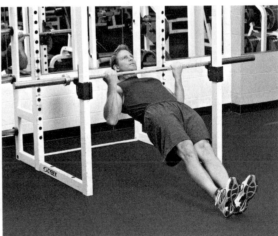

CHINUP

Set an empty bar on the highest supports of a rack or cage. Next, bend your knees and hang from the bar using a supinated, shoulder-width grip. Cross your feet behind you and pull yourself up as high as you can—your chin should go over the bar. Pause, then lower yourself until your arms are almost completely straight.

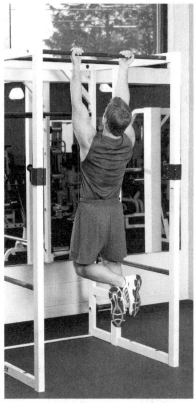
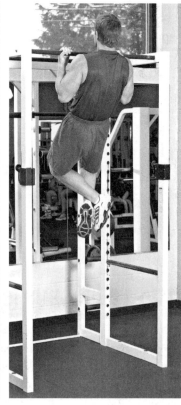

REVERSE PUSHUP (PRONATED GRIP)

Secure a bar 3 to 4 feet above the floor in a squat rack or cage. Lie under the bar and grab it with a shoulder-width, pronated grip. Hang at arm's length from the bar with your body in a straight line from your ankles to your shoulders. Keep your body rigid and pull your chest to the bar. Pause, then lower yourself back to the starting position. You can make this exercise more challenging by placing your feet on a bench instead of the floor.

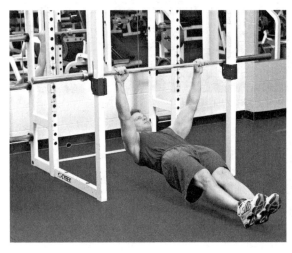
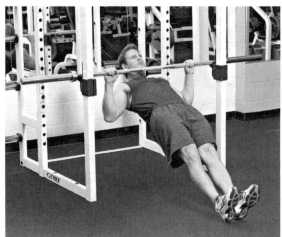

FIXED-BAR TRICEPS EXTENSION

(MUSCLES TRAINED: TRICEPS, CORE)

Set a bar on the supports of a squat rack or cage set at about waist level. (The higher the bar, the easier the exercise is to do—the lower it's set, the harder it is.) Grab the bar with a pronated grip that's just inside shoulder-width. With your body and arms completely straight and your weight on the balls of your feet, begin by slowly bending your arms and lowering your entire body head-first toward the bar. When your forehead is about an inch or two from the bar, pause for a second, then push back up to the starting position.

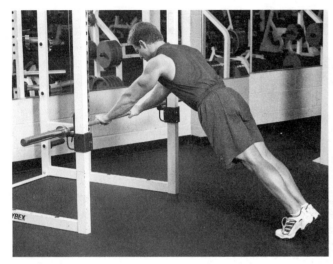 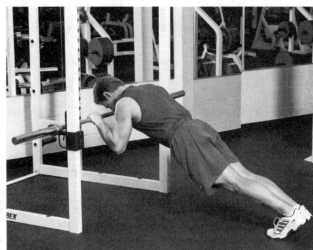

PULLUP

(MUSCLES TRAINED: UPPER BACK, BICEPS, BRACHIORADIALIS)

Set an empty bar on the highest supports of a rack or cage. Next, bend your knees and hang from the bar using a pronated shoulder-width grip. Cross your feet behind you and pull yourself up as high as you can—your chin should go over the bar. Pause, then lower yourself until your arms are almost completely straight.

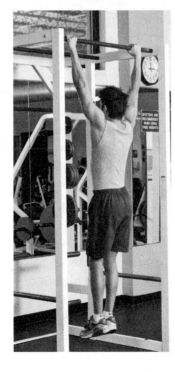 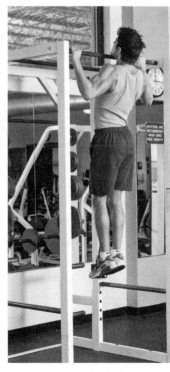

CHAPTER TWELVE

STANDARD MACHINATIONS

Getting to Know Some of the More Common Machines in the Gym

UP TO THIS POINT, WE'VE MADE a pretty strong case for the use of free weights. So much so, in fact, that you may be wondering whether strength-training machines are in fact even necessary. After all, given the fact that they have more application to real-world activities and often offer a better stimulus for the development of size, strength, and muscular coordination, free weights are pretty tough to beat. Yet despite their apparent superiority, good old-fashioned barbells and dumbbells will never render machines obsolete for a variety of reasons.

For starters, there's the intimidation factor. We could tout the benefits of free weights until we're blue in the face and some of you still wouldn't go anywhere near them. Whether it's born out of a bad past experience or just an uncertainty as to the proper way to use them, some folks just flat out refuse to work with the heavy iron. Another popular reason for avoiding free weights is a fear of becoming "too bulky." For decades now there's been a belief that the mere act of touching a loaded barbell will somehow transform people into hulking behemoths almost overnight. Take it from two guys who've trained very hard for every ounce of muscle we've ever gained—it ain't that simple!

In addition to fear and preconceived notions, practicality

is also another good reason for using machines. Certain exercises like leg curls and calf raises, for instance, are awkward, if not downright impossible to do with free weights. Lat pulldowns are another great example. Not everyone is strong enough to do pullups, but that doesn't mean you shouldn't do anything to strengthen your lats. There's also a lot to be said for the increased training variety machines allow for. We flat out love free weights, but even a couple of hardened gym rats like us can admit that once in a while it's nice to change things up a little with some machines. It lets us hit our muscles from different angles and can often be just the ticket for breaking through training plateaus.

Last but not least, perhaps the biggest reason to accept machines is that they're not going anywhere anytime soon. Gym owners absolutely love them because they make an impressive statement to prospective members. No one's going to want to plunk down several hundred dollars for a membership if all they see is a bunch of free weights and assorted benches strewn all over the place. Now show these same people a gym full of state-of-the-art machines with upholstery that matches the gym's decor, and their eyes will practically glaze over. It's a fact of life—glitz sells.

THE USUAL SUSPECTS

Now that you have a better understanding and appreciation of their value, it's time we get you acquainted with some of the more common machines you'll find on the gym floor. We'll go over some of the more specialized machines by specific manufacturers in the chapters to follow.

MULTI-PURPOSE MACHINES

CABLE CROSSOVER STATIONS
(MUSCLES TRAINED: MULTIPLE)

As we mentioned in Chapter Nine, the cable crossover stations offer perhaps the most versatility of any machine in the gym. Thanks to both high and low pulleys, you can do a wide variety of upper-body, lower-body, and core exercises. And if the pulleys happen to be adjustable to a number of different levels, the list of exercises you can do grows exponentially. For a list of all the exercises you can do, along with pictures and complete descriptions, check Chapter Nine.

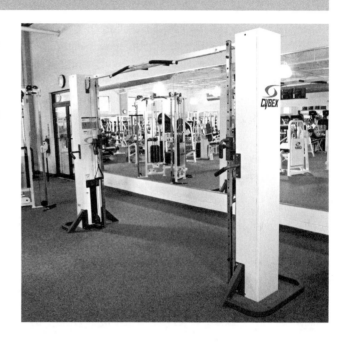

THE SMITH MACHINE
(MUSCLES TRAINED: MULTIPLE)

This is easily one of the most common and most controversial pieces of equipment you'll find on a gym floor. It's extremely versatile, allowing you to perform a seemingly endless array of exercises. Its built-in safety mechanism makes it possible to train without a spotter. Whether you're doing squats, bench presses, or virtually any other exercise you can think of, a simple turn of the wrists will set the weight down safely anywhere in the range of motion. These two features have undoubtedly made it one of the more popular machines in the gym.

The controversial downside is that because the bar is suspended by cables and follows a set, linear path, it makes for some unnatural movement patterns. Because our bodies move in a series of arcs, the linear motion the bar is forced to travel through can often cause unnecessary strain on certain key joints like the knees, shoulders, and lower back. Still, though, there are many who are willing to overlook potential orthopedic discomfort in the interest of safety. In the end, whether you choose to use it or not really comes down to a matter of personal preference.

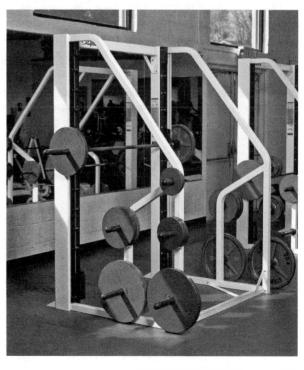

CORE MACHINES

CRUNCH MACHINE
(MUSCLES TRAINED: ABDOMINALS)

There are actually several versions of these put out by different manufacturers. No matter which brand you use, though, the basic premise is the same: Lie back, put up your feet, and grab the handles behind your head as you crunch your chest toward your pelvis. Be sure not to tug on the handles, though. Instead, focus on using your abdominals to lift yourself up.

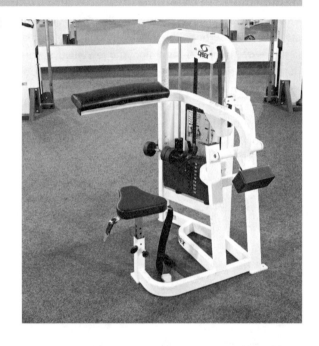

ROTARY TORSO
(MUSCLES TRAINED: ABDOMINALS, OBLIQUES)

Here's a classic example of a machine that looks like it's straight out of a medieval torture chamber. To begin, adjust the seat height so that the pad is right in the middle of your chest. Then, sit down and press your legs against the pads to hold them in place as you gently grab hold of the handles and use your core muscles to rotate as far as you can in one direction. Once you've finished all the reps on one side, a simple pull of a pin will set the weights in position to work your other side.

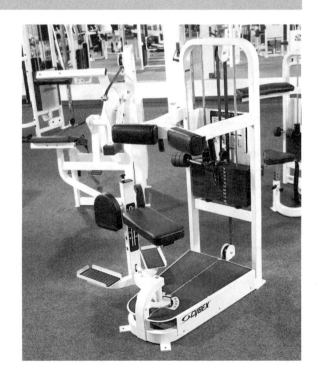

BACK EXTENSION

Mixed in among all the ab machines, you'll find this simple-looking device designed to target the lumbar extensors (lower back muscles). All you have to do is set the seat height so the pad rests on your upper back and then simply fold your arms across your chest as you extend backward until your shoulders are past your waist.

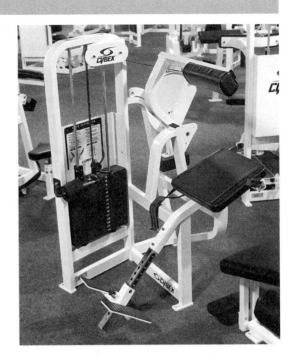

CHEST AND BACK EQUIPMENT

FLAT BENCH PRESS

(MUSCLES TRAINED: CHEST, SHOULDERS, TRICEPS)

There are usually two options here: a lying press, or an upright seated press. Both versions work the same muscles, but depending on which grip you use, you can slightly change the focus of the exercise. Most types will offer both a parallel and a horizontal grip. While the parallel grip will isolate the pectorals a little better, it can also be tough on the shoulder joint. Opting for the horizontal grip will still allow you to train your chest while easing strain on this oft-overworked joint.

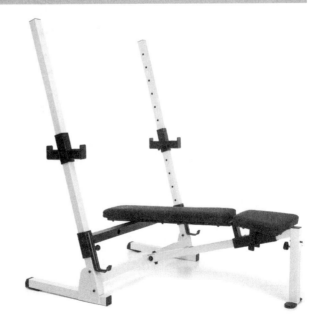

Whichever version of the machine or grip you choose, just make sure that the handles are lined up with your armpits. Working with the handles either too high or too low can throw even more stress on your shoulders. From there, you simply press the handles out until your arms are straight and then lower the weight back to within a couple of inches of your shoulders.

INCLINE PRESS

Unlike the flat bench press, the incline press usually only comes in one style—an angled bench with handles suspended above each shoulder. These too usually offer two types of grips and, regardless of which you choose, should be positioned in line with your armpits. Also be sure to keep your feet on the floor and avoid excessively arching your lower back while performing the lift. Press out until your arms are straight and then lower the weights back to the starting position.

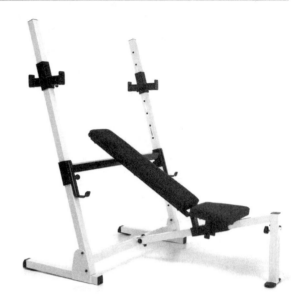

PEC DECK

Here's another machine that comes in two versions. While both are completely upright, one requires the arms to be bent 90 degrees, while the other keeps the arms almost completely straight. The difference between the two is that the straight-arm version is much harder due to the longer lever arm used to lift the weight. With both versions, however, range of motion is a real issue. Care should be taken not to allow the arms to drift back too far behind the torso. This holds especially true for the bentarm version, as the combination of the 90-degree bend and taking the arms back too far can be extremely stressful to the shoulder joint.

When setting the seat height, make sure your shoulders are in line with, or slightly above, the level of the handles. This will help ease strain on your shoulders and direct most of the work to your chest. With the bent-arm version, position your elbows against the pads and lightly grasp the handles. If you're using the straight handles, simply grab the handles. Then contract your chest to bring your arms across the front of your body before slowly returning the weight to the starting position.

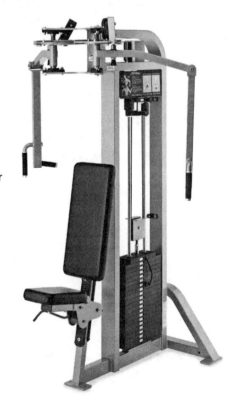

REVERSE FLY

Certain types of Pec Decks (aka fly machines) can also be used to work your upper back. This unique machine is one of them and allows you to switch from working your chest to your back with just the pull of a pin. To work your chest, simply follow the setup instructions described previously. To work your back, turn around so your chest is facing the pad and set the arm handles all the way around to the back by pulling the locking pin out and pivoting them on the flywheel. Then, set the seat height so your shoulders are in line with or slightly above the handles, as you take your choice of one of the two grips. The vertical handles will place more stress on the upper back, while the horizontal handles will increase the emphasis on the rear deltoids. Whichever handle you choose, make sure you work the weight back by pinching your shoulder blades together and keeping your elbow slightly bent.

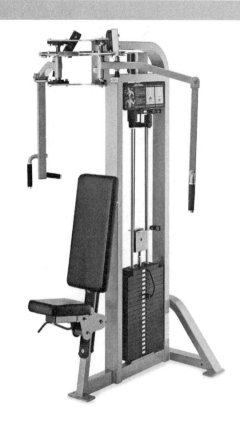

PULLOVER

Not as common nowadays, but still a machine that pops up from time to time, the pullover basically works all the large muscles of the upper body in one smooth movement. Begin by sitting on the machine with the seat height set so that your shoulder joint is lined up with the rotational axis of the machine. From there it's just a matter of grabbing the handles and driving with the elbows as you push the weight down until the crossbar reaches your waist. Pause, then return the weight to the starting position.

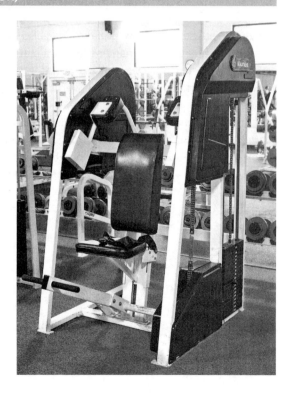

LAT PULLDOWN

Every gym in creation has one of these. With this one it's just a matter of selecting your handle (see "Get a Handle on This" on page 190) and pulling the weight down, hence the name. In setting the seat, be sure that you can fit your legs comfortably below the leg supports, but are still locked in tightly enough so you don't fly up with the weight. This can easily be done by pulling on the lock pin and adjusting the leg pads to hold you in place.

With most versions of the pulldown, regardless of what handle you choose you'll be pulling the weight down toward your chest in an effort to strengthen your lats and upper back. The lone exception is the behind-the-neck pulldown, where the bar is pulled to the base of your neck. This is an advanced maneuver, however, and is best left to those with good shoulder girdle flexibility and no history of shoulder problems.

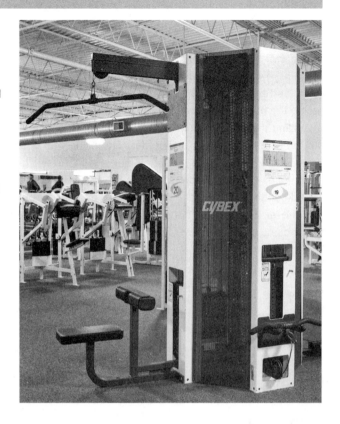

CABLE ROW

Like the lat pulldown, the low cable row can also be done with a wide variety of handles to direct more emphasis to certain muscles. However, since it involves a horizontal as opposed to a vertical pulling motion, it works the scapular retractors of the upper back more than the lat pulldown, which, as the name suggests, targets the lats more. After choosing your handle, simply sit up straight with your shoulders over your hips and use your upper back and arms to pull the weight back until it touches your torso. Avoid leaning back to get the weight back further, as this can place strain on the lower back.

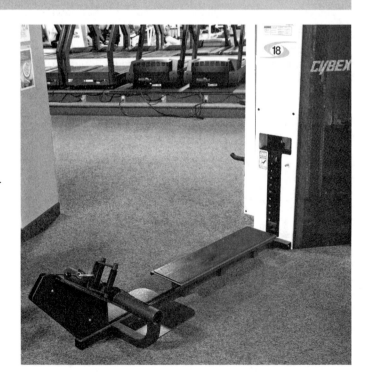

SEATED ROW

The difference between the cable row and the seated row is the latter usually offers a chest support so that you don't have to use your core muscles as much. Here, you simply sit down and set your chest against the support pad, making sure the seat height is set so the pad hits you in the middle of the chest. Then, take a choice of either the horizontal (more scapular retractor emphasis) or vertical (more lat emphasis) handles and pull the weights back toward your torso.

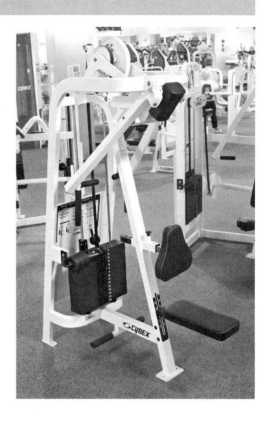

ASSISTED CHIN/DIP

(MUSCLES TRAINED: CHIN: UPPER BACK, BICEPS; DIP: CHEST, SHOULDERS, TRICEPS)

This towering machine allows those of you who aren't strong enough to perform these exercises with your own body weight to include them in your routine. It does, however, work a bit differently than other weight stack machines. Usually, the lower you place the pin on the stack, the more weight you get and the harder the exercise becomes to do. With this machine, the lower the pin, the more of an assist you get, making the exercise easier to do—so make sure you're aware of that going in. Once you set the weight, simply kneel on the support pad and either pull yourself up until your chin clears the bar for pullups, or grab the dipping handles and lower yourself until your upper arms are parallel to the floor and then press back up.

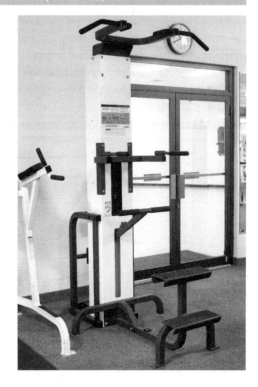

SHOULDER AND ARM MACHINES

SHOULDER PRESS
(MUSCLES TRAINED: SHOULDERS, TRICEPS)

Like the chest presses and rows, most shoulder press machines offer two handles—a horizontal and a vertical grip. Both work the shoulders and triceps, but the horizontal handles can often be more stressful on the shoulder joint. In setting the seat height, make sure your shoulders are slightly below the level of the handles and your feet are flat on the floor. You then simply press the weights up until your arms are straight and then lower them back down to the starting position.

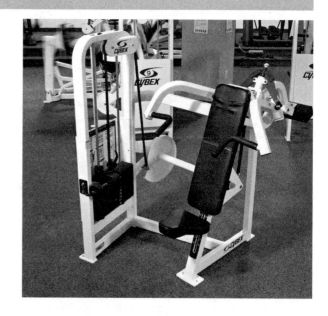

LATERAL RAISE
(MUSCLES TRAINED: SHOULDERS)

This machine simulates one of the more popular exercises in the gym—the dumbbell lateral raise. Set the seat height so that your shoulders are lined up with the rotational axis of the machine. Placing your elbows firmly against the pads, grasp the handles and use your shoulders to work the weights up until your arms are parallel to the floor. Be sure to keep your elbows on the pads and avoid leading with your wrists.

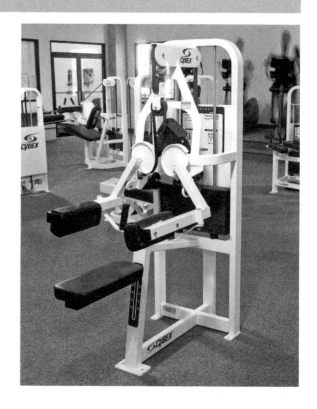

PREACHER CURL

(MUSCLES TRAINED: BICEPS, FOREARMS)

The unique angled bench makes this one a real killer for the biceps. Set the seat height so that when your arms are forward over the pad your elbows are in line with the rotational axis of the machine. Grab the handles and, keeping your back flat and feet firmly on the ground, curl the weight up toward your shoulders. When lowering the weight back down, be sure to keep a slight bend in your arms to avoid straining your elbows.

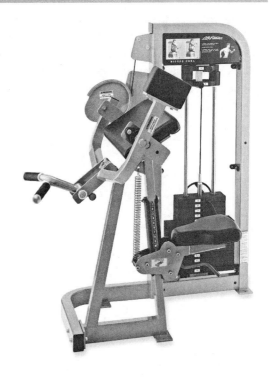

SEATED CURL

(MUSCLES TRAINED: BICEPS, FOREARMS)

A pretty straightforward machine, all this one asks you to do is sit down, grasp the handles, and start curling. As long as you make sure your elbows are lined up with the rotational axis, you're good to go. Whether you curl both arms together or take turns alternating, you're sure to get a killer pump.

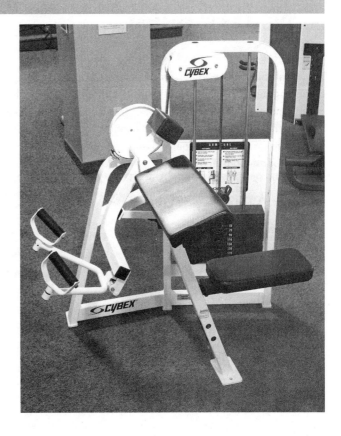

TRICEPS PUSHDOWN

(MUSCLES TRAINED: TRICEPS)

This one's right up there with the lat pulldown in terms of popularity. After choosing from any number of handles, simply keep your elbows tucked in toward your sides as you push the weight down from about chest level until your arms are completely straight. Some models even come with a back pad to lean against to steady yourself, although most simply hang off the side of a multipurpose cable station.

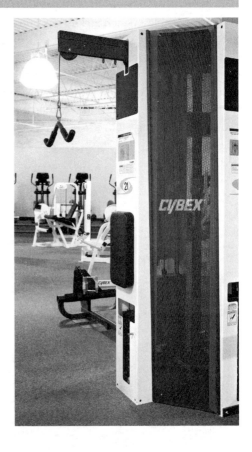

OVERHEAD EXTENSION

(MUSCLES TRAINED: TRICEPS)

The difference between this machine and the pushdown is that extending the arms overhead places the triceps under a stretch and directs more focus to the long head (located on the very back of your arm). With this machine, you set the seat height so that your shoulder blades are firmly against the pad and you can easily reach the handles behind your head (once again you will have a variety of handles to choose from). You then simply extend your arms while keeping your elbows as close to your head as possible.

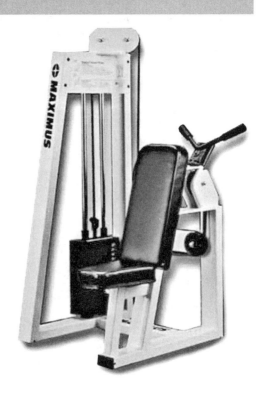

SEATED EXTENSION
(MUSCLES TRAINED: TRICEPS)

Yet another extension movement aimed at targeting the triceps. Position yourself in the machine so that your elbows are in line with the rotational axis of the machine. You'll also want to make sure that the seat height is set so that your shoulders are in line with your elbows. Next, keeping your upper arms firmly against the pad, grab the handles and extend your arms until they're straight. Pause, then return the weight to the starting position.

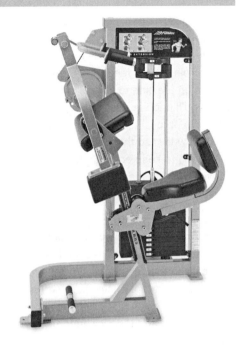

LOWER BODY MACHINES

LEG PRESS (45 DEGREE)
(MUSCLES TRAINED: QUADRICEPS, GLUTES, HAMSTRINGS)

Another extremely popular piece, this plate-loaded machine allows you to get many of the benefits of squats without supporting the weight on your back. To begin, adjust the seat height so that your torso is at an approximate 45-degree angle to the force plate. Next, place your feet up on the plate and press your lower back into the pad. From there it's just a matter of pushing the weight up and turning the handles to free it from the supports and then lowering it down until your thighs are parallel to the footplate. Pause slightly before pressing the weights back up.

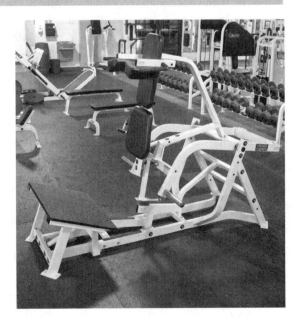

Depending on where you position your feet, it is possible to direct more stress to certain muscle groups. Placing your feet high on the plate and pushing through your heels, for instance, will target the glutes and hamstrings more. Placing them down lower and pressing more through the ball of your foot will increase the stress on the quadriceps. Whichever version you choose, be sure not to go too deep (past parallel) and never to bounce the weights out of the bottom position, as this can place the lower back and knees at risk.

LEG PRESS (HORIZONTAL)

(MUSCLES TRAINED: QUADRICEPS, GLUTES, HAMSTRINGS)

A slightly less intimidating yet equally effective way to work your legs, this machine uses a weight stack rather than free weights. Simply lie down with your back on the pad and place your feet on the force plate, then use the lock pin on the side to set the sled to the desired height. Since you'll once again be going to a point where your thighs are parallel to the ground, set the height just one level below that so that when in the parallel position, you're able to keep constant tension on the muscles involved. As with the 45-degree press, you can also change the way the exercise feels by altering your foot position.

Placing the feet higher will once again direct more focus to the hamstrings and glutes, while a lower foot position will increase the demand on your quadriceps. Once your seat height and foot position are set, simply push the weights up by extending your legs until they're straight but not locked and then lowering back down to the starting position.

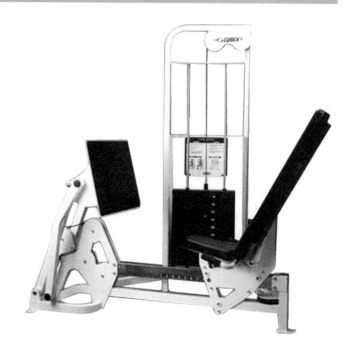

HACK SQUAT

(MUSCLES TRAINED: QUADRICEPS, GLUTES, HAMSTRINGS)

This one is very much like the 45-degree leg press, except that the more upright position directs more emphasis to the quadriceps regardless of foot position. Here you simply lie back on the pad and get your shoulders under the supports. Then it's just a matter of extending your legs and turning the handles on the sides of the sled to free the weight. Once there, you set your foot position and lower the weights down under control until reaching the parallel position and pushing back up. After completing the desired number of reps, simply turn the handles back in toward you and rest the weight down on the supports.

You can slightly alter the feel of the exercise by positioning your feet the same way you did on the leg press (high = more glutes and hams; low = even more quads), but the difference in feel won't be as great. The hack squat is pretty much a quadriceps builder.

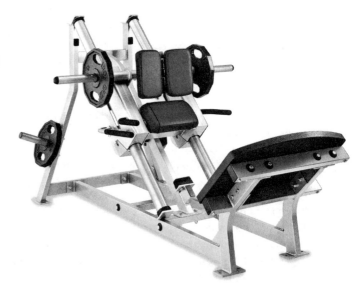

LEG EXTENSION

Another extremely popular machine, this one allows you to isolate your quadriceps like nothing else. Simply sit on the seat, making sure that your knees are lined up with the rotational axis of the machine and the leg pad is set just above the front of your ankle. Some types even allow you to control how far back you want the lever arm to start. We suggest starting with your feet just slightly behind your knees so that your quads are under a slight stretch. Setting the feet back too far under the seat can often result in unnecessary strain on the knees. From there all you do is extend your legs up until they're parallel to the floor.

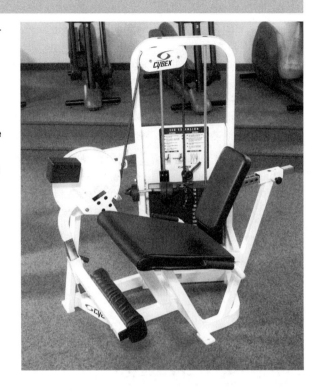

LEG CURL (SEATED)

(MUSCLES TRAINED: HAMSTRINGS, CALVES)

This antagonist to the leg extension helps you keep your leg development balanced by isolating the hamstrings, with a little help from the calves. Once again, sit on the seat, making sure your knees are lined up with the rotational axis of the machine. This time, though, the leg pad will be out in front of you, slightly higher than parallel to the ground. After adjusting the leg pad so that it hits you just above the Achilles tendons, on the lower part of your calves, lock yourself into place with the lap bar and curl the weights down until your feet get slightly behind your knees. Pause for a second and then return the weights to the starting position.

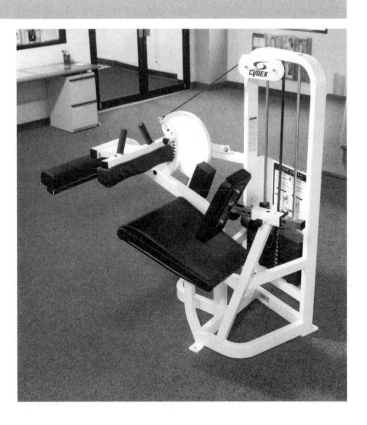

LEG CURL (LYING)

(MUSCLES TRAINED: HAMSTRINGS, CALVES)

The only major difference between this and the seated leg curl is that it's easier to cheat here by lifting your butt up off the pad. With this exercise you lie facedown on the pad, once again making sure your knees line up with the rotational axis of the machine. Just as with the seated leg curl, set the leg pad so that it rests on the lower calves, just above the Achilles tendons.

From there, hold on to the support handles as you use your hamstrings and calves to bring the weight up as close to your butt as possible. Be sure to avoid using momentum by flinging the weight up, and keep your hips pressed down into the pad.

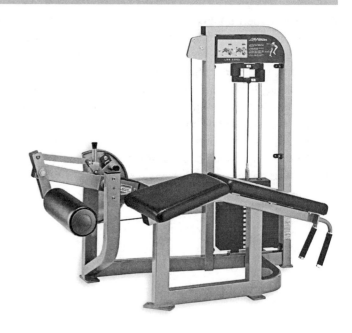

STANDING CALF RAISE

(MUSCLES TRAINED: CALVES—SPECIFICALLY THE GASTROCNEMIUS)

They don't get much simpler than this one. Simply step underneath the shoulder supports and place the balls of your feet on the calf block. In doing so, make sure the height is set so that it's not too difficult to get under and your calves are getting a good stretch in the standing position. Begin by straightening your legs and dropping your heels below the level of the block. Once there, pause and then press back up until your heels are well past the block and you're standing on the balls of your feet. Pause, lower, and repeat.

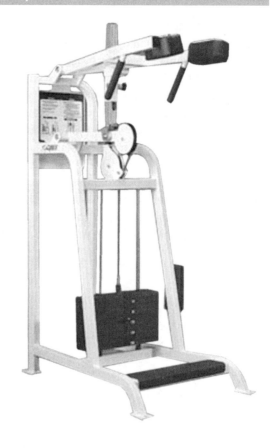

SEATED CALF

This calf raise allows you to direct more of the stress to the soleus—the muscle located deep below the gastrocnemius that is visible along the sides of your calves. Sit down and place your knees under the pads, once again using the lock pin to ensure that in doing so, your calves are placed under a stretch in the bottom position. After selecting your weight, keep your torso straight and tall as you push with the balls of your feet until your heels come up past the block. Pause, lower, and repeat.

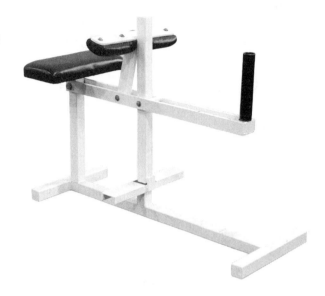

ABDUCTOR

Certainly not among the best-designed machines in the gym, this piece, along with the Adductor, looks more like something you'd find in a gynecological office. That being said, they do get the job the done. After selecting your weight, sit down and position your legs inside the pads—whether your gym offers the bent leg or straight leg version, you'll find that the pads are located right at the outside of the knees. From there all you have to do is use your outer thighs to push the weight out as far as possible. Pause for a second, and then return the weight to the starting position.

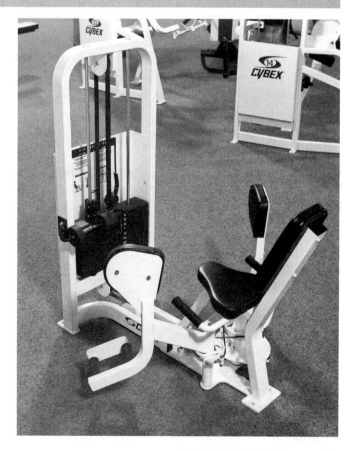

ADDUCTOR

(MUSCLES TRAINED: INNER THIGHS)

Here you start in the opposite position as you did with the abductor—with your legs spread out to the sides. Use the lock pin to adjust the range of motion so you're not beginning in too much of a stretch position. Then place your knees behind the pads and sit up straight as you bring your legs together. Pause for a second, and then return the weight to the starting position.

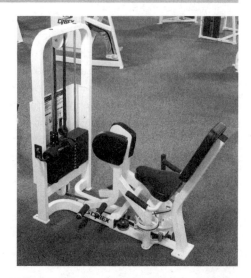

GET A HANDLE ON THIS

The following bars can be attached to either the lat pulldown/low cable row or triceps pushdown stations to vary which muscles get utilized more.

LAT/CABLE ROW

- Angled Bar: The most widely used, this bar allows you to use a variety of grips, which will affect your back development in different ways:
  - Supinated grip (palms facing you), shoulder-width apart: More lat and biceps involvement.
  - Pronated grip (palms facing away from you), shoulder-width apart: More upper back and lats.
  - Pronated grip (hands on the bent part of the bar): Increases lat emphasis.
- Neutral-Grip Straight Bar: Increased range of motion/easier on shoulders.
- Triangular Bar: Slightly decreases range of motion/allows heavier loads to be used.
- Rope: Increases emphasis on grip strength/really targets rear delts when pulled to face instead of chest on both exercises.
- Stirrup Handle: Even greater range of motion than neutral grip handle.
- Unilateral Stirrup Handle: Allows you to work unilaterally (one side at a time).

TRICEPS

- V Bar: More comfortable for wrists than straight bar.
- E-Z Bar: Allows for even greater wrist comfort, as well as the use of both close and wider hand positions.
- Rope: Increases grip strength and allows for more intense contraction by pulling apart at the end of each rep/requires slightly lighter loads to be used.
- Small Straight Bar: Manageable, but often uncomfortable to wrists.
- Rotating Straight Bar: More comfortable for wrists.
- Unilateral Stirrup Handle: Allows you to train unilaterally and with different hand positions (such as palms facing up) for added variety.

CHAPTER THIRTEEN

PUT THE FUNCTION INTO FITNESS

New Ways to Get In the Best Shape of Your Life!

WITHOUT QUESTION, ONE OF THE BIGGEST changes to the gym landscape over the past decade or so is the advent of what's come to be known as "functional training." Rather than isolating specific body parts with various free weight and machine-based exercises á la Arnold Schwarzenegger, more and more folks these days are opting for moves that work more muscles in less time. Using a wide array of what are more often than not decidedly low-tech tools, today's gym rats are twisting, slamming, bending, and heaving their way to the bodies of their dreams. They're pushing weighted sleds across turf, hoisting what look like bowling balls with handles up over their heads, and performing various gyrations with long pieces of dock rope—all in their quest to burn fat and build muscle. And you know what? They're on to something here because the approach definitely works!

Not only are they becoming leaner and fitter than ever, but those who favor this more functional approach to fitness tend to see their hard work carry over into other aspects of their lives. Whereas before, a lean sculpted body didn't necessarily mean you'd be any better at sports or able to meet the sudden challenges of daily life, now just the opposite is true. Whether it means jumping higher and running faster in your regular pickup game or being better able to scoop up your toddler and carry him

up a flight of stairs to bed, the perks of training your body as a functional unit are undeniable. Not to mention the fact that it's a whole lot of fun to boot!

Just in case any of this is news to you or you've seen some of the functional training tools but are not quite sure how to use them, fear not because you've come to the right place! In this chapter we break down the multitude of functional training gadgets and gizmos you now see in the gym on a regular basis, but just may not know how to use. Not only will we show you how to get the most out of them, but we'll even show you how you put these various tools together to give you some of the most challenging, yet fun workouts that you've ever tried! (See the chapter Sample Workouts and Training Logs).

So let's get right down to work and meet some of the featured players.

POT, MEET KETTLE: BANISH BELLY FAT WITH THIS INCREDIBLY VERSATILE TOOL!

Granted, they may look a little weird and even somewhat intimidating, but trust us when we tell you that kettlebells can give you one of the best workouts imaginable. By bringing together elements of cardio, strength training, and flexibility (quite often in the same exercise), they'll give you a whole new opinion of what it means to pump iron! Not only are they great for getting stronger and challenging your muscles and connective tissues in ways that traditional free weights can't, but some of the exercises you can do with them will take your fat loss efforts to new heights. And if it's better mobility you're after, then look no farther because training with kettlebells will challenge your range of motion in ways you never thought possible. Whether it's the traditional kettlebell swing that will get your heart rate revving like crazy, the demanding windmill exercise that will challenge the limits of your flexibility, or the torturous "bottom up" press for wrist and shoulder stability, kettlebells truly offer something for everyone.

What makes kettlebells so uniquely versatile is their design. That "cannonball with a handle" look didn't happen by accident. Kettlebells are designed that way because having the handle positioned where it is extends the weight's center of mass beyond the hand. This makes them perfect for ballistic and swinging movements that work lots of muscles simultaneously and as a result burn tons of calories. They're also a great way to challenge stabilizing muscles in the upper body (not to mention the core) on various types of pressing movements. Plus, the handle also makes for a great way to challenge the body in ways that traditional free weights simply can't—like rapidly switching a swinging weight from one hand to the other during certain exercises, or seamlessly passing the weight between your legs or around your torso during others. Who knew such a relatively simple looking device could be so complex?

It's also worth mentioning that kettlebells just flat out look cool! It's hard not to feel like a badass when you're repeatedly swinging one of these behemoths up and down, or hoisting it over your head with your fist pumped into the air like some sort of conquering warrior. And although that may not be the deciding factor when determining what type of equipment to use in the gym, it certainly doesn't hurt. Because whether you're trying to intimidate the guy who stole your favorite locker or impress that little hottie who's always checking you out while she uses the StairMaster, training with kettlebells makes you pretty hard to miss.

KETTLEBELL TWO-ARM SWING

(MUSCLES TRAINED: GLUTES, HAMSTRINGS, SPINAL ERECTORS, CORE, UPPER BACK, SHOULDERS)

Place a kettlebell on the floor about a foot in front of you. With a shoulder-width stance, hinge at the waist and with your arms extended, pick up the kettlebell, maintaining a rigid torso. Begin by swinging the kettlebell underneath your legs, similar to a center hiking a ball to the quarterback. Next, use your hips to rapidly reverse the motion and swing the weight forward, as you come out of the hip hinge to an upright stance with the kettlebell out in front of you at shoulder's height. Immediately swing the weight back down between the legs by hinging at the hips until you've completed 15 to 20 repetitions.

Training tip: Keep just a slight bend in the knees and rigid spine to execute a true hip hinge and avoid any rounding of the lower back.

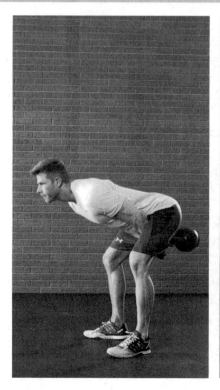
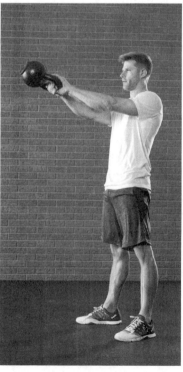

KETTLEBELL ONE-ARM SWING

(MUSCLES TRAINED: GLUTES, HAMSTRINGS, SPINAL ERECTORS, CORE, UPPER BACK, SHOULDERS)

A variation of the two-arm swing. The same muscles are trained and the execution is similar to the two-armed version, just using a little less weight.

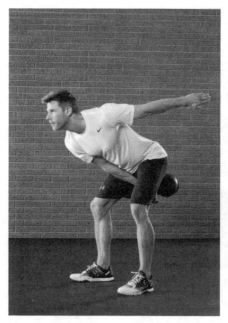
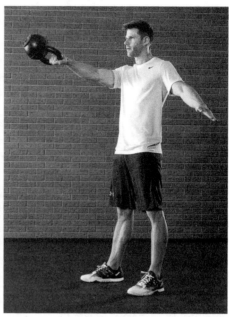

KETTLEBELL WINDMILL

(MUSCLES TRAINED: CORE, LATS, SHOULDERS, SPINAL ERECTORS, HAMSTRINGS, GLUTES)

Stand holding a kettlebell in your right hand and adopt a shoulder-width stance with your feet rotated about 45 degrees to the left. With the kettlebell positioned in front of your shoulder, press it up overhead. Hold it there, with the weight resting on the back side of your forearm, keeping your knees slightly bent, and drive your hips out to the right and reach your left hand down toward the inside of your left foot. In the bottom position, your arms should be vertically stacked with your torso approximately parallel to the ground. Pause there for a second, then keep your arm straight as you return to the standing position. Repeat for 6 to 10 reps per side.

Training tip: Stay rigid in the torso and keep the shoulder locked in place to stabilize the load in the bent-over position. Avoid allowing the elbow to bend.

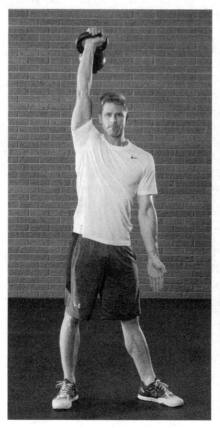
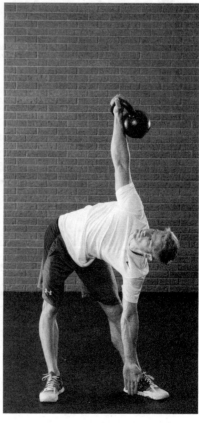

KETTLEBELL TURKISH GET-UP

(MUSCLES TRAINED: GLUTES, HAMSTRINGS, QUADS, CORE, SHOULDERS, UPPER BACK)

Begin by lying on your back holding a kettlebell with your right arm outstretched vertically over your chest. With your right knee bent and foot flat on the floor and your left leg straight, initiate a diagonal situp toward your left, making sure to keep your right arm straight. Continue holding the weight vertical with your right arm, as you prop up onto your left forearm and hand in a continuation of the situp. Next, simultaneously push into the ground with your left hand and right foot as you bridge your hips off the ground. From this position, sweep your left leg under your body until your left knee makes contact with the ground, then shift your weight to your right leg while you stand up, continuing to hold the weight vertically the entire time. Reverse the steps and lie back down on the ground. Repeat for 5 to 8 reps per side.

Training tip: Avoid using momentum to initiate the situp and be sure to keep the arm holding the kettlebell vertical at all times.

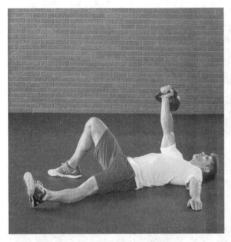
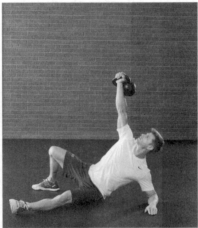
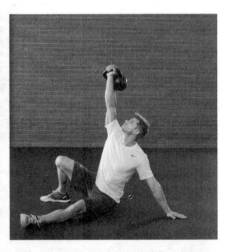

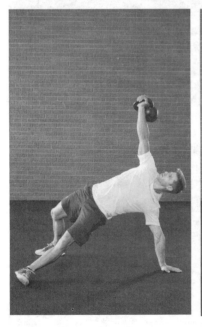
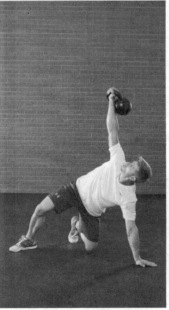
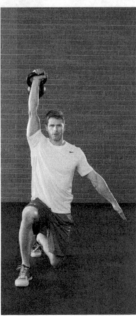
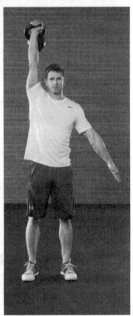

KETTLEBELL GOBLET SQUAT

(MUSCLES TRAINED: GLUTES, HAMSTRINGS, QUADS, CORE, BICEPS, UPPER BACK)

Stand holding a kettlebell by the handle directly in front of your chest. With a stance slightly wider than shoulder width, keep a rigid torso as you push your hips back and descend into a squat. Once the tops of your thighs are parallel to the ground and your elbows are just inside your knees, pause for a second before pressing back up to the starting position. Repeat until you've completed 10 to 12 reps.

Training tip: Keep the kettlebell close to your chest throughout the movement and focus on "tearing the floor open" with your feet to activate your glutes.

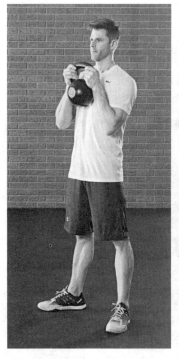 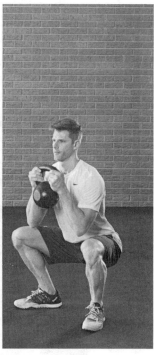

KETTLEBELL REVERSE LUNGE AND PRESS

(MUSCLES TRAINED: GLUTES, HAMSTRINGS, QUADS, CORE, SHOULDERS, TRICEPS)

Stand holding a kettlebell in the racked position with your hand just in front of your shoulder. Begin by striding back into a reverse lunge with the leg on the same side as the arm holding the weight. Simultaneously press the weight overhead until you end up with your back knee just a couple of inches from the ground and your arm holding the weight fully extended. Pause for a second, then return to the starting position as you lower the weight. Repeat for 8 to 10 reps per side.

Training tip: Keep your core lightly braced and avoid excessively arching your lower back to get the weight up overhead.

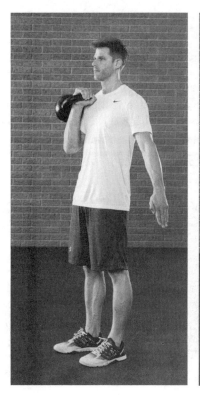 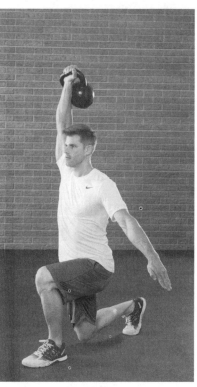

KETTLEBELL SINGLE-ARM SNATCH

(MUSCLES TRAINED: GLUTES, HAMSTRINGS, QUADS, UPPER BACK, CORE)

Begin holding a kettlebell by its handle in front of the middle of your body. Start by dipping into a quick quarter squat and then rapidly reversing the movement by extending your ankles, knees, and hips. As you do this, start shrugging the weight up toward your chest and once there, snatch it up overhead to a straight arm as you catch the weight behind your forearm, in that same quarter-squat position. Lower the weight back down and repeat for 3 to 6 reps per side.

Training tip: Avoid yanking the weight with your arm—let the extension of the lower body joints and shrugging movement create the power to hoist the weight overhead.

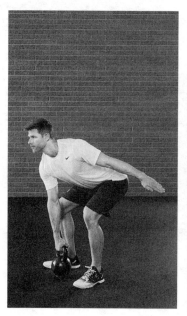 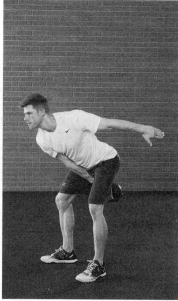 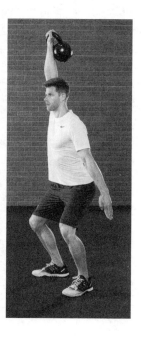

KETTLEBELL RENEGADE ROW

(MUSCLES TRAINED: CORE, UPPER BACK, BICEPS)

Position two kettlebells on the ground and place your hands on top of the handles as you assume a pushup position. With your feet approximately shoulder-width apart, brace your core and initiate a rowing movement with one arm, as you press the other kettlebell into the floor to create more stability in the shoulder. Once your elbow is just past your torso, pause for a second and then lower the weight back down and switch sides. Repeat until you've done 6 to 8 reps per side.

Training tip: Keep your core braced and hips balanced—avoid allowing them to rock from side to side when rowing the weights.

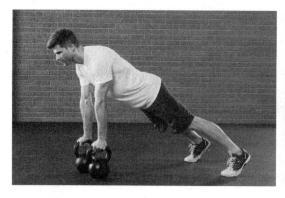 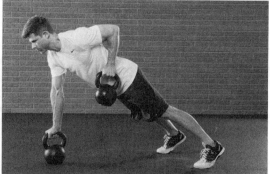

KETTLEBELL BOTTOM UP PRESS

From a half-high kneeling position, grab hold of a kettlebell and lift it up in front of your shoulder so that the flat underside of the bell faces the ceiling. Brace your core and press the weight overhead, making sure not to allow the weight to change position. Your forearms and all of the stabilizing muscles around the shoulder will be working extremely hard here. Pause for a second at the top and then lower and repeat until you've completed 8 to 10 reps per side.

Training tip: Go a little lighter than you would for a regular dumbbell press to ensure you can properly stabilize the weight.

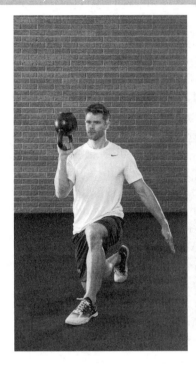
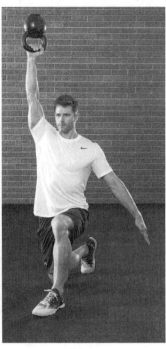

KETTLEBELL HALO

Stand holding a kettlebell by the handle directly in front of your chest. Begin by taking the weight up and over your head by lifting one elbow up toward the ceiling—similar to the act of putting on a jacket. Continue the movement all the way around your head until you've brought it back to the starting position. Repeat to the opposite side and continue until you've done 6 to 8 times per side. This one requires good range of motion in the shoulders.

Training tip: Keep your ribcage down to avoid hyperextending your lower back to complete the range of motion.

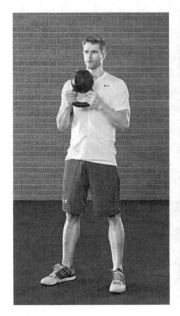
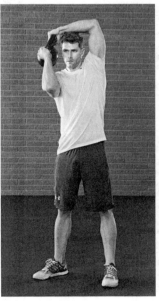
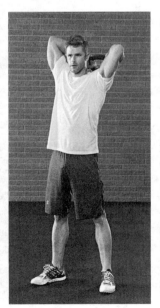
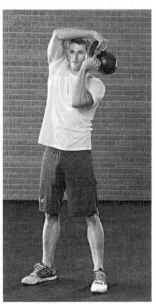

NO DAY AT THE BEACH: DISCOVER THE POWER OF SANDBAG TRAINING!

When you were a little kid, playing with sand was a fun, relaxing pastime. Now that you're an adult who's trying to keep fit, sand takes on an entirely different meaning in your life. Sure, you know that running in sand is pretty tough (why else would Apollo make Rocky do it?), but did you know that lifting sand is also one hell of a workout? Not the individual grains—that would just be tedious and make a huge mess. However, filling sturdy sacks with sand that also have strategically placed handles can take one of your favorite childhood playthings and turn it into the bane of your fitness existence. That's because training with sandbags is a relatively inexpensive, incredibly time-efficient way to burn fat, build muscle, and get in fantastic cardiovascular shape. What makes such a seemingly simplistic tool so great, you ask? Let's "dig" a little deeper to find out. (You see what we did there?)

Sandbag training is great for a variety of reasons. First and foremost it enables you to build "real world" strength. Unlike a barbell that may be perfectly positioned in a squat rack for you to just walk up and start curling (on a side note: you should never do this! They're called squat racks and power cages for a reason. And no part of that reason involves weenies who are too lazy to use the premade barbells for their sacred curls—but we digress), sandbags have to be lifted off the floor in order for you to get them into the proper position. This involves an incredible amount of grip, core, and leg and upper body strength. It also mimics the same way we often have to pick things up in real life. No convenient handles, no symmetrical load—just weight, often in inconvenient positions that we have to pick up and move.

Secondly, sandbag training makes it easy for you not only to work multiple muscle groups, in multiple ranges of motion at the same time, but also to switch easily from one exercise to the next, taking a regular strength training workout and turning it into a fat-burning cardio bonanza! So, if you're looking to challenge your grip and core, recruit more motor units, and become more athletic or just take your workout to new heights in general, we wholeheartedly recommend you give sandbag training a try.

SANDBAG LUNGE WITH ROTATION

(MUSCLES TRAINED: CORE, GLUTES, HAMSTRINGS, QUADS, SHOULDERS)

Stand holding a sandbag by the two inner handles in the rack position in front of your chest. Begin by striding into a lunge with your right leg, bending both knees until they're approximately at 90 degree angles. In the bottom position the back knee should only be a couple inches off the ground. As you stride into the lunge, allow your arms to straighten as they swing the sandbag down and outside of your right knee. Keep your torso erect and use your core to stop the momentum of the bag when it gets outside your right hip. Then immediately press back up to the standing position as you return the sandbag to the rack position in front of your chest. Repeat until you've done 6 to 8 total reps and then repeat on the left side.

Training tip: Avoid allowing the weight to rotate your torso—remain upright at all times.

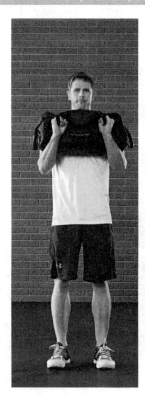 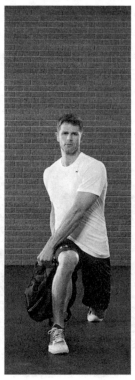 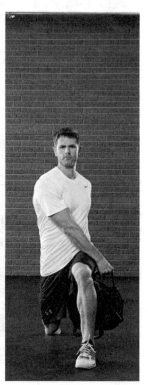

SANDBAG ZERCHER SQUAT

(MUSCLES TRAINED: QUADS, HAMSTRINGS, GLUTES, UPPER BACK, CORE, BICEPS)

Stand holding a sandbag up in front or your chest with your arms bent at 90 degrees and the weight resting in the crook of your elbows. Maintain a nice upright torso as you lower your hips into a squat until your thighs are parallel to the ground. Pause there for a second, then press back up to the start position. Repeat for 8 to 10 reps.

Training tip: Inhale as you descend with the weight to help keep the torso rigid and don't exhale until you're more than halfway back up.

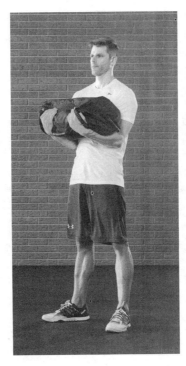
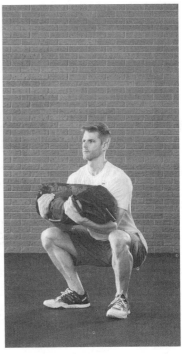

SANDBAG FRONT-LOADED GOOD MORNING

(MUSCLES TRAINED: HAMSTRINGS, GLUTES, SPINAL ERECTORS, CORE, BICEPS, UPPER BACK)

Stand with your feet shoulder-width apart, holding the sandbag in the Zercher Squat standing position against your chest. With a slight bend in your knees, execute a hip hinge by driving your hips back as you maintain a rigid torso and lean forward at the waist. When your shoulders are even with your hips and your torso is parallel to the ground, pause for a second before pressing your heels firmly into the ground and standing back up. Continue until you've completed 6 to 10 reps.

Training tip: Maintain a rigid spine and slight knee bend to keep strain off the lower back.

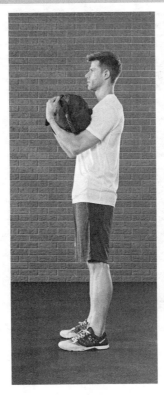
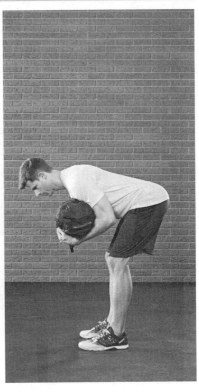

SANDBAG ROMANIAN DEADLIFT

(MUSCLES TRAINED: HAMSTRINGS, GLUTES, CORE, SPINAL ERECTORS, UPPER BACK)

Stand with your feet shoulder-width apart and hold a sandbag by the side handles in front of your hips. Begin by hinging at the hips and leaning your torso over toward the ground. Maintain a slight bend at the knees, keep your shoulders packed and your torso rigid as you drive your hips back, and lean over until your torso is approximately parallel to the ground. Pause for a second and then drive back up through your heels to the start position. Repeat until you've completed 6 to 10 reps.

Training tip: Avoid allowing the weight to pull your shoulder blades apart as you lean forward. Keep your shoulder blades packed together.

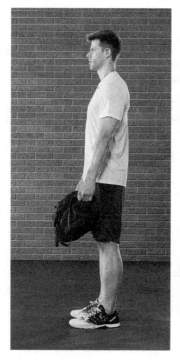 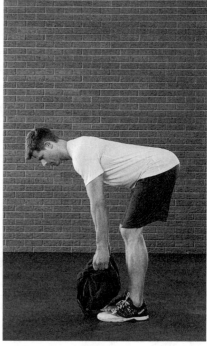

SANDBAG ALTERNATING OVERHEAD PRESS

(MUSCLES TRAINED: SHOULDERS, TRICEPS, CORE)

Stand with your feet shoulder-width apart and knees slightly bent. Begin by holding a sandbag just over one shoulder with a neutral grip (palms facing each other). Brace your core as you press the bag up overhead and lower down until it's positioned just over your opposite shoulder. Continue repeating in this fashion until you've completed 6 to 8 reps per side.

Training tip: Avoid locking your knees and flaring your ribcage up and out to reduce strain on the lower back as you press.

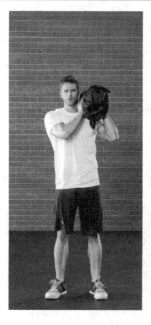 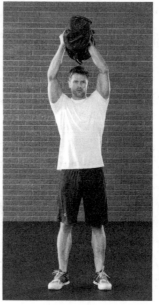 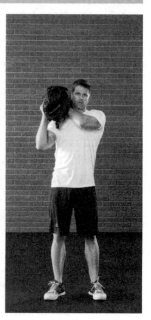

SANDBAG DUCK UNDER SQUAT

(MUSCLES TRAINED: QUADS, GLUTES, HAMSTRINGS, GROIN, UPPER BACK, BICEPS)

Basically a moving variation of the Zercher Squat, this challenging version taxes the groin and helps improve hip mobility by adding in a lateral component. Adopt the same setup as you would for a regular Zercher Squat, with your feet a little bit closer together. Next, stride out to the left side a bit as you simultaneously drop into a squat and shift your weight toward your right leg. Press up using your left leg primarily and once again bring your feet together. Repeat to the right side by striding out to the right. Continue alternating sides until you've completed 6 to 8 reps per side.

Training tip: Go lighter than you would on a regular Zercher Squat due to the extra movement required.

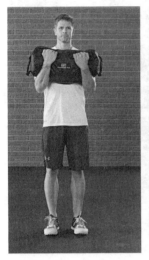 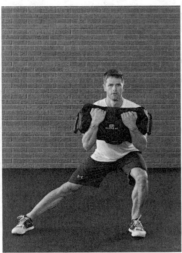 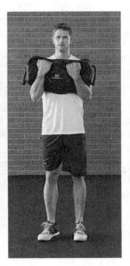 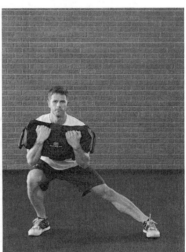

SANDBAG PLANK WITH ALTERNATING PULL THROUGH

(MUSCLES TRAINED: CORE, SHOULDERS, TRICEPS, BICEPS, LATS, HIP FLEXORS)

Get into a pushup position with a sandbag placed at arm's reach in front of you. With your feet about shoulder-width apart, brace your core and without losing balance, reach forward with one arm to grab hold of the sandbag. Pull it until it's right under your chest, then maintain a nice flat back as you crawl backward a few steps until the sandbag is once again at arm's reach in front of you; repeat with the other arm. Continue for a specified distance, or until you've done 6 to 10 reps per side.

Training tip: Keep your core braced to take strain off the lower back when holding the plank position.

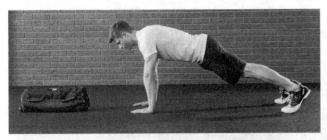 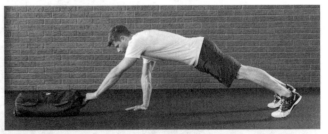

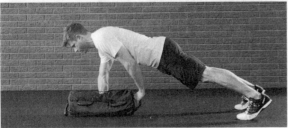 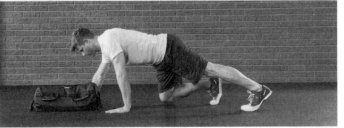

SANDBAG SHOVELING

(MUSCLES TRAINED: GLUTES, HAMSTRINGS, CORE)

Stand with your feet shoulder-width apart and torso erect, and hold a sandbag by the inner handles. Start the bag just outside of your left knee so that your torso is slightly rotated to the left and your right hip is rotated toward your left side. Next, use your hips and core to swing the sandbag over to your opposite side, straightening out your left leg and pivoting your right as you do so. Continue in this manner, initiating the movement with the hips and core until you've done 10 to 15 reps per side.

Training tip: Maintaining an upright torso and hinge from the hips. Avoid rounding the back at any point.

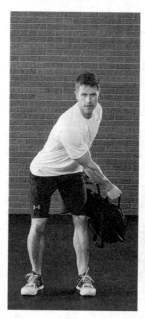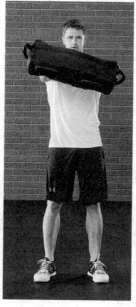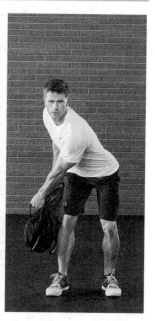

SANDBAG BENT-OVER ROW

(MUSCLES TRAINED: UPPER BACK, BICEPS, SPINAL ERECTORS, HAMSTRINGS, GLUTES, QUADS, CORE)

Stand holding a sandbag by the end handles horizontally across the front of your hips. Begin by bracing your core and leaning forward at the waist until your torso is just short of parallel to the ground with your arms fully extended toward the ground. Maintaining a slight bend in your knees and a rigid spine, pinch your shoulder blades together to lead the pull as you row the weight up to your waist. Pause there for a second, then lower and repeat for 10 to 12 reps.

Training tip: Emphasize using the upper back to lead the pull by bringing the shoulder blades together and not just yanking with your arms.

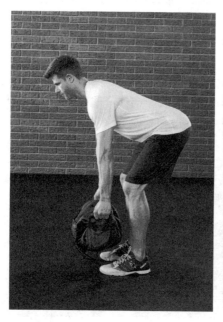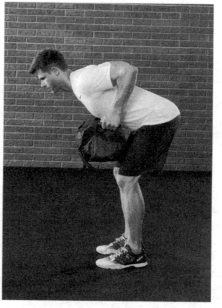

ON THE PROWL: THE BENEFITS OF TRAINING WITH PROWLER SLEDS

It used to be that pushing weighted sleds was something reserved just for football players. How times have changed! These days, you'd be hard-pressed to walk into your local gym and not see someone doing some variation of a sled push—and with good reason! If you're looking for one of the toughest, most grueling exercises you can possibly do in a gym, prowler pushes would be right up at the top of the list. Pushing one of these bad boys loaded up with plates not only looks megacool, but it also will give your legs, lungs, and upper back one hell of a serious burn. And that's just if you push it, mind you; there are actually lots of different ways you can use this particular torture device/piece of gym equipment. Besides being pushed, prowlers can be towed, rowed, pressed, and even used to thrash your core. Looking for a tough finisher to top off a great workout? Try some heavy prowler pushes! Tired of regular rowing exercises to strengthen your back and want to try something different? Try some prowler rows! If you're really feeling ambitious, you could even try some prowler sprints! Talk about an ass kicker!

Regardless of how you use it, though, the prowler is guaranteed to become that one piece of gym equipment you love to hate. You know the type: The one you dread doing all day before you even get to the gym, but just wouldn't feel right about skipping out on. In fact, once you get used to it (well, at least as used to nearly vomiting as a person can get), you'll wonder how you ever got by without it. Whether you use it as a strength builder, as a conditioning tool, or just as a way to breathe some much-needed life into your workouts, the prowler sled is pretty hard to beat. So, let's go ahead and take a look at some of its many uses.

PROWLER PUSH

(MUSCLES TRAINED: QUADS, CALVES, GLUTES, HAMSTRINGS, CORE, UPPER BACK)

Stand behind a prowler sled and place your hands a few inches down on the upright poles. Next, straighten your arms and get your feet placed behind you so that you're getting a good lean into the sled. Keep your arms straight and your core braced as you drive with your legs and push the sled for a specified distance. Depending on how much weight is on it and how much room you have, this usually ends up being about 20 to 40 yards. Once you've pushed the sled for the distance you've chosen, you can either push it right back to the starting point (for shorter distances), or take a quick break before bringing it back (longer distances).

Training tip: Brace your core to maintain a rigid torso.

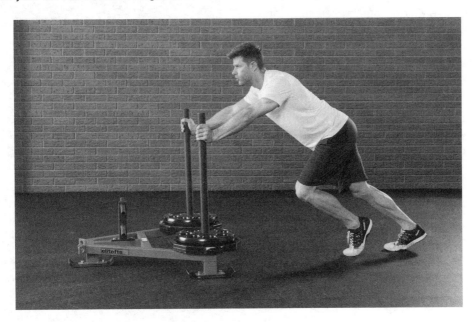

PROWLER DRAG

Attach a battle rope or a suspension trainer to a prowler sled and grab hold of the handles. Next, you have the choice of either facing the sled and doing a backward drag (more quads), or turning your back on it and dragging it behind you (more glutes and hamstrings). Drag the sled for the predetermined distance, making a conscious effort to push into the ground and use your lower body. You can then either drag it right back or take a short break (60 to 90 seconds) before doing so.

Training tip: Even though you're "pulling," or dragging the sled, make sure the bulk of your effort is coming from driving with your legs.

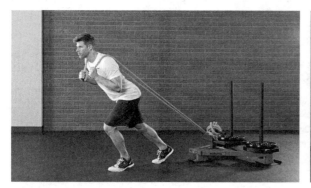 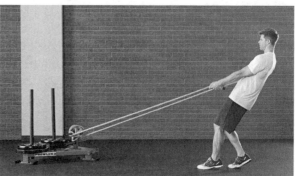

PROWLER CROSSOVER DRAG

Stand aside a prowler sled with a battle rope or suspension trainer attached to it. Grab hold of the handle with one arm and lean your body away from the sled to create the proper pushing angle into the ground. With both feet facing straight ahead, begin by taking the leg closest to the sled and striding across your body in a crossover motion, dropping into a 90-degree squat with that same leg. Leaning heavily away from the sled, push into the ground with that lead leg and press back up to an angled standing position (don't lose your lean away from the sled). Continue in this manner until you've covered the predetermined distance and repeat back the other way.

Training tip: Keep the toes pointed straight ahead throughout the movement and avoid turning them toward the direction you're stepping in with the crossover leg.

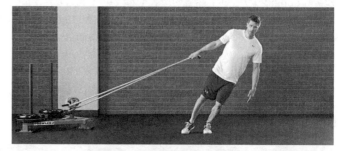

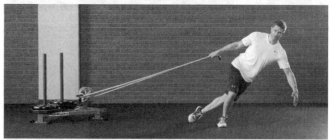

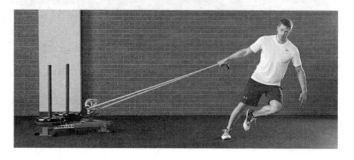

PROWLER TRAVELING PRESS

Stand behind a prowler sled and place your hands a few inches down on the upright poles. Next, get into a split stance so that your elbows are bent slightly more than 90 degrees and you have a good forward lean so that your nose is positioned over the toes of your lead foot. Brace your core and push the sled away until both arms are straight. Then bring the opposite leg forward and repeat the pressing moment for the desired number of reps.

Training tip: Keep your core braced to avoid hyperextending the lower back when pressing the sled forward.

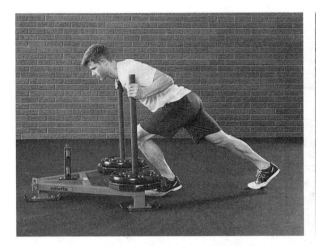 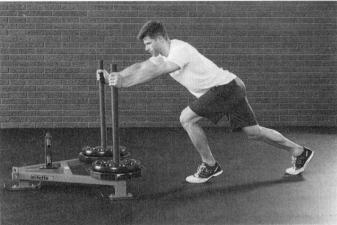

PROWLER TRAVELING ROW

Attach a battle rope or suspension trainer to a prowler sled and stand facing the sled. With your arms fully extended, sit back into a squat position with your hips back and chest up. Next, bring your shoulder blades together and down to initiate the movement and pull the sled toward your feet, until your arms are just past your torso. Then stand up and take a few steps back until your arms are straight again and repeat for the desired number of reps.

Training tip: Keep your chest up as you initiate the pull with your upper back; avoid allowing it to cave in.

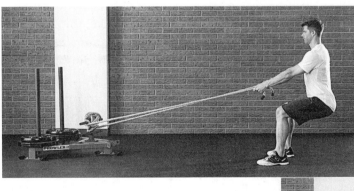

PROWLER SPRINT

(MUSCLES TRAINED: QUADS, HAMSTRINGS, GLUTES, CALVES, CORE, UPPER BACK)

Stand behind a prowler sled and place your hands a few inches down on the upright poles. Next, get into a ready sprint position by placing your feet behind you to get a good lean and bend both legs by crouching down a bit. Once you're ready, keep your arms straight and your torso braced as you fire into a sprint for a specified distance (15 to 30 yards). Rest for 15 to 30 seconds and repeat for 6 to 8 repetitions.

Training tip: Focus on putting force into the ground by extending the back leg and driving the lead knee forward.

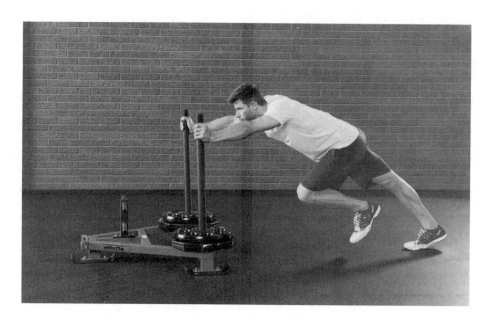

FIT TO BE TIED: BEHOLD THE POWER OF BATTLE ROPES

As you can see, thus far, most of the equipment featured in this functional training chapter is decidedly pretty low-tech. After all, no one is going to confuse kettelbells, sandbags, or a prowler sled with some of the fancy machines you see littering the floor of most commercial gyms. However, if you think the items we've featured to this point have been somewhat primitive, get ready to have your mind blown. This next piece is probably the most simplistic of the lot, but that doesn't stop it from packing one hell of a punch! We're talking about battle ropes—aka those oversize pieces of dock rope you often see sitting off in the corner tethered to a squat rack. They may not look intimidating, but pick up the ends and start moving them around a bit, and before too long they'll have you wishing you never had. Available in a variety of

lengths and thicknesses, these seemingly harmless pieces of twine will give you the cardio workout of your life.

Whether you slam them, swirl them, shimmy them, or climb on them (yes, they can be used for that, too), you're bound to get your heart pounding like never before. They'll also tax your wind and your grip and at some point will have you convinced that your shoulders and arms are actually on fire! They're also a great core workout, too, as moving the ropes in different directions and rapidly accelerating and then decelerating them will light up your midsection like a Christmas tree. Not bad for something you could find down at the local pier. Just don't use the ones you come across there—the fishermen tend to frown on that. All kidding aside, though, we can honestly say that the battle ropes are one serious conditioning tool. Especially when you consider all of the different exercises you can do with them!

BATTLE ROPE REPEATED SLAM
(MUSCLES TRAINED: UPPER BACK, BICEPS, TRICEPS, CHEST)

Stand in an athletic stance holding the battle ropes in front of your hips with your palms facing each other. Maintaining a slight bend in your knees, keep your torso erect as you lift the rope to about shoulder height and then rapidly slam them down into the ground. Immediately lift them back up and then continue to slam them repeatedly for the desired time interval (usually about 30 seconds).

Training tip: Avoid rounding your back as you slam the ropes. Maintain an upright torso.

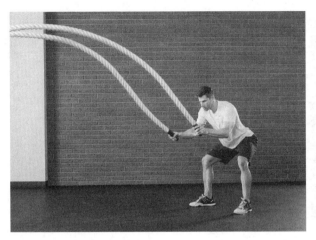 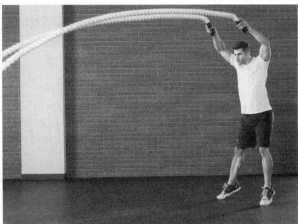

BATTLE ROPE DRUM
(MUSCLES TRAINED: SHOULDERS, BICEPS, TRICEPS, CORE)

Stand in an athletic stance holding the battle ropes in front of your hips with your palms facing each other. Begin by making a drumming motion with your arms, lifting the ropes and slamming them down one arm after the other. Attempt to make rippling waves with the ropes that roll all the way back to their anchor point. Continue for the desired time interval (usually about 30 seconds).

Training tip: Use your core! Maintain a rigid torso and avoid rocking side to side to get the ropes moving.

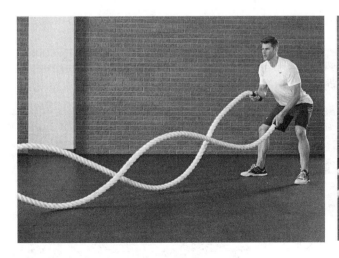 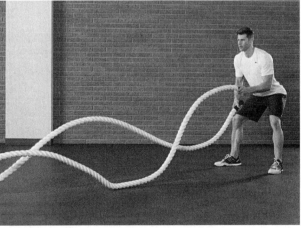

BATTLE ROPE SNAKE

Stand in an athletic stance holding the battle ropes in front of your hips with your palms facing each other. Lower yourself into a good squat position so that your hands are hanging down close to the floor and begin bringing your arms apart and then together in a rapid motion. The ropes should remain close to the ground and their movement should resemble that of a couple of snakes slithering across the floor. Continue for the desired time interval (usually about 30 seconds).

Training tip: Stay low into the legs to keep the ropes close to the ground.

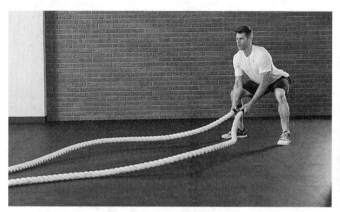 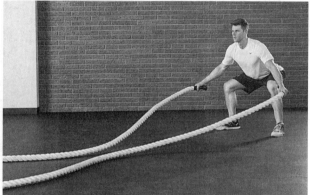

BATTLE ROPE INSIDE CIRCLE

Stand in an athletic stance holding the battle ropes in front of your hips with a thumbs-up grip. Begin by bringing your arms down and out to the sides in a wide, circular motion. As your hands pass your hips, bring your arms up and around in a wide arc, just above your shoulders, until finally brining your hands back in toward each other to complete the circle. Continue cycling your arms in this manner for the desired time interval (usually about 30 seconds).

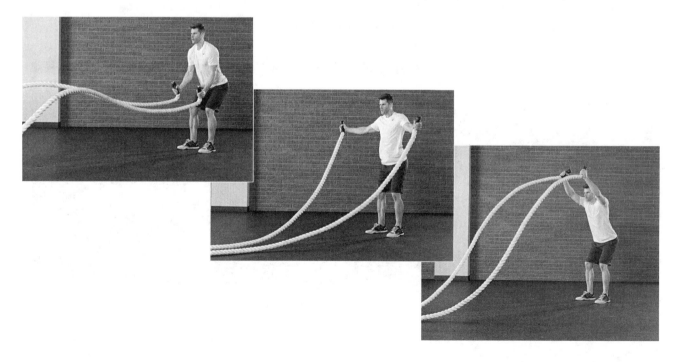

BATTLE ROPE OUTSIDE CIRCLE

(MUSCLES TRAINED: SHOULDERS, UPPER BACK, CHEST, CORE)

Same execution as the Inside Circles, just reversed. Start your arms going up and out to the sides in a wide arc above your shoulders and then bringing them back in and around once they pass your hips.

Training tip for both: Use the large muscles of your upper back and shoulders to get the ropes moving. Don't just throw your hands.

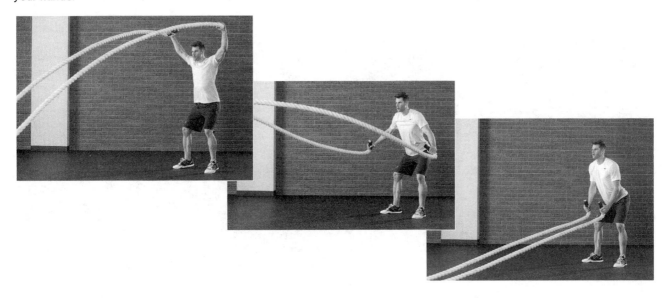

BATTLE ROPE HIP FLIP

(MUSCLES TRAINED: CORE, UPPER BACK, BICEPS, HIPS)

Stand in an athletic stance holding the battle ropes in front of your hips with a thumbs-up grip. Begin by using your core and hips to "flip" the ropes over to one side, pivoting the opposite side leg as you do; that is, if flipping the ropes to the right, pivot the left hip. As soon as the ropes make contact with the ground, immediately flip the ropes over to the left, this time pivoting the right side as you do. Repeat for the desired time interval (usually about 30 seconds).

Training tip: Generate the power to flip the ropes from your core and hips and think of your arms as extensions of the ropes.

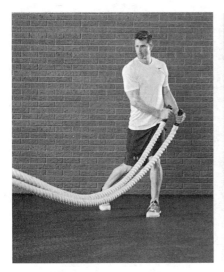 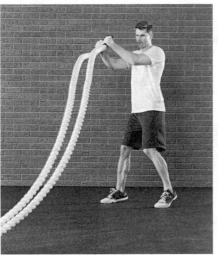 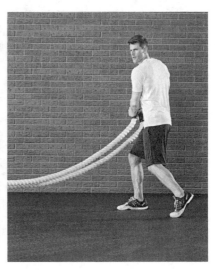

BATTLE ROPE CYCLONE

(MUSCLES TRAINED: HIPS, CORE, BICEPS, UPPER BACK)

Stand in an athletic stance holding the battle ropes in front of your hips with your palms facing each other. Begin by using your core, hips, and upper body to get the ropes going in a circular motion. After the desired time interval (usually about 15 to 20 seconds), quickly reverse direction and complete the drill in the opposite direction.

Training tip: Once again, try and generate most of the power from your core and hips as opposed to just moving the ropes with your arms.

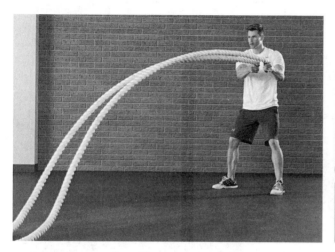 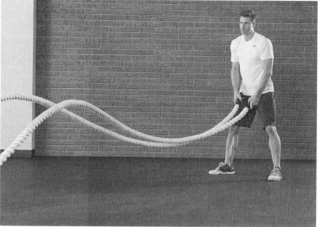

BATTLE ROPE JUMPING JACK

(MUSCLES TRAINED: SHOULDERS, LEGS, CORE)

Stand in an athletic stance holding the battle ropes at your sides with a thumbs-up grip. Begin by executing a basic jumping jack by bringing your arms up over your head while holding the ropes. Continue for the desired time interval (usually 30 to 45 seconds).

Training tip: Land as lightly as you can. Do not allow the extra weight provided by the ropes to jar your lower back.

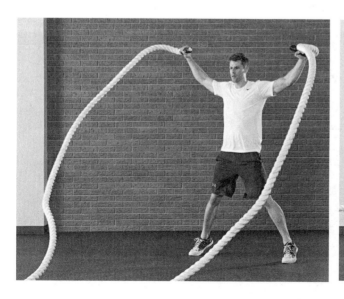 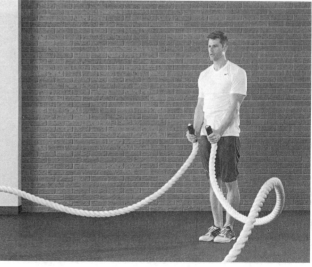

BATTLE ROPE SEATED ROTATION

(MUSCLES TRAINED: CORE, BICEPS, SHOULDERS)

Sit on the ground facing an outstretched pair of battle ropes, holding them with a thumbs-up grip. Begin by lifting your feet off the ground, bracing your core and leaning back slightly. From this position, rapidly bring the ropes over from one hip to the other, using your core to rotate your upper body. Continue for the desired number of reps (usually about 30 seconds).

Training tip: Keep your core braced to protect your lower back.

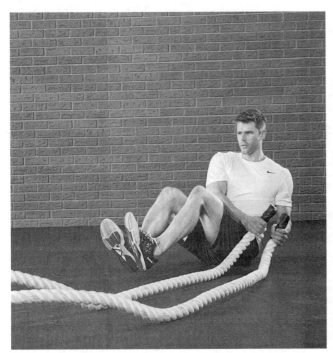
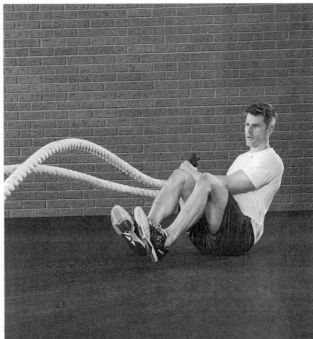

FLIPPING OUT! BUILD SERIOUS STRENGTH WITH TRUCK TIRES

A decade ago, the site of a truck tire inside a gym would have garnered its share of raised eyebrows and confused looks. Fast forward to today, though, and it's odd not to see one among the array of other equipment. That's because tire flipping has become the new darling of the strength set. After all, why do exercises as passé as bench presses and squats when you can unleash your inner NFL lineman and turn plenty of heads in the process! Be forewarned, though—tire flipping is easily one of the hardest exercises you can do in the gym. It requires a strong grip, unbelievable core strength, good hip mobility, strong legs, and a powerful upper body as well. Trans-

lation: It's not for everyone! Even if you can't flip the tire, though, there are plenty of other ways to use it.

If your gym has a sledgehammer lying around (and good luck finding one that doesn't these days), you can blast your core with sledgehammer tire hits. Or maybe you're the more nimble type. In that case, try some tire in-and-out jumps to build explosive lower body power. Or for you outdoor enthusiasts, there're always tire stepups to provide an unstable surface for you to get up and down on—great for those of you who are into hiking and other activities that require a mixture of leg strength and balance. The point being, even though tires are most often used for flipping, there are other exercises you can do with them that can add some nice diversity to your workouts.

TIRE FLIP

Stand with a wide stance (outside shoulder's width) about a foot or so behind a truck tire that's lying on its side. Begin by squatting down and leaning forward to grab the base of the tire with your arms positioned out wide to the sides, and place your chest and collarbone against the top of the tire. In this position, your torso should be angled forward slightly—kind of like an offensive lineman ready to fire out of his stance. Next, drive with your legs as you simultaneously begin to lift the tire up and forward to stand it up. As soon as you have enough clearance, get one knee up under the tire to "bump it up" toward your chest, as you rotate your arms into a pressing position. Finally, use your upper body to push the tire over onto its opposite side. Repeat for 5 to 6 repetitions.

Training tip: Avoid excessive strain on the biceps and lower back by dropping your arms straight down under your shoulders and attempting to lift the tire with a rounded back. The wide stance and grip will allow you to use your lower body more and get a more powerful drive off of the ground.

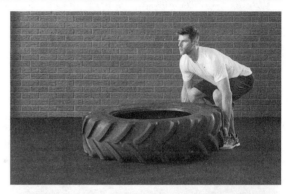

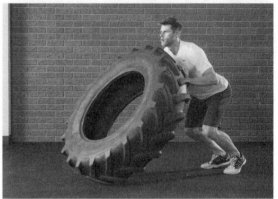

TIRE SLEDGEHAMMER HIT

Stand a foot or so behind a truck tire, holding a sledgehammer with your left hand positioned at the base of the hammer and right about halfway up its neck. Begin by bracing your core and lifting the hammer up and over your right shoulder, then quickly change direction and swing the hammer down from over your head to strike the tire. As you do this, slide

your right hand down the handle until it's on top of your left and bend your knees as you strike the tire to help absorb the force of the strike. Reposition your hands and continue until you've completed 10 to 12 repetitions and repeat with the other side.

Training tip: Make sure to use your legs both as you wind up and then strike the tire by keeping a slight bend in your knees.

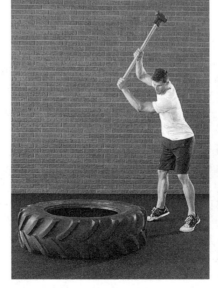

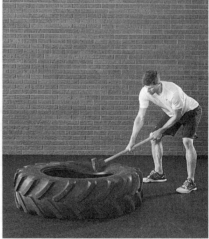

TIRE JUMP IN AND OUT

(MUSCLES TRAINED: QUADS, CALVES, GLUTES, HAMSTRINGS, CORE)

Stand behind a truck tire that's positioned on its side with your feet about shoulder-width apart. Begin by rapidly dipping down into a quarter squat, as you swing your arms slightly behind your torso. Quickly reverse directions and swing your arms forward as you jump up into the air and land in the middle of the tire. As soon as you contact the ground, dip your knees quickly and jump back out of the tire. Make a quick turn while on the ground and repeat the drill going back the way you came from. Continue until you've completed 10 reps total (5 each way).

Training tip: Try to rebound quickly off the ground when jumping out of the tire.

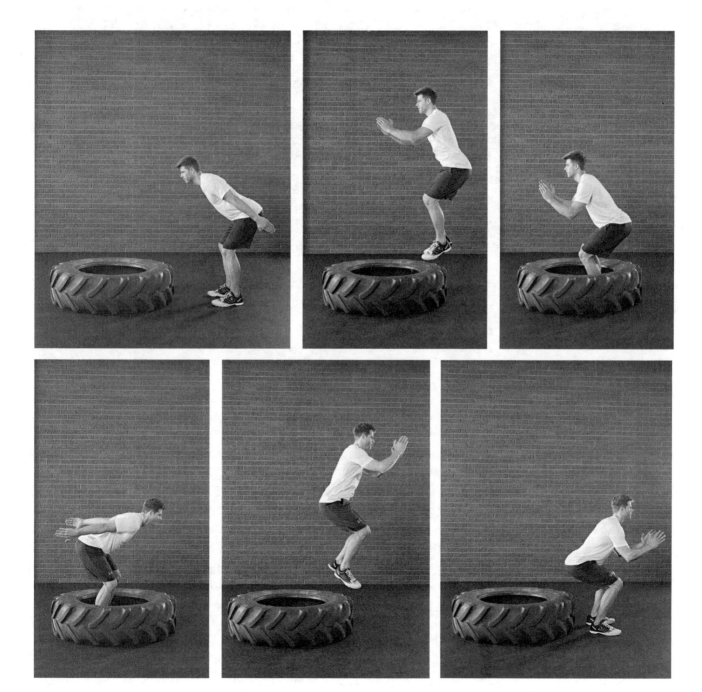

TIRE STEPUP

(MUSCLES TRAINED: GLUTES, QUADS, HAMSTRINGS, CALVES, CORE)

Stand behind a truck tire that's lying on its side. Begin by stepping up on the tire with your entire foot—emphasizing pushing through the heel—until you're standing on top of the tire. Then lower yourself slowly back down, making sure that the last leg up is the first one back to the ground. Continue until you've completed 10 to 12 reps and then repeat with the other leg.

Training tip: Maintain an upright torso and avoid using the back leg to help propel you up too much. Focus on "crushing" the tire with your lead leg.

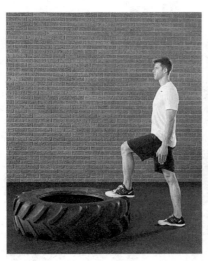 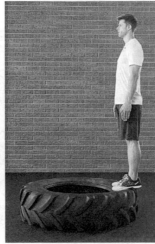 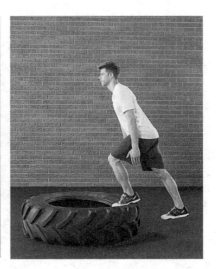

THE SUSPENSE IS KILLING ME: MAKE YOUR BODY YOUR MACHINE WITH SUSPENSION TRAINING

A few years ago, if someone told you that a couple of nylon straps hanging from a squat rack, or a chinup bar could give you an amazing workout, you'd probably think they were nuts! Now, it's nearly impossible to walk into a gym and not see one or more TRXs tethered to some overhead anchor point. That's because suspension training provides gym goers with a versatile (there are literally dozens of exercises you can do), self-limiting (you control the difficulty based on how you position your body in relation to the anchor point), and incredibly time-efficient workout. In fact, you could easily work your entire body in 30 minutes or less by simply adopting different positions with the straps. All you need to do is decide whether you want to grab the handles or place your feet in the cradles and adjust the straps to the

appropriate length—and you're good to go!

Want to blast your core and upper body in one shot? Try the Atomic Pushup. Looking for a kick-ass leg exercise? Suspension Pistol Squats will definitely fit the bill. Or why not just attack your upper back and work on that desk-jockey posture of yours with some suspension Rows? As great as these exercises are on their own, one of the biggest benefits to suspension training is the ease in which you can switch from one drill to the other with no elaborate setups or having to wait for someone to get off the equipment. Just change position and you're good to go! Of course, you can also just sprinkle them in here and there to your existing workout—the choice is yours. Either way, just know that you have the benefit of one of the most versatile tools in the gym at your disposal— perfect for a quick lunchtime circuit or mixed in among one of your more elaborate torture sessions.

TRX ROW

Stand facing a suspension trainer and take hold of the handles. Walk your feet toward the anchor point as you gradually lean back until your arms are straight. At this point your body should be at an angle to the ground with your arms extended out in front of your shoulders. For more resistance, bring your feet closer to the anchor point and increase your lean; for less, back your feet up slightly.

Begin your pull by bringing your shoulder blades together and down toward your waist as you simultaneously pull with your arms. Once your elbows are slightly past your torso, pause for a second before lowering back down to the starting position—making sure that your body forms a straight line and your hips don't sag. Do 10 to 12 repetitions.

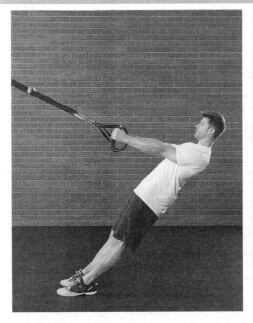 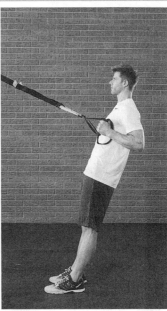

Training tip: Keeping palms facing each other and elbows in near the torso will target the lats more; having the palms facing the floor and elbows flared away from the body will hit more of the rear deltoids, traps, and rhomboids.

TRX SINGLE-ARM ROW

Begin by threading the handles of the suspension trainer through each other so they don't slip. Next, grab hold of one handle as you begin to position your feet near the anchor point as with a two-armed Row. Once in position, place your other hand on your hip and lower yourself down into position—for more resistance, move your feet closer to the anchor point, and for less, move them further away. Next, initiate the pull by bringing your shoulder blade down and back as you simultaneously pull with your arm. Do 10 to 12 repetitions per side.

Training tip: Keeping your palm facing your torso and elbow tucked close will target the lats more; having the palm facing the ground and elbow flared away from the body will hit more of the rear deltoid, trap, and rhomboid.

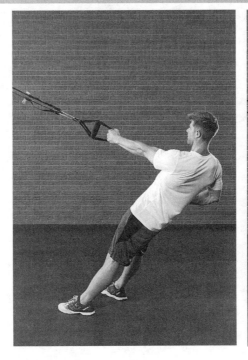 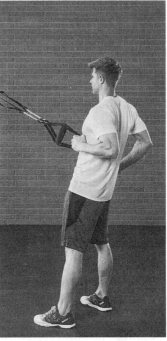

TRX YTW

Face a suspension trainer and grab hold of the handles. Bring your feet toward the anchor point as you gradually lean back until your arms are straight. For more resistance, bring your feet closer to the anchor point and increase your lean; for less, back your feet up slightly. To start executing the Y raise, with your arms extended out in front of you and palms facing down, use your upper back muscles to lift your arms overhead as you keep the straps tight. At the top of the movement, your arms should form the letter Y with your torso and your entire body should be in a straight line from your heels to your head. Lower back down to the starting position and repeat until you've done 6 to 8 reps of the Y raise.

Next, turn your palms to face each other and maintain a slight bend in your elbows as you execute the T raise by squeezing your shoulder blades together and down as you bring your arms out to the sides for 6 to 8 reps.

Finally, go back to the hand position you used for the Y raises and back your feet a little farther away from the wall. Begin the W raise by pulling into position as if about to do a row, but stop just a little short of your elbows being even with your torso. Next, keep your upper arms still as you pivot at the elbow and bring your forearms into as close to a vertical position as possible. Lower slowly and repeat; making sure not to let your body deviate from a straight line at the bottom of each rep. Do 6 to 8 repetitions.

Training tip: You may have to alter your foot position for each part of the exercise, going from feet farther from the wall for the Y raise, a little closer for the T (the strongest position), and finally in again for the W.

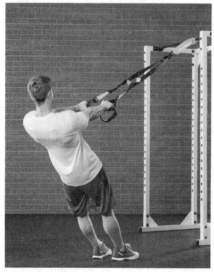
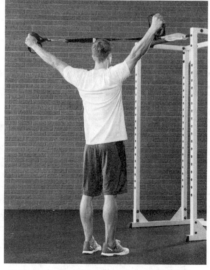
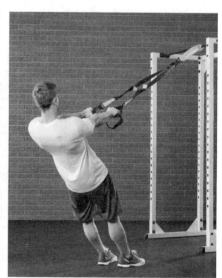

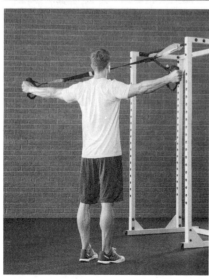
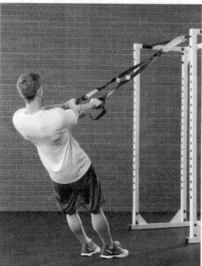
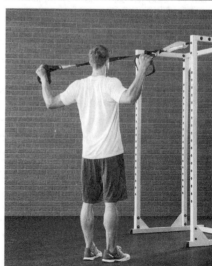

TRX BICEPS CURL

Stand facing a suspension trainer and take hold of the handles. Walk your feet toward the anchor point as you gradually lean back until your arms are straight. Begin with your palms facing the ceiling and arms extended out in front of your shoulders. Keeping your upper arms still, pull with your biceps by bringing your hands toward the top of your head. Make sure to avoid allowing your upper arms to drop toward the floor as you do. Pause at the top and squeeze your biceps for a second, before lowering back down to the starting position. Repeat until you've completed 10 to 12 repetitions.

Training tip: Starting with your palms facing down and then rotating them up as you curl can give the biceps an even more intense contraction.

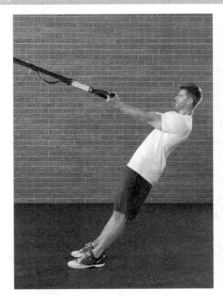
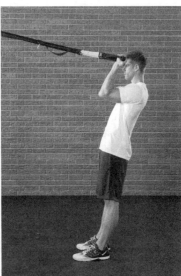

TRX TRICEPS EXTENSION

Grab the handles of a suspension trainer and turn away from it. Move your feet toward the anchor point as you extend your arms out in front of you until you adopt a position similar to Superman in flight. For more resistance, bring your feet closer to the anchor point and increase your lean; for less, walk your feet forward slightly. To begin, balance your weight on the balls of your feet and brace your core as you keep your upper arms still and use your elbow as a hinge by lowering your body toward your hands (forehead first). Just before your forehead touches your hands, use your triceps to extend your arms as you push back up to the starting position. Repeat until you've performed 10 to 12 repetitions.

Training tip: Be careful not to let your lower back cave in as you perform the exercise. Brace your core and keep your torso rigid throughout movement.

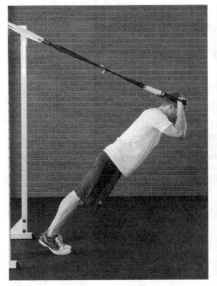
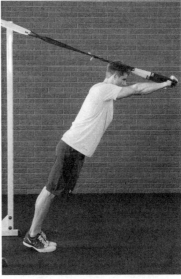

TRX PUSHUP (FEET ON GROUND)

(MUSCLES TRAINED: CHEST, SHOULDERS, TRICEPS, CORE)

Grab the handles of a suspension trainer and turn away from it. Move your feet toward the anchor point as you extend your arms out beneath your shoulders. Begin by bracing your core as you bend at the elbows and lower yourself down into a pushup position. Once your elbows are slightly past your torso, pause for a second before easing back up to the starting position. Perform 10 to 12 repetitions. For more resistance, move your feet closer to the anchor point; for less, walk them slightly forward.

Training tip: Keep your core braced and elbows positioned approximately 45 degrees in relation to your torso.

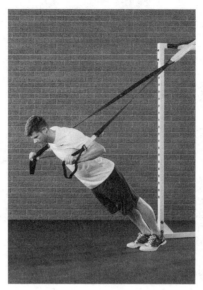 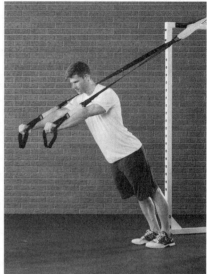

TRX ATOMIC PUSHUP (FEET IN FOOT HOLDERS)

(MUSCLES TRAINED: CHEST, SHOULDERS, TRICEPS, CORE)

From a kneeling position, place your feet into the foot cradles of a suspension trainer. Once secured, get up onto your hands into a pushup position. Next, brace your core as you lower yourself down toward the ground. When your arms are just past your torso, pause for a second before pressing back up to the starting position. Before executing another pushup, use your core to bring your feet in toward your face by bending your knees. Hold that position for a second before allowing your legs to extend back out and repeat the sequence until you've completed 10 to 12 repetitions.

Training tip: Be careful not to use momentum when executing either motion.

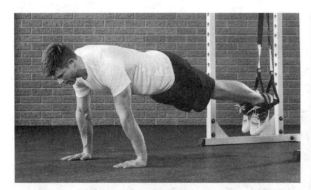
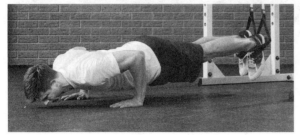
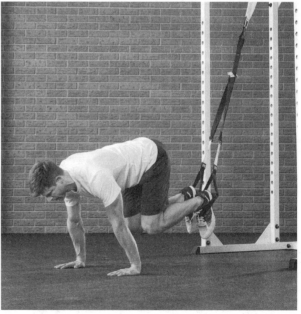

TRX PISTOL SQUAT

(MUSCLES TRAINED: QUADS, HAMSTRINGS, GLUTES, CORE, CALVES)

Stand facing a suspension trainer and grab hold of the handles. Next, walk your feet toward the anchor point as you gradually lean back until your arms are straight. Once you've found a comfortable position, begin by lifting one foot off the ground and extending your leg out in front of you. Next, keeping an upright torso, squat down by sitting your hips back and lowering yourself with a controlled descent until your leg forms a 90 degree angle. Pause there for a second before pressing back up. Continue until you've done 8 to 10 repetitions per leg.

Training tip: Make sure to keep the heel of the working leg pressed into the ground and your torso upright throughout the movement.

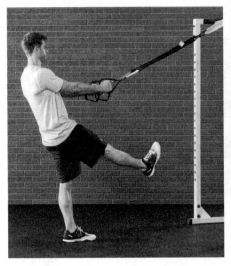 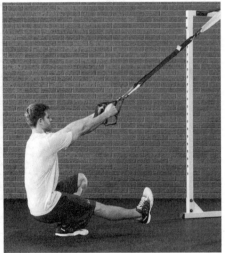

TRX LEG CURL

(MUSCLES TRAINED: HAMSTRINGS, CALVES, CORE)

Lie down with your feet facing a suspension trainer anchored to an overhead object. Place your heels in the foot cradles and lie flat on your back. Begin by bridging your hips so that your body forms a slight diagonal line from your head to your heels. From this position, brace your core as you bring your heels in toward your butt as you simultaneously continue bridging your hips. In the top position your knees would be bent about 90 degrees, with your body forming a nice straight line from your knees to your shoulders. Slowly extend your legs and repeat until you've done 10 to 12 repetitions.

Training tip: Be careful not to use momentum when bringing your feet in toward your body and raising your hips to avoid unnecessary stress on the lower back.

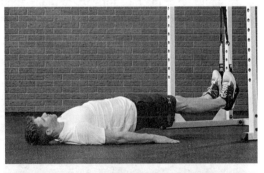

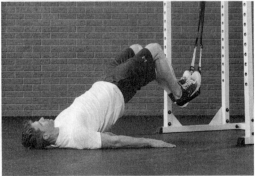

TRX SIDE PLANK

Get down on the ground and position the sides of your feet into the foot cradles of a suspension trainer as you turn onto one side. Next, prop your body up onto your underside elbow and forearm making sure to brace your core and straighten your legs; allowing your feet to line up one behind the other with your top leg in front of the bottom one. Once in position, simply hold for time—making sure to keep a nice straight line from your feet to your head and not letting the underside of your torso sag toward the floor. Hold for 20 to 40 seconds and repeat with the other side.

Training tip: Keep your core braced tight to avoid lower back strain.

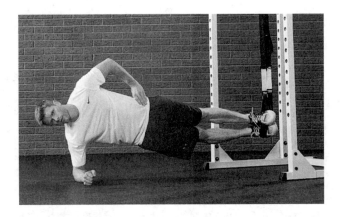

TRX ROLLOUT

Kneel down beneath a suspension trainer facing away from the anchor point. Grab hold of the handles and brace your core tight, as you begin with your hands slightly in front of your hips. Initiate the movement by driving the glutes forward and keeping the core braced, as you extend your arms out in front of you. It's imperative that you use your knees as the fulcrum and drive the hips forward to really engage the core. Only go out as far as you can, holding on to a core neutral position (no excessive arching or rounding of the lower back). Pause at your farthest point before using your core to return to the starting position. Repeat for 8 to 10 repetitions.

Training tip: Inhale as you descend into the rollout to keep the torso rigid and protect your spine.

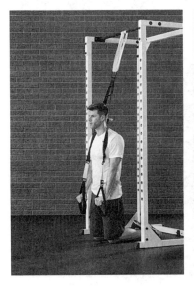
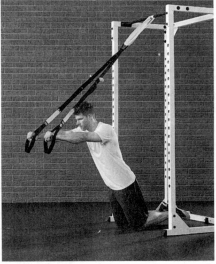
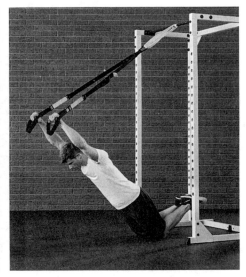

TRX ALLIGATOR

(MUSCLES TRAINED: UPPER AND LOWER TRAPS, LATS, REAR DELTOIDS, RHOMBOIDS, TRICEPS)

Stand facing a suspension trainer and take hold of the handles. Walk your feet toward the anchor point as you gradually lean back until your arms are straight. At this point your body should be at an angle to the ground with your arms extended out in front of your shoulders and your palms facing each other. For more resistance, bring your feet closer to the anchor point and increase your lean; for less, back your feet up slightly. Begin by keeping both arms straight and using your upper back muscles to bring one arm up overhead and the other down next to your hip. In the finish position, both palms should be facing straight ahead. Pause for a second before lowering back to the starting position. Then alternate arms for the next repetition. Continue until you've done 6 to 8 repetitions per side.

Training tip: Avoid using momentum by driving your hips toward the anchor point before your chest. Use a slow, controlled motion when bringing your body toward the anchor point.

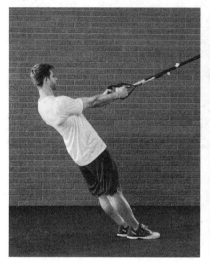 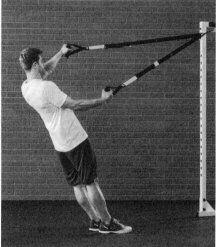 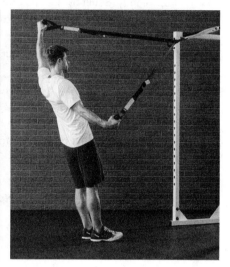

TRX BULGARIAN SPLIT SQUAT

(MUSCLES TRAINED: QUADS, HAMSTRINGS, GLUTES, CALVES, CORE)

Begin by threading the handles of the suspension trainer through each other so they don't slip. Next, turn your back to the anchor point and position one foot in the foot cradle so that the sole faces behind you. From this position where you are now balancing on one leg, maintain a rigid torso as you bend at the knee, hip, and ankle and descend into a squat, by allowing both knees to bend, until the working thigh is parallel to the ground. Pause there for a second before pressing back up. Repeat until you've completed 10 to 12 repetitions per side.

Training tip: Because of the intense stretch on the back leg, be especially careful not to bounce or use momentum to get out of the bottom of the squat.

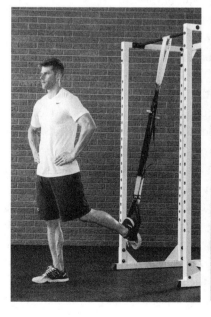 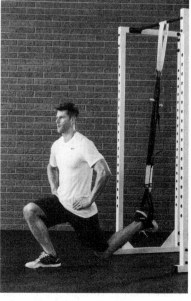

TRX SQUAT AND ROW

(MUSCLES TRAINED: QUADS, GLUTES, HAMSTRINGS, CALVES, UPPER BACK, BICEPS)

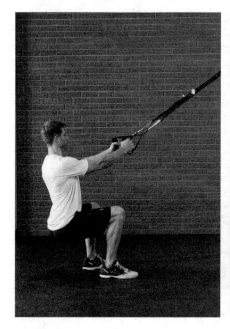
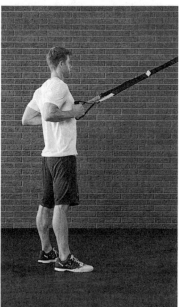

Stand facing a suspension trainer and take hold of the handles. Walk your feet toward the anchor point as you gradually lean back until your arms are straight. At this point your body should be at an angle to the ground with your arms extended out in front of your shoulders. For more resistance, bring your feet closer to the anchor point and increase your lean; for less, back your feet up slightly. Begin by holding on to the handles and with your feet positioned a little wider than shoulder-width apart, descend into a squat position. Once your thighs are parallel to the ground, press back up as you simultaneously execute a row. In the top position your legs are straight and arms are bent just as with a regular suspension row; just descend back into a squat as your arms straighten. Do 15 to 20 repetitions.

Training tip: Try to make the motion as integrated as possible, with the ascent from the squat and row flowing together as one piece.

HALFING A BALL! THE DOUBLE-SIDED THREAT OF THE BOSU BALL

You've definitely seen them before. Sometimes they're out on the gym floor near the abdominal mats and stability balls, while other times they're stacked up one on top of the other in a rack in the corner of the aerobics room. So you obviously take one look at the BOSU ball—that weird half stability ball with the one flat side—and think to yourself "definitely a chick thing." Well, Hercules, turns out you couldn't be further from the truth. In fact, there are a lot of very challenging exercises that can be done on the BOSU, many of which would have the most hardened gym rat sweating bullets before too long. So before you go and judge its admittedly less than masculine looking exterior, just know that the BOSU ball has a lot to offer a workout program that's suffering from a major case of stale! By offering you the opportunity to work with either side up (blue or black), this incredibly versatile piece takes just about any exercise you can imagine and cranks up the core contribution immeasurably!

Tired of doing the same old routine every time you hit the gym? Trade in some of those chest presses for a BOSU pushup and work toward improving shoulder stability and core strength. Or maybe you're looking for a change of pace from traditional free weight squats and want to try something that will challenge your balance and coordination? Simply flip the blue side of the BOSU down and watch your legs tremble as you descend into a set of BOSU squats. Even black side down, the BOSU allows you to challenge yourself in ways that more traditional gym equipment can't. Think we're kidding? Try the Lateral Bound drill for explosive power, or the Side Plank to torch your core. No matter how you use it though, the BOSU is bound to change your opinion of functional exercise equipment. Just because it may not look like much doesn't mean it's not worth your consideration.

BOSU PUSHUP

(MUSCLES TRAINED: CHEST, SHOULDERS, TRICEPS, CORE)

Position a BOSU with the round side down and grab it with both hands on the side. Assume a pushup position and keep your core braced. Begin lowering yourself toward the surface of the BOSU by maintaining a plank position and bending your arms. When your elbows are slightly past your torso and your chest is just a few inches away from the surface of the BOSU, press back up to the starting position, being sure to keep balanced the entire time.

Lower and repeat until you've completed 10 to 12 reps.

Training tip: Keep your core braced to avoid arching your lower back.

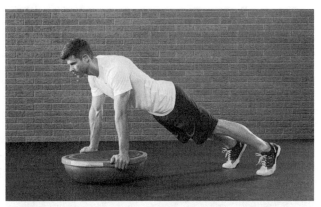

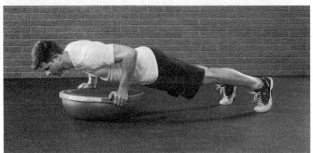

BOSU SQUAT

(MUSCLES TRAINED: QUADS, HAMSTRINGS, GLUTES, CORE)

Position the BOSU with the round side down and place one foot on one side as you brace your core and step up to place your other foot on the opposite side. Stand with your feet shoulder-width apart for a moment and get used to balancing on the BOSU. Next, sit your hips back and bend your knees as you descend into a squat, as you simultaneously raise your arms out in front of you as a counterbalance. When the tops of your thighs are parallel to the surface of the BOSU, pause for a second before pressing back up to the start position. Repeat for 10 to 12 repetitions.

Training tip: Use a slow, controlled motion and maintain a rigid torso throughout the squat.

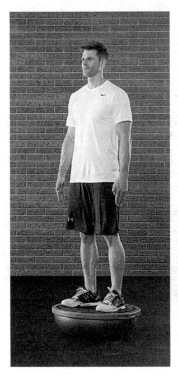

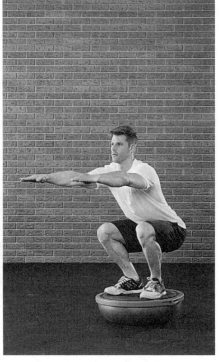

BOSU ONE-LEG SQUAT

(MUSCLES TRAINED: QUADS, HAMSTRINGS, GLUTES, CALVES, CORE)

Position the BOSU with the blue side down and step up onto it, placing one foot in the middle. Keeping one knee bent behind you at a 90-degree angle, stand and get used to balancing on the BOSU for a moment. Next, bend at the hip and knee as you descend into a squat, making sure to keep your torso as upright as possible. Once the top of your thigh is parallel to the surface of the BOSU, pause for a second and then press back up to the start position. Repeat until you've completed 8 to 10 reps and then switch sides.

Training tip: Keep your weight equally distributed across the sole of your balancing leg's foot—avoid sitting too far back on the heel or leaning forward toward the toes.

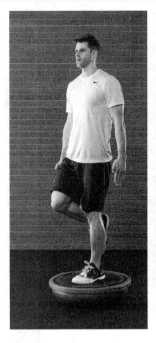
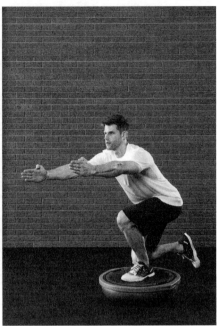

BOSU PLANK

(MUSCLES TRAINED: CORE, UPPER BACK, SHOULDERS, QUADS)

Place a BOSU on the ground blue side up and kneel down onto the floor with it positioned in front of you. Place your forearms on the ball and get up onto the balls of your feet as if getting ready to do a pushup. Brace your core, pack your shoulder blades together, and hold your body in a straight line from your head down to your feet for the desired time interval (usually 30 to 60 seconds).

Training tip: Keep your core braced and shoulders packed together to avoid your lower back caving in or upper back rounding.

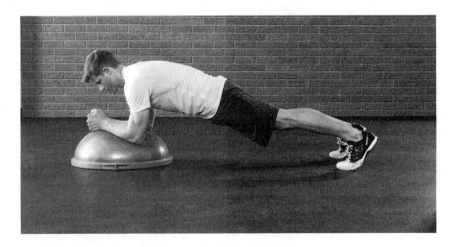

BOSU SIDE PLANK

Place a BOSU on the ground blue side up and lie on the ground next to it. Begin by placing one forearm on the BOSU and turning to one side so that your shoulder is stacked vertically above the arm on the BOSU. Next, engage your core as you lift your hips and thighs off the ground. In the top position, only the sides of your feet should be touching the ground, with your forearm on the BOSU and everything from your underside armpit down to your calf hovering above the ground. Hold for the desired time interval (usually 30 to 60 seconds) and repeat on the other side.

Training tip: Place one foot behind the other for better balance. Or you can stack your feet one on top of the other for added difficulty.

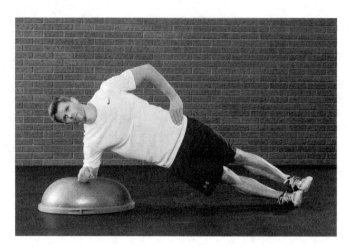

BOSU LATERAL BOUND

(MUSCLES TRAINED: CALVES, QUADS, GLUTES, HAMSTRINGS, CORE)

Position a BOSU blue side up against a sturdy object that you know isn't going to move and stand a foot or two beside it. Begin by bounding out to the side by pushing off the leg furthest from the BOSU and landing about halfway up the side of it with your inside leg. Quickly absorb that landing by bending at the knee, hip, and ankle and then use the elasticity of the BOSU to bound back to the starting position. Try to stick the landing on your outside leg. Pause for a second and repeat. Continue until you've completed 6 to 10 reps. Repeat on the other side.

Training tip: Try to land softly on both jumps by bending at the ankles, hips, and knees. To make the exercise more challenging, you can try bounding continuously from one side to the other without the stick.

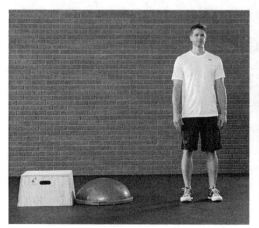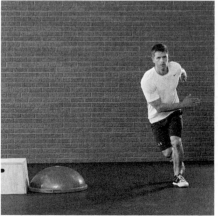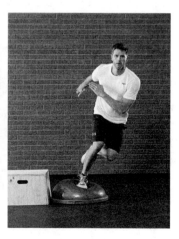

BOSU SPLIT SQUAT

Place a BOSU with the round side down and place one foot flat on the top of the platform. Next position your other leg about 2 feet behind you and balance on the ball of your back foot. Keeping your torso erect, begin by bending both knees and dropping down into a split squat until your top of your lead thigh is parallel to the ground. Maintain your balance and press back up to the top. Continue for 8 to 10 reps and repeat on the other side.

Training tip: Try to keep your weight equally distributed across the sole of the foot on the BOSU and only the ball of the back foot in contact with the ground throughout the exercise.

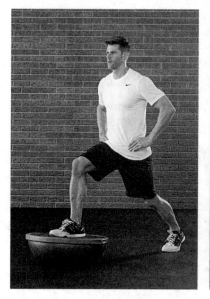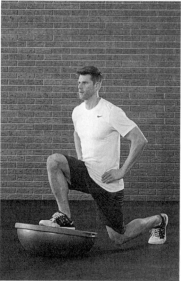

BOSU HIP BRIDGE

Place a BOSU on the ground blue side up and lie down behind it. With your hips close to the base of the BOSU, place your feet on the top of the dome with both knees bent at approximately 90 degrees. Begin by bracing your core and driving your heels down into the BOSU to emphasize the use of your glutes and hamstrings. At the top of the movement, your body should form a straight line from your knees down to your shoulders. Hold for a second and repeat until you've completed 12 to 15 reps.

Training tip: Keep your core braced and avoid distending your abdominals or arching your back excessively in an attempt to get your hips off the ground.

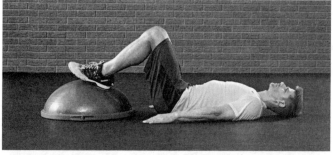

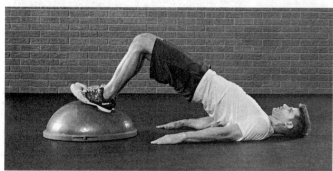

A SLIPPERY SLOPE: SLIDEBOARD TRAINING FOR YOUR WHOLE BODY

Okay, admit it. If you thought that prowler sleds and truck tires were just for football players, you must look at the slideboard and think you have to be a hockey player to use it. Not so! In fact, there are tons of ways to use the slideboard that have absolutely nothing to do with ice hockey and everything to do with giving you an awesome workout! That's because the slippery surface of the board provides a nice way to challenge your body through different ranges of motions that it's accustomed to when doing more traditional forms of strength training. When was the last time you were able to throw a chest fly in, *as you were doing* a set of pushups? Or, challenge the limits of your lower body flexibility while also training strength as with the sideboard Lateral Squat? You can do exercises like these and plenty more, because the slideboard offers such tremendous versatility. So if you're the type who's pressed for time and never seems to leave enough for things like mobility or core work, you might want to give it a try. Especially when it allows you to do the types of exercises featured here.

SLIDEBOARD REVERSE LUNGE

(MUSCLES TRAINED: QUADS, GLUTES, HAMSTRINGS, CORE)

Stand with the backs of your heels touching the end of a slideboard facing away from it. Place the ball of one foot on the board behind you and leave your other fully in contact with the ground. Begin by maintaining an erect torso and bending your lead leg to descend into a squat, as your back leg also bends and slides back behind you. In the bottom position your torso should remain erect, with your lead knee forming a 90-degree angle and your other foot a couple of feet behind you on the sideboard. To get back up, press your lead leg into the ground as you simultaneously pull with the back hip to get back up to the starting position. Continue until you've completed 8 to 10 reps per side.

Training tip: Make sure to bend both knees as you descend. Avoid keeping the back leg straight and overstretching the hip flexor.

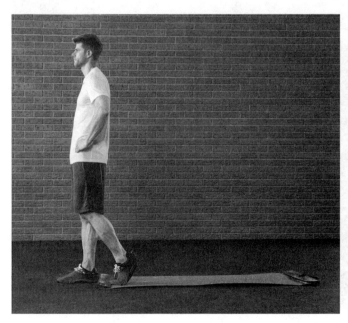
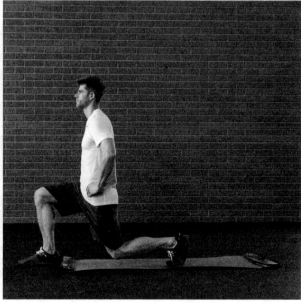

SLIDEBOARD PLANK BODY SAW

(MUSCLES TRAINED: CORE, QUADS, UPPER BACK, SHOULDERS)

Get down on the ground with a slideboard positioned behind you. Begin by placing your forearms on the ground just in front of the edge of the board, while pacing the balls of your feet onto it as you get into a plank position. Starting with your face positioned directly above your hands where you feel your core working fairly hard, rock back (while maintaining the same neutral spine position) to the point where your face is above the space between your arms. Pause there for a second and then use your core and upper body to "pull" yourself back to the start position. Repeat until you've completed 8 to 10 reps.

Training tip: Only rock back as far as you can without altering the position of the plank—this might only be a couple of inches initially.

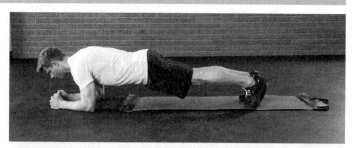

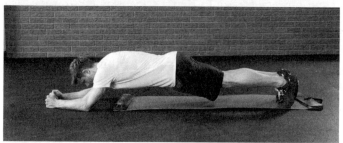

SLIDEBOARD PUSHUP WITH LATERAL REACH

(MUSCLES TRAINED: CHEST, SHOULDERS, TRICEPS, CORE)

Position your body perpendicular to a slideboard wearing the boots on your hands. Begin by assuming a pushup position on the board with your arms slightly wider than shoulder-width apart and core braced tight. Next, execute a pushup with one arm as you reach out to the side with the other by sliding it along the board. Pause for a second in the bottom position and then simultaneously push with one arm and pull with the other to get back up to the start position. Repeat to the other side and continue until you've done 6 to 10 reps per side.

Training tip: Only go out as far as you can without altering the position of your core.

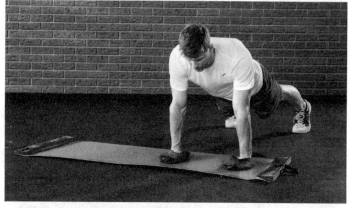

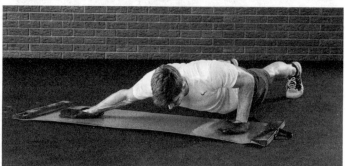

SLIDEBOARD FLY

(MUSCLES TRAINED: CHEST, SHOULDERS AND CORE)

Position your body perpendicular to a slideboard wearing the boots on your hands. Begin by assuming a pushup position on the board with your arms slightly wider than shoulder-width apart and core braced tight. Next, slowly allow both arms to drift out to the sides as you maintain a neutral spine position with your core. Once you've reached your farthest point holding that position, use your pecs to pull your hands back to the start. Repeat until you've completed 8 to 12 reps.

Training tip: Keep your core braced tight and avoid allowing the hips to sag as you near the end range at the bottom of each rep.

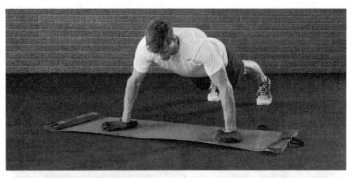

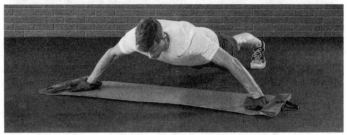

SLIDEBOARD MOUNTAIN CLIMBER

(MUSCLES TRAINED: CORE, HIPS, UPPER BODY)

Get down on the ground with a slideboard positioned behind you. Assume a pushup position with your hands just in front of the edge of the board on the ground and the balls of your feet resting on the board. Next, brace your core and slide one foot up toward your waist, while keeping the other straight. As soon as you get it there, push that leg back as you simultaneously bring the other leg forward. Continue "sawing" your legs back and forth in this fashion, while maintaining a neutral spine position, for the desired time interval (usually about 30 seconds).

Training tip: Keep your upper body and core still as you pump your legs back and forth.

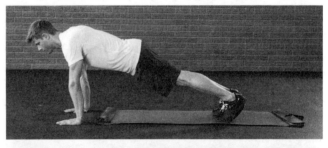

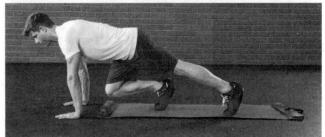

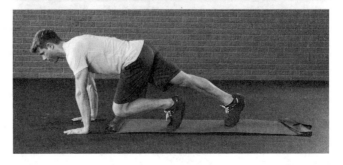

SLIDEBOARD SKATER

Stand on the end of the slideboard with both feet on it and the outside of one foot up against the support. Next, adopt an athletic position and push off with your outside leg as you glide across to the other side of the board. Once your opposite foot makes contact with the support on the other side, push off again to return to the starting position. Continue for the desired time interval (usually 30 to 60 seconds).

Training tip: Stay low and get into your hips as you push off and absorb each repetition. Staying up tall will increase likelihood of your falling off the board.

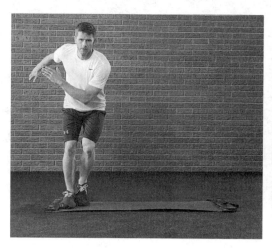 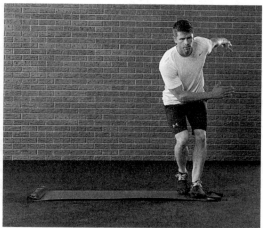

SLIDEBOARD LATERAL SQUAT

Stand aside a slideboard with a couple of dumbbells in your hands. With one foot positioned on the slideboard and the other on the ground, begin by allowing your leg to slide out to the side as you descend into a squat with the leg that's on the floor. When you reach the point where the top of your working thigh is parallel to the ground, pause for a second and then press back up to the starting position. Continue until you've done 10 to 12 repetitions and repeat on the other side.

Training tip: Maintain a controlled speed on the descent to protect your groin.

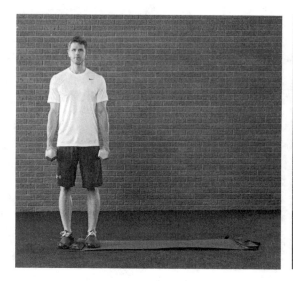 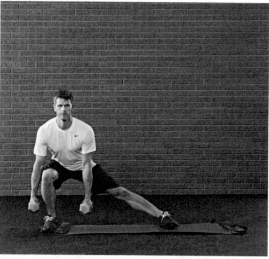

SLIDEBOARD PIKE

Begin by getting into a pushup position with your hands positioned on the floor, just in front of one end of the slide-board and your feet on it. Bracing your core and keeping your legs straight, bring your feet toward your hands as your butt rises up toward the ceiling. Once you've gotten your feet as close to your hands as possible, pause for a second and descend back to the starting position. Continue for 10 to 12 repetitions.

Training tip: Exhale as you use your core to draw your feet toward your hands and maintain a neutral spine (no heavy arch in the lower back or rounding of the upper) in the bottom position.

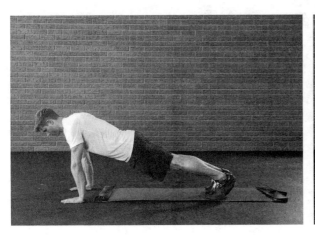
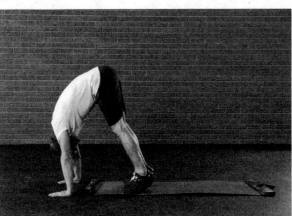

CHAPTER FOURTEEN

USING IT ALL TO YOUR ADVANTAGE

Learning How to Use the Equipment to Reach Your Goals

IF YOU'VE EVER SPENT TIME TRYING to build or fix something, you know that having the right tools makes the job a heck of a lot easier. You might actually be able to accomplish your goal without having everything you need from the get-go; it'll just be a longer, more frustrating process. Well, when it comes to your body, you're now in possession of the ultimate toolbox. By simply joining a gym you've made it infinitely easier to get results, regardless of what your goals may be. So now that you know how everything works, what say we teach you how to put it to use to reach your individual goals?

The workouts in this section have been designed with four specific results in mind: losing fat, building muscle, getting stronger, and improving overall fitness. These are complete programs that have been designed to get you where you want to go in the quickest, most efficient way possible. We mention this because these are specialized programs and they're meant to be followed the way they were designed.

They're also based on the assumption that your gym allows you access to all of the equipment we've included. If that's not the case, you could always substitute other exercises in place of something you don't have, or refer to the back of the book where there are even more of these types of workouts based on different equipment scenarios.

THE ULTIMATE LOSER: 6-WEEK FAT-LOSS WORKOUT

We might as well start with one of the most popular goals. After all, you would have an easier time shooting pool with a rope than trying to find someone in a gym who isn't interested in burning fat. Hold on to your hat, though; the fat-loss workouts featured here will likely be quite a departure from what you're used to. When it comes to fighting flab, we eschew the typical low-intensity cardio, lightweight/high-repetition strength-training approach in favor of something far more combustible. This high-intensity program is so effective for shedding those unwanted pounds you might be tempted to use it year-round. It's best handled in small, 4- to 6-week doses so that your body doesn't totally adapt to it and stop producing the desired results. Besides, after a month on this baby, you'll be glad to take a break.

Before we lay out the actual exercise prescription, here are a few take-home points on why we set things up the way we did:

- There's a lot of strength training in this workout. This is to help you retain muscle mass and keep your metabolism revving high. Also, contrary to popular belief, strength training burns LOTS of calories, both during and, even more so, after your workout.

- All the cardio work is of the interval type, meaning that instead of drudging away at one set intensity, you'll alternate between brief periods of high-intensity effort and active recovery. This might entail running at a near sprint on the treadmill for 20 to 40 seconds and then lowering your intensity to a fast-paced walk for double that time interval (a 20-second run followed by a 40-second brisk walk, and so on). We chose intervals because they burn more calories in less time and pose a more potent cardiovascular stimulus.

- All of the exercises will be noncompeting supersets, whereby you alternate between upper-body and lower-body lifts. This will allow one muscle group to recover while the other is working. Additionally, you'll find that most of the exercises are big, compound lifts like squats, bench presses, and rows, with little if any direct arm work. We did this because these types of exercises require the greatest energy expenditure and are more effective for fat loss.

- You'll have very little downtime during the workout. Unlike typical strength training where you rest for 1 to 2 minutes between sets, the exercises here are to be performed in pairs—alternating between upper- and lower-body lifts. After completing each pairing, you'll then get only a 30-second break before moving on to the next pairing. Once you've completed all of the exercises in order, you'll then do an intense 5 to 7 minutes of interval cardio work before going around for a second time.

The Workout

Perform the following workout two or three times per week for 6 weeks, allowing at least 1 full day of recovery between training sessions. If you work out twice, do Workout A one day and Workout B the next time you train. If you work out three times, alternate the workouts each week:

Week One: A/B/A

Week Two: B/A/B

You may also incorporate 1 or 2 additional days of interval cardio work for 15 to 20 minutes on off days if you like.

WORKOUT A

A-1 Squat or Leg Press × 10–12

A-2 Pushup × Max Reps

B-1 Chinup or Lat Pulldown × 8–10

B-2 Dumbbell Lunge × 8–10 per leg (alternating)

C-1 Dumbbell Stepups × 10–12 per side

C-2 Dumbbell or Machine Shoulder Press × 8–10

D-1 Dumbbell Woodchopper × 8–10 per side

D-2 Back Extension × 10–12 per side

WORKOUT B

A-1 Bench Press × 10–12

A-2 Romanian Deadlift × 8–10

B-1 Cable Row × 10–12

B-2 Dumbbell Thruster × 10–12

C-1 Cable Upright Row × 8–10

C-2 Dumbbell Sumo Deadlift × 10–12

D-1 Kettlebell Windmills × 6–8 per side

D-2 Pushup Position Row × 8–10 per side (alternating)

INTERVAL CARDIO 5 TO 7 MINUTES

Work to Recovery Ratio = 1:2

Rower, stationary bike, elliptical machine, or stairclimber: 30-second burst (near all-out), followed by 60 seconds of lower intensity continuous exercise × 4 to 6 intervals—or 6 to 9 minutes.

- Treadmills wouldn't work well here with the short intervals, as too much time would be wasted constantly changing to the proper speed and grade.

THE INCREDIBLE BULK: 6-WEEK MUSCLE-BUILDING WORKOUT

So, you say you want to put on some size, eh? Well, you've come to the right place. The workouts contained in this section of the book are specifically designed to help you increase muscle mass. Before we go a step farther, however, we'd be remiss if we neglected to mention that in order to do that you're going to have to follow a sound nutritional approach. We don't care how much effort you put into your training—if you're not providing your muscles with a sufficient amount of calories from quality food sources, you'll never achieve that well-muscled physique you've been wishing for. Seeing as how nutritional guidance is beyond the scope of this book, we will provide you with some resources where you can find out everything you need to know about eating to gain size.

1. JohnBerardi.com: As the name of the site suggests, this is the home of Dr. John Berardi, a noted sports nutritionist and our go-to guy when it comes to muscle building nutrition. In addition to his academic credentials, Dr. Berardi is a sought-after speaker at various nutritional conferences and also runs his own training/nutritional consultation firm that boasts dozens of professional and amateur athletes.

2. *Scrawny to Brawny:* One of the most comprehensive books to date on muscle-building training and nutrition. Cowritten by Dr. Berardi, this book contains shopping lists, meal plans, and even recipes and would be an excellent addition to anyone's training library.

Nutritional needs aside for the moment, let's get back to the business of training. This program will have you working out four times per week by doing different upper- and lower-body workouts. We chose 4 days because many experts now feel that it's a muscle's frequency of exposure to a training stimulus, rather than just the intensity of that stimulus, that leads to greater improvements in hypertrophy (muscle growth). Don't get us wrong—you still have to train hard! It's just that you'll probably see better results working your chest moderately hard twice per week, as opposed to obliterating it once every 7 to 9 days.

In addition, these four weekly workouts will allow you to include a substantial amount of training volume (total number of sets, reps, and exercises), yet still keep the workouts relatively brief. This is important because keeping your workouts in the 45- to 60-minute range has been shown to bring about a greater increase in anabolic (muscle building) hormones than longer, more drawn-out training sessions. In fact, the latter can even increase your body's secretion of cortisol—a catabolic, or "muscle wasting," hormone. These workouts were therefore designed to be relatively quick and intense. Don't worry if they seem quite different from what your fellow muscle-heads are doing. You can rest assured that you're the one on the right path.

As we did with the fat-loss workout, we'd like to lay out some parameters before you start:

- You'll be doing two different styles of training for both your upper- and lower-body workouts. Your first upper-body workout will be comprised of antagonistic supersets—or exercises that involve muscles that work

in direct opposition to each other, such as a bench press and a cable row. This will allow for improved recovery between sets, since one set of muscles must relax in order for the others to work.

- Your second upper-body workout, which will come later in the week, will involve compound, or giant, sets. These are essentially supersets in which two or three exercises for the same muscle groups are strung together into one long set. An example here would be a bench press followed by an incline dumbbell press, finished off with a cable crossover. This technique brings about a much deeper state of fatigue and can often serve as the catalyst for new growth.

- Your lower-body workouts will follow a much different format. Because most of the exercises involve all of the major lower-body muscles working together, antagonist supersets are pretty much out of the question. We've therefore set it up so that you'll be doing straight sets: One day you'll work your legs with heavy loads and higher reps and the next will test your endurance to a far greater extent. This will provide your lower body with two unique yet extremely effective types of stimuli for muscle growth.

- Because we want to maximize the secretion of anabolic hormones during the workout, you're going to keep your rest intervals relatively brief—60 seconds after each exercise. So if you're supersetting a bench press and a cable row, you'd rest 60 seconds after the bench press, then go immediately to the row. After resting another 60 seconds, it would be back to the bench press, and so on. This protocol will make sure the workouts are completed in a very time-efficient manner. For your lower-body workouts, rest a full 2 minutes between sets on your heavy day (Workout B) and only 60 seconds between sets on your lighter day (Workout D).

- Seeing as how the goal of this phase is to gain muscle mass, you won't want to get too carried away with the cardio. A couple of brief interval workouts lasting 15 to 20 minutes in duration should help you maintain cardiovascular fitness without cutting into your muscle gains—provided, of course, you account for the added energy expenditure in your daily caloric consumption.

The Workout

Perform the following workout four times per workout on a nonrotating schedule: A/B/C/D, allowing at least

48 to 72 hours between workouts for the same muscle groups. (Upper- and lower-body workouts can be performed on back-to-back days if your schedule dictates.) Please note that while the upper-body exercises will be comprised entirely of supersets, the lower-body workouts will be done as straight sets.

Note: You can throw in a couple of different core exercises at the end of these workouts, or on off days, three times per week. Try and keep it to no more than two or three exercises per workout, and keep the sets (1 to 2) and the reps (8 to 20) manageable.

WORKOUT A

A-1 Bench Press or Machine Chest Press 3 × 6–8
A-2 Cable Row 3 × 6–10

B-1 Bulgarian Split Squat 4 × 6
B-2 Pullup or Lat Pulldown 3 × 6–8
B-3 Military or Machine Shoulder Press 3 × 6–8

C-1 Barbell Upright Row 3 × 6–8
C-2 Dip 3 × 6–8

WORKOUT B

A-1 Front Squat 5 × 5
A-2 Romanian Deadlift 5 × 5

B-1 Glute Ham Raise 4 × 6

WORKOUT C

A-1 Incline Barbell or Incline Machine Press 2 × 4–6
A-2 Flat Dumbbell Press 2 × 6–10

A-3 Cable Crossover 2 × 12–15
A-4 Cable Pull Through 3 × 10–12
B-1 Neutral Grip Pullup or Lat Pulldown 2 × 4–6
B-2 Dumbbell Prone Row 2 × 6–10
B-3 Reverse Fly 2 × 12–15

C-1 Barbell Hang Clean 2 × 4–6
C-2 Dumbbell Shoulder Press 2 × 6–10
D-1 E-Z Barbell Preacher Curl 2 × 8–10
D-2 Dumbbell Overhead Triceps Extension 2 × 8–10
D-3 Lateral Raise 2 × 12–15

WORKOUT D

Barbell Squat 4 × 10–12
Leg Curl 4 × 8–10
Dumbbell Lunge 3 × 10–12 per side
Standing Calf Raise 3 × 8–12

THERE'S STRENGTH IN NUMBERS: 6-WEEK STRENGTH-BUILDING PROGRAM

Who cares about being strong anyway? It's not as if you want to be like those big, brutish guys who strut around the gym in cutoff flannel shirts, wearing work boots and screaming their heads off as they lift ridiculously heavy amounts of weight. Besides, between your interval cardio and supersetting from one exercise to the next, you're doing everything you can to ensure a better quality of life through regular exercise. Or are you? If you never train with the express goal of trying to become stronger, how can you truly say you're covering all of your physiological bases?

We know what you're going to say, " . . . but the lifting I do now has got to be making me stronger." Agreed. You'll get no argument from us that lifting on a regular basis will improve strength to some degree. It will certainly improve strength endurance, or the ability to lift submaximal weights repeatedly.

This can come in awfully handy when you're loading a bunch of stuff into your car or walking bags of fertilizer across the yard. What happens, though, when you need to lift something with a little more heft to it? Like loading a heavy suitcase onto the luggage rack of your SUV or lifting a keg up off the ground? Do you really think doing the typical 3 sets of 10 reps is going to help with tasks like that?

We're not saying you have to become a powerlifter or anything like that. All we're suggesting is that you occasionally work with some heavier loads to both boost your body's performance potential and enhance your appearance. Oh sure, that got your attention! Well, you read it right—working with heavy loads can lead to greater increases in size for two reasons: 1) Heavy loads in the 1 to 5 repetition range target your type IIb fast twitch fibers, the ones with the greatest potential for growth, and 2) strength builds endurance. Let's say for instance that you can press 50-pound dumbbells for 10 reps. Then, after a 6-week strength program like the one featured here, you can suddenly press the 60-pound dumbbells for the same 10 reps. Do you suppose that keeping your muscles under a heavier load for the same time frame might lead to some increased growth?

Now, before you go around the gym testing how much you can lift, let's first establish a few ground rules.

- Because lifting maximal weights can be extremely tough (not to mention potentially dangerous without a spotter), you'll be sticking mainly in the 3 to 5 repetition range during this phase of your training.
- Working with heavy loads means you'll need more

recovery time between sets. The stored chemical energy in your body that provides the bulk of the fuel for these brief, albeit high-intensity, efforts, takes a few minutes to replenish. So count on taking a full 2- to 3-minute rest intervals between sets.

- Don't be afraid to ask for a spot if you need one. Most of your fellow gym members would be happy to oblige. Just be ready to return the favor when they ask.

- Since your cardiovascular system doesn't exactly get taxed during a typical strength program, a little extra cardio wouldn't hurt during this phase. Plus, you'll be dropping your number of lifting days from 4 down to 3, so a little extra activity would probably be a good thing. Therefore three to four interval workouts per week should work well.

The Workout

Perform this workout three times per week, doing each of the three workouts in succession: A/B/C, with at least 24 hours rest between training sessions. Rest a full 2 to 3 minutes between sets of the first three exercises of the workout and 90 seconds between sets of the last two, which focus on smaller, yet extremely important muscles like those of the rotator cuff. Cardio can be done either after your workout or on off days from lifting.

WORKOUT A
Squat 5 × 3–5
Pullup 5 × 3–5
Military Press 5 × 3–5
*Russian Twist 2 × 10–12
Back Extension 2 × 10–12
WORKOUT B
Bench Press 5 × 3–5
Romanian Deadlift 5 × 3–5
One-Arm Row 5 × 3–5
Weighted Situp 2 × 8–10
*Cable External Rotation 2 × 10–12
WORKOUT C
Deadlift 5 × 3–5
Dip 5 × 3–5
Split Squat 5 × 3–5
*Saxon Side Bend 2 × 8–10
Standing Calf Raise 2 × 10–12
*Perform that number of reps to each side.

FIT FOR LIFE:
8-WEEK TOTAL-FITNESS WORKOUT

Okay, so maybe your goals aren't quite as specific as the others we've covered so far. You like the idea of burning fat, wouldn't mind adding some extra muscle tone, and appreciate the importance of being strong. What you're not necessarily on board with is the idea of devoting a set time frame to one specific goal. After all, who says you can't have it all—strength, flexibility, cardiovascular fitness, and a butt you could bounce a quarter off? So if you're more into overall fitness, the following workout should be just what you're looking for.

Because this is a workout that includes various aspects of fitness in a single training session, at somewhat lesser intensities than the previous more specified programs, the need for recovery won't be as great. You'll therefore be able to train anywhere between four to six times per week, depending on your schedule. Before you begin, though, here are a few things to keep in mind.

- Because you'll be looking to achieve a variety of objectives with your strength training, you'll be working with a variety of repetition ranges during your workout. This will mean alternating between lower and higher rep work to stimulate different types of muscle fibers.

- Similar guidelines should also be followed with your cardio workouts. While intervals are still the preferred way to go, sprinkling in a few longer, lower-intensity workouts will offer a nice change of pace.

The Workout

Do the following three workouts on a rotating schedule regardless of how many times per week you train. Workouts can be done on successive days; just be sure you rest at least 1 or 2 days per week. Perform Workout A as supersets, doing the 6-rep load for each exercise and then resting 60 seconds before doing the 12-rep load. Then proceed on to the next pairing. This will be followed by a core circuit and a brief interval workout. Workout B will be done as a circuit, where you go immediately from one exercise to the next until you finish them all. You'll then rest 60 to 90 seconds before going around again. This will be followed by 30 minutes of steady-state cardio. Finally, in Workout C your goal will be increased mobility.

All of the exercises will have a heavy flexibility component, yet still emphasize strength and cardiovascular fitness. The exercises here will once again be performed as paired supersets. This time, though, you'll go immediately from one exercise to the next and rest 60 seconds after each pairing. As far as cardio goes, this time you'll do a form of interval training that's more taxing to your aerobic energy system and lasts somewhat longer than the interval training in Workout A.

WORKOUT A	WORKOUT B	WORKOUT C
Squat or Leg Press × 6/× 12	Dumbbell Thruster × 15–20	Overhead Squat × 10–12
Pullup or Lat Pulldown × 6/× 12	Dumbbell Stepup × 1 minute per leg	Rotational T-Pushup × 10–12
Rowing machine × 2 minutes	Barbell Reverse Lunge × 12 per leg (alternating)	Bulgarian Split Squat × 8–10
Lunge × 6/× 12	Vertical Knee Raise × 12–15	Saxon Side Bend × 8–10
Dumbbell Incline Bench Press × 6/× 12	Elliptical Machine × 2 minutes	Pike Walk × 6
Dumbbell or Machine Bench Press × 12–15	Chinup or Lat Pulldown × 10–12	Stability Ball Leg Curl × 8–10
Leg Curl × 6/× 12	Rest 60–90 seconds and repeat	Russian Twist × 10–12
Military Press × 6/× 12		
Interval Cardio 15–20 minutes		
Work to Rest Ratio 1:3 (i.e., 20 seconds high intensity: 60 seconds low intensity)		
Cable Woodchopper × 10–12 per side		Bent-Over Row with Back Extension × 8–10
Lateral Raise × 15–20		
Core Circuit: 2 rounds		
Incline Board Reverse Crunch × 10–12		
Dumbbell Russian Twist × 10–12		
Back Extension × 10–12		
Interval Cardio 15–20 minutes	Steady Paced Cardio × 30 minutes	Cardio: Interval Training 28–32 minutes
Work to Rest Ratio 1:3 (i.e., 20 seconds high intensity: 60 seconds low intensity)		Work to rest ratio 1:1 (i.e., 2 minutes work: 2 minutes active recovery 7–8 intervals)

CHAPTER FIFTEEN

CARDIO EQUIPMENT DEMYSTIFIED

Pick and Choose the Right One for You

FINDING THE CARDIO AREA OF ANY gym is easy. Just keep walking until you find yourself in what looks like an assembly line of sweat.

Stare down the chorus line of rows and rows of cardiovascular machines and you'll see rows and rows of out-of-breath exercisers. Whether they're plugged into their iPods, texting on their phones, putting their nose in a magazine, or pulling a neck muscle watching TV as they exercise, they all have one thing in common. They all hope that when their time is up, they'll be getting off whatever cardio machine they've been huffing and puffing on just a few ounces lighter in the body fat department.

Walking into that arena can be pretty intense and intimidating for the first-time gym goer, especially since most decent gyms offer you a selection of cardio machines to choose from—such as treadmills, stationary cycles, stairclimbers, etc. Seeing all those machines—and all those choices—can make it difficult to decide which one to pick. But knowing your way around cardio machines in your gym isn't as hard as you think it is.

Here's lesson #1: The more options your gym offers, the more of a mix of different manufacturers you will probably end up seeing that may confuse you. That's

because most manufacturers only specialize in certain types of cardio machines, but may not manufacture all types. Precor. Life Fitness. Landice. ProForm. Star Trac. Cybex. StairMaster. Did we mention any brand you recognize in your gym? The good news is that as a gym member, it really doesn't matter.

Maybe the machine you're starting on has a built-in touch screen and a wireless heart rate monitor. In that case, lucky you! Maybe the cardio equipment in your gym barely has room to hold a water bottle or even a magazine. If that's your situation, then that's okay—we'll make that work for you, too.

Look, it really doesn't matter what brand or type of cardio equipment your gym invested their money into. The only thing that counts is making sure that you're prepared for every possible situation. That's why we're going to teach you how to use any machine—no matter whom it's made by or what its price tag was—so you always know what you're doing, and more important, always burn the most calories in the least amount of time.

TREADMILLS

Great for: Burning the most calories in less time. Because of the full-body effort it requires, running is one of the most effective ways to burn calories, especially when you compare it to most cardio machine exercises. (To see the difference, see the sidebar about calorie expenditure at the end of this chapter.)

THE 3 RULES OF CARDIO EQUIPMENT

No matter which machine you decide to start with, there are several important things to remember when using any piece of aerobic equipment.

1. WARM UP FOR 5 MINUTES BEFOREHAND

You may be anxious to lose fat, but your body's not anxious to get hurt. That's why you need to warm up your muscles before you start. Set the machine at a low level or slow setting and exercise for 5 minutes. On the treadmill, that may mean a brisk walk before running. On the cycle, stair-climber, or elliptical machine, that means placing the machine on level 1 or 2. On the rowing machine, that equates to setting the tension on its lowest setting or rowing at a much slower speed than usual.

2. GIVE EVERY MACHINE A 2-WEEK TEST DRIVE

Most cardio machines offer a certain amount of preprogrammed workouts built in. With the push of a button, you can change the speed, level, incline, etc., of a machine, depending on which one you're using. These programs vary from manufacturer to manufacturer—some of the names run from "heart rate hill," "fat burn," and "speed interval jogger"—so it's hard to say which ones you may encounter. Still, these can be terrific ways to change up your workouts, so we encourage you to try them eventually.

However, before trying any of the built-in programs, use the machine on your own for a few weeks to get a hang of the controls. Most machines have a button that just reads "START" or "QUICK START" on it. Hit this button, then apply the advice offered in this chapter on how to vary your workout intensity. After a few weeks, you should feel familiar enough with the machine—and its buttons—to give its programs a shot.

3. SWITCH MACHINES EVERY 3 TO 4 WEEKS

If you are looking to burn calories long-term and stay injury-free, mix up which machine—or activity—you use every 3 to 4 weeks. Too many people get stuck in a rut when they stick with the same piece of cardio equipment every time they exercise. Besides the boredom factor, there are two other reasons why this is never a good idea:

The first reason is that doing the same routine every time you exercise will eventually cause you to burn fewer and fewer calories as your body learns to work more efficiently to perform those specific movements. Just as they do during resistance training, your muscles—including your heart—will quickly adjust to the demands you place on them when training them aerobically. Eventually, they adjust accordingly and improve only the muscle fibers necessary for performing an activity. Increased speed and effort level are the only components that help you continue to burn calories. The rest of your body never gets a chance to work as hard or burn excess fat and calories.

The second reason is that using the same muscles over and over again overuses them—or makes them stronger than other muscles, causing a muscular imbalance. Both situations can lead to aches, pains, and possible injury—just the thing to shorten or stop your future workouts altogether.

Bad for: Anyone with a knee problem. Every time your foot hits the ground, the impact places pressure on your leg that's equal to up to five times your body weight. Running on a quality treadmill can lessen that slightly, but not by much. According to research from the American Academy of Orthopaedic Surgeons, in-shape runners without knee problems rarely suffer from repetitive injuries, but those with knee problems who run only increase the damage to their knees.

Master the controls: The majority of treadmills give

you two options to change your workout intensity: speed (shown in miles per hour—raised in 1/10 mph increments, such as 5 mph, 5.1 mph, 5.2 mph, etc.) and incline (broken down typically in half-point degrees, such as .5 percent, 1 percent, 1.5 percent, 2 percent, etc.). Raising or lowering either one—or both—of these options as you run increases or decreases the intensity of your workout.

Make the right adjustments: Even if you have no intention of raising the height of the treadmill during your workout, studies have shown that you should at least set the incline at 1 percent as you run. A treadmill pulls the ground underneath you, plus being indoors means your body doesn't feel any wind resistance, two factors that make running indoors on a treadmill slightly easier. This tweak in elevation compensates for that loss, making it just as effective as running outdoors.

Check your form: Keep your head and chest up, your shoulders back, and your abs flat. Maintaining an upright position at all times will keep your weight distributed evenly as you move, preventing you from fatiguing certain muscles that could tire out before the rest of you is ready to stop. Also, pump your arms back and forth to help propel your body forward. The faster you move your arms, the faster your feet will move, so as you speed up, make sure your arms move just as vigorously.

Each time your foot hits the treadmill, try to land softly on each heel, roll forward on your foot, and push off with your toes. This helps to absorb the shock while it adds more push-off to your stride. Finally, don't worry about the length of your stride. If your stride feels normal and you're not noticing any unusual pain or discomfort, you're probably moving in the right way. Instead, just allow your feet to land where they want to—or else you can easily shift your natural body mechanics off center, making the exercise less effective and increasing your risk of injury.

Try Out These Workouts for Size
BEGINNER

1. Set the incline at a 1-percent grade and warm up at a low-intensity speed (3.5 to 4.5 mph) for 5 minutes.

2. Increase your speed to a higher pace until you reach a point that makes it uncomfortable to talk and run at the same time. Maintain this pace for 1 to 2 minutes.

3. Reduce your speed back down to a lower level that's easy for you to maintain. Continue for 4 minutes.

4. Bring the speed back up to the previous higher pace for another 1 to 2 minutes.

5. Continue flipping back and forth for the length of your workout.

6. Complete your workout with a cooldown walk, setting the machine at 2.5 to 3 mph.

INTERMEDIATE

1. Warm up for 5 minutes at a low-intensity speed (3.5 to 4.5 mph).

2. Set the treadmill at a comfortable pace you could normally maintain for 30 minutes (5.5 mph, for example) and run for 1 minute.

3. Raise the incline by 1 percent and run for another minute.

4. Continue raising the incline by 1 percent every minute until your treadmill is set at a 5 percent incline, and run for 2 minutes. Lower the level of incline by 1 percent, while increasing your speed by 2/10 mph. (For example, if you were running at 5.5 mph at a 5 percent incline, you should now be running at 5.7 mph at a 4 percent incline.)

5. Run at this new setting for 1 minute, then repeat the process, lowering the incline 1 percent while increasing your speed by 2/10 mph. Keep decreasing the level of incline by 1 percent and raising your speed 2/10 mph every minute until your treadmill is back at a 1 percent incline. Run at this new setting for 2 minutes.

6. Finally, increase the incline by 1 percent, lowering your speed by 2/10 mph. Run at this new pace for 1 minute. Continue increasing the incline 1 percent while lowering your speed by 2/10 mph every minute until you're back running at a 5 percent incline.

7. Run for 2 minutes, then lower the incline 1 percent each minute, leaving the speed where it's at as you go, until you're back running at a 1 percent incline.

8. Run for another 3 minutes, then end your workout with a 5-minute run at a low-intensity speed (3.5 to 4.5 mph).

ADVANCED

1. Set the incline at a 1 percent grade and warm up at a low-intensity speed (3.5 to 4.5 mph) for 5 minutes.

2. Adjust the speed to 5 mph and run for 1 minute.

3. Raise your speed by 2/10 mph and run for 3 minutes.

4. Continue to raise your speed by 2/10 mph every 3 minutes until you reach a speed you could only maintain for 5 to 10 minutes.

5. Keep running at this speed for 3 minutes, then lower your speed back down to 5 mph and run for 1 minute.

6. Raise the incline to 3 percent and begin increasing your speed 2/10 mph every 3 minutes until you reach a pace that you could maintain for 5 to 10 minutes.

7. Keep running at this speed for 3 minutes, then lower your speed back to 5 mph and run for 1 minute.

8. Increase the incline to 5 percent and raise your speed 2/10 mph.

9. Continue to raise the incline every 3 minutes until you reach a speed that's difficult to maintain for more than 5 minutes.

10. Run at this pace for 3 minutes, then return your speed back to 5 mph.

11. Run for 3 minutes, then lower your incline 1 percent each minute until you're once again at a 1 percent incline.

12. End your workout with a 5-minute run at a low-intensity speed (3.5 to 4.5 mph).

STATIONARY BIKE

Great for: Balancing out the muscles of the legs and/or for the heavier exerciser. Because the treadmill tends to be the number one choice of many exercisers, most people end up with imbalanced legs. That's because running strengthens your hamstrings—the muscles behind your thighs—instead of the quadriceps, the muscles in front of them. Over time, having stronger hamstrings and weaker quadriceps can cause a muscular tug-of-war with your kneecaps, which can lead to knee pain and/or injury. Cycling focuses on the quadriceps, helping you balance out your leg muscles so both sets are good and strong. Plus, it's not a load-bearing activity like running, so your legs—mainly your knees, ankles, and feet—are spared any unnecessary pounding.

Bad for: Those looking to lose weight fast. Whether you're using a regular stationary cycle or a recumbent one—the type with a backrest on it—there's still no way to get your arms involved in the exercise. That prevents your upper body from getting any type of workout, which is why you burn fewer calories per hour than other machines that force you to use your entire body.

Master the controls: There are two ways to change the intensity of your ride: You can raise the level, which increases the amount of resistance on the pedals—or you can pedal faster. Your pedal speed shows up as rpms (rotations per minute) on the bike's monitor—if it has one.

Make the right adjustments: First, adjust your seat height. Your legs should never be entirely straight in a locked-knee position. Your seat should be low enough—or back far enough, if you're in a recumbent bike—to allow for a slight bend in your knees, even when you have your leg fully extended by pushing all the way down on the pedal. Once you have the height right, check how even it is. The angle of the seat should be level. If it's tilted too far up, it can put pressure in places between your legs that don't need impinging. If it's tilted too far down, it can cause your body to shift forward, a position that can add stress on your knees (and well as your arms and hands if you use the handlebars).

Finally, slip your feet through the foot straps. They let you pull the pedals up as you ride, instead of just pushing them down. This gets all your leg muscles involved, so you'll have the energy to work out longer and burn more calories.

Check your form: Keep your back straight and your head lifted and look forward over the handlebars—this keeps your neck in line with your spine so you can breathe easier for more energy. As you pedal, focus on

MAKE YOUR MUSIC WORK FOR YOU

Don't just hit shuffle on your media player. First, make a playlist of all your favorite songs—enough to last a minimum of a week's worth of cardio workouts (at least 5 hours worth). Next, take the time to listen to them for a few seconds each and keep only those with a tempo between 90 and 110 beats per minute or higher—just tap your foot to each song, count how many times you tap your foot in 10 seconds and times that by 6! Finally, arrange them from your least favorite tune to your most coveted songs. Why? As you exercise, each song you hear will be more motivating than the next, giving you a boost as you begin to lose steam.

cycling in circles rather than mashing your feet down on each pedal. Instead, you want to concentrate on pushing down with one foot as you simultaneously pull the other foot in—that way, you'll work both legs with every rotation.

Once you get moving, focus on, well, what's moving! Your upper body should remain still as you ride. If it's rocking from side to side, you could be putting excess stress on your lower back. Another helpful trick: Try to breathe in sync with your pedaling. Instead of just cycling away, concentrate on breathing in for a four-count (or four full rotations) and breathing out for a four-count. If you pick up the pace, you can speed up your breathing to a three- or two-count—so long as it's in rhythm with your pedaling. Keeping them synced ensures you'll get plenty of oxygen for energy, whether you're looking to use that energy to exercise for a longer period of time, or, need that stamina for more intense, shorter duration workouts.

Try Out These Workouts For Size
BEGINNER

Start with a long warmup of 5 minutes, setting the bike at level 3 to 4. Keep your rpms (rotations per minute) between 80 and 100.

1. Raise the resistance to a level that feels challenging for 15 seconds. Keep your rpms at 90.

2. Lower the resistance to a comfortable level (3 to 6) and cycle for 45 seconds. Raise your rpms to 100.

3. Keep the resistance at a comfortable level but lower your speed to 90 to 100 rpms and continue for 1 minute.

(Repeat 10 times for a 20-minute workout; 15 times for a 30 minute workout.)

INTERMEDIATE

Start with the same 5-minute warmup in the beginner's plan.

1. Raise the resistance to level 7 to 9, increasing your rpms to 110 to 120. Hold this speed for 20 seconds.

2. Decrease your speed to 80 to 100 rpms and pedal for another 20 seconds.

3. Increase your speed to 110 to 120 rpms and pedal for 40 seconds.

4. Lower the speed to 80 to 100 rpms and continue for another 40 seconds.

5. Increase your speed to 110 to 120 rpms and pedal for 1 minute.

6. Lower the speed to 80 to 100 rpms and continue for another minute.

7. Increase your speed to 110 to 120 rpms and pedal for 40 seconds.

8. Lower the speed back down to 80 to 100 rpms and continue for another 40 seconds.

9. Increase your speed to 110 to 120 rpms and pedal for 20 seconds.

10. Lower the speed to 80 to 100 rpms and continue for another 20 seconds.

11. Lower the resistance to level 4 or 5 for 1 minute (80 to 100 rpms).

(Repeat the 11-part cycle three times for a 20-minute workout; four times for a 30-minute workout.)

ADVANCED

Start with the same 5-minute warmup in the beginner's plan.

1. Raise the resistance to the highest level you can handle and pedal for 30 seconds, keeping your rpms at 80.

2. Lower the resistance one level, pedal for 30 seconds, raising your rpms to 90.

3. Lower the resistance one level, pedal for 30 seconds, raising your rpms to 100.

4. Lower the resistance one level, pedal for 30 seconds, raising your rpms to 110.

5. Lower the resistance one level, pedal for 30 seconds, lowering your rpms to 90.

(Repeat the 5-part cycle eight times for a 20-minute workout; 12 times for a 30-minute workout.)

STAIRCLIMBER

Great for: Building quality muscle as you burn calories. Aptly named, stairclimbers mimic actual stair climbing, an activity that helps build lean muscle throughout your hips, thighs, buttocks, and calves. That alone can save you from having to train your legs as hard in the weight room. In addition, the machine is designed in a way that places less impact and pressure on your knees, so it's less abusive to your body than the real thing.

Bad for: Those with self-esteem issues. Because most people associate the stairclimber as being great for shaping the butt muscles, some people have a hang-up using them, for fear that other exercisers might think they're on one to reshape their rear end. If that's you, we say, "Get over it!" That's just a side perk that comes with using this effective, calorie-burning machine. Even though, let's face it, most people could benefit from building a better butt regardless.

Master the controls: There's really only one way to adjust most stairclimbers and that's by level. The higher the level, the less tension you'll feel on the footpads—which makes them drop faster under your own body weight. The faster they drop, the faster you're forced to step to keep up the pace.

Make the right adjustments: The good news is that whether you're 5 foot 2 or 6 foot 8, one size fits all with a stairclimber, so just step on and start sweating. Just make sure your entire foot is on each step—letting your heels hang off can cause a numbness and/or discomfort in your feet as you go.

Check your form: As you exercise, keep your head and chest up and your back straight. Bending your neck to look down at your feet can tire you out much faster by limiting your air flow—if you have to look down, you're more than likely going too fast for your level of expertise.

Each step should be slow and deep as you push through with your entire foot—the deeper you step, the more muscles you'll use, which in turn burns more calories. If you find yourself taking smaller, shorter, quicker

DON'T SKIP THIS OPPORTUNITY!

That jump rope in your gym may not have a built-in TV screen, 35 preprogrammed routines, and a long line waiting to use it, but there's one thing it does have—and that's respect. Skipping rope burns serious calories, lets you exercise practically anywhere you want, and strengthens your legs, all while improving your agility, eye-hand coordination, and foot/hand speed.

Just don't make the mistake of thinking that the higher you jump, the better your workout will be. It's not how high you jump, but for how long that makes the greatest difference. So when you're ready to show off your skills in the gym, hop only as high as needed—**about an inch or two**—and land on your toes to absorb the shock throughout your calf muscles. Leaping any higher than that—or coming down flatfooted—only places excess stress on your knees and slows down your pace, burning less calories while increasing your risk of injury.

steps, you're probably pushing down only with the balls of your feet, which puts more effort onto your calves and uses less of your leg muscles. This technique will make your smaller calf muscles tire out much faster than your larger legs muscles (quadriceps, hamstrings, and glutes), causing you to quit sooner and burn fewer calories.

Also, don't expect to have your body in perfect alignment from head to toe. Even though you should be standing upright, it's entirely natural to be leaning slightly forward, which will prevent you from placing undue stress on your knees and lower back.

Finally, don't make the mistake of supporting yourself with the railings on your stairclimber. Leaning on the machine takes away a percentage of your body weight from the workout, which can cause you to burn up to 30 percent fewer calories than usual. If you absolutely have to hold on, try placing your fingertips lightly on either the side rails or the bar in front of you. If you find that you need to grip either tightly or can't seem to step without putting a lot of weight onto your fingers, the machine is most likely set on a higher level you may not be ready for just yet. Try lowering the level and speed of your steps until you can manage without needing to hold on to anything.

Try Out These Workouts For Size
BEGINNER

Warm up at a low level (2 or 3 to start) for 5 minutes.

1. Raise the level to a setting that feels comfortable and step for as many minutes as you can. Try to build yourself up to a total of at least 20 minutes each session.

INTERMEDIATE

Start with the same 5-minute warmup in the beginner's plan.

1. Raise the level one notch and step for 30 seconds.

2. Keep raising the level one notch every 30 seconds until you reach a level that's hard to maintain for an entire 30 seconds.

3. Lower the level back down to your warmup level (2 or 3) and step for 30 seconds.

(Repeat this three-part routine for the length of your workout.)

ADVANCED

Start with the same 5-minute warmup in the beginner's plan.

1. Raise the level two notches and step for 30 seconds.

2. Keep raising the level two notches every 30 seconds until you reach a level that's hard to maintain. Try to maintain this level for as long as you can.

3. Lower the level down three notches and step for 1 minute.

(Keep repeating steps 2 and 3 over again for the length of your workout; you should end up exercising at an even higher level toward the middle of this cycle.)

ELLIPTICAL TRAINER

Great for: Runners with knee problems. An elliptical machine offers the same type of workout that running does by challenging primarily the same muscle groups. But what makes it better is that because your feet stay on the footpads, there's no stress on your knees to worry about. It's also capable of burning up to 700 calories an hour, improving your overall balance, and toning your muscles from head to toe (including your legs, glutes, chest, back, shoulders, arms, and core) simultaneously.

Bad for: Those with balance issues. There's a certain "glide" to elliptical machines that takes a little practice to master. If you're the type that doesn't like to feel silly, you may want to try getting the hang of the machine when fewer gym members are around.

Master the controls: Most machines offer you only two ways to up your intensity. You can increase the level of resistance—which makes it more difficult for the pedals to rotate—or you can simply try moving your legs faster. Some elliptical machines also have poles attached that let you grab hold and pump with your arms at the same time—this advantage can get your heart pumping even faster. More high-end ellipticals even let you adjust the incline like a treadmill—which can range from 0 percent to 10 percent. Because that's not a feature that's as common on most machines, the workouts suggested in this chapter work whether you have that option or not.

Make the right adjustments: Most ellipticals are like stairclimbers, designed for anyone to jump aboard. Still, if you have very long legs—or short ones—you may need to adjust the stride length on the machine a few times until you get the best length for your body

(16 to 19 inches works best for most people).

Next, step up onto the machine and place your feet flat on the center of each pedal to start. Your feet don't have to stay centered, but it's a smart starting point. So if they feel more comfortable more forward or back further on the pad as you use the machine, just do what feels best for your body.

Lastly, grab the arm poles at the height of your shoulders. If you're a shorter guy, this may mean grabbing the poles below the handles, but don't sweat. You'll be doing your form a favor by placing your arms at a height that will help your stride when you finally get moving.

Check your form: Your stride should be similar to how you would run on a treadmill. As you go, stand straight and always look forward (never at your feet). Also, keep your feet flat on the pedals at all times—this isn't just for safety reasons, but it also splits up the workload more evenly throughout your legs, so you use more muscle fibers—and burn more calories—as you glide.

As you glide, avoid hunching forward—your shoulders should be back with your body in an upright position in line with your hips. Also, keep your weight on your heels and focus on rolling through your foot (instead of keeping your heels off the pad the entire time) to give your legs more of a workout (and keep your calves from becoming exhausted before the rest of your leg muscles).

When holding the handles, try not to grip them too loosely. The best way to incorporate more upper-body muscles (and burn more calories) is by grabbing them firmly and pumping your arms back and forth the same way you would when running. You'll improve your balance, engage more of your core, and burn more overall calories by involving more upper-body muscles.

Finally, no matter how tempted you may be to do it, avoid looking down at your feet. Instead, focus straight ahead—at either something directly in front of you or on the screen—since looking down will only impair your breathing (so you have less energy) and throw off your balance.

Try Out These Workouts For Size
BEGINNER

Warm up at a low level (2 or 3 to start) for 5 minutes.

1. Raise the level to a setting that feels comfortable and glide for as many minutes as you can. Try to build yourself up to a total of at least 20 minutes each session.

Note: If you feel yourself bouncing as you glide, then add a little more resistance.

INTERMEDIATE/ADVANCED

Start with the same 5-minute warmup in the beginner's plan.

1. Raise the level one notch and glide for 30 seconds.

2. Reverse the motion—so that you're gliding backward instead of forward—for 30 seconds.

3. Keep repeating steps 1 and 2 so that you glide 30 seconds forward and 30 seconds backward at a level one notch higher than the last time. Once you reach a level that's hard to maintain for an entire 30 seconds—either forward or backward—lower the level back down to your warmup level (2 or 3) and glide for 30 seconds.

(Repeat this three-part routine for the length of your workout.)

ROWING MACHINE

Great for: Getting a full-body workout. Indoor rowing pulls off what most cardiovascular machines can't, which is to train your upper and lower body at the same time, as well as your core. It's the reason why—on average—it can burn up to 800 calories an hour. It's also a nonimpact activity that's much easier on the knees than most cardio machines and activities.

Bad for: Those with lower back problems or poor coordination. The rowing machine is a great exercise for strengthening the lower back, but it's a fast way to aggravate it if you already have problems. Also, it's a machine that requires more coordination between your upper and lower body, so if you're easily frustrated, be warned—it may take a few tries to master the motion.

Master the controls: There are only two ways to change the intensity on most rowing machines. You can increase the tension, which makes it harder to pull back the bar, or you can simply row faster.

Make the right adjustments: Strap your feet into the footrests and make sure the straps are tight enough that your feet are secure and don't move when you begin to row. Grab the handle firmly, but not too tight, with both hands, palms facing down. Your butt should sit flat in the sliding seat; keep your ankles almost perpendicular to the floor. Your head should be up, with your arms straight in front of you.

LEARN HOW TO BURN!

Whether your reason to jump on a cardio machine is to burn fat, strengthen your heart and lungs, reduce your risk of developing heart disease—or pull off all three—then you need to understand one simple fact: **To see results, on average, it requires exercising at a pace that keeps your heart rate elevated at a certain level for at least 20 minutes or more.**

It's a smart strategy to stick with, but for many, it's not always easy to put in practice, especially if you're unclear about what exactly your "maximum heart rate" even is in the first place. That's where we can help.

1. FIND OUT YOUR MHR

What's an "MHR"? It's short for your maximum heart rate, which is the maximum number of beats per minute that your heart can beat in a single minute. To find that number, the easiest way to do it is to simply subtract your age from 220. (For example, if you're 40, then your MHR is 180.)

2. GET IN THE ZONE

The most common way to make the most from aerobic exercise is to elevate your heart rate so that it's beating between a range of 60 to 80 percent of your MHR for at least 20 minutes.

How do you figure out that range? Multiply your MHR by 0.6 (this is your minimum training pace). Then, multiply your MHR by 0.8 (this is your maximum training pace). The range between these two numbers is your target heart rate zone. For example, if you're 30, then your MHR would be 190. So, you would exercise at a pace that keeps your pulse between 114 (190 x 0.6) and 152 (190 x 0.8) beats per minute.

3. STAY IN THE ZONE

The easiest way to keep an eye on your pulse is by using either a heart rate monitor or a fitness tracker that can measure your pulse. Or, just do the math yourself by taking your pulse for 6 seconds as you exercise—if possible—then multiply that number by 10 to give yourself a rough estimate

---

Before you start your workout, set the machine at a low resistance, then row for a few strokes to see if the setting is right. If it's too heavy at the start, it could compromise your form early in your routine. If it's too light, it may cause you to have to interrupt the flow of your workout several times to get it right. Instead, start low, then row, then tweak the resistance until you find the perfect setting.

Check your form: Done right, the entire exercise should feel like one fluid, flowing motion. On the pulling stroke, keep your upper body leaning slightly forward and push back with your legs first. As you go, lean back slightly and pull the handle toward your midsection or directly below your chest.

On the return stroke, let the bar pull your arms straight in front of you, then bend your knees and lean slightly forward. Don't make the mistake of bending your knees up until after your hands pass them—or else you'll have to lift the bar over your kneecaps and break form. You should feel the exercise working your upper back, butt, and legs—if your lower back and/or arms get tired first, you're not doing the strokes correctly.

Don't make the mistake of just pulling with your arms. This not only robs you of burning as many calories as possible, but it also makes your upper body do all the work, placing extra stress on your lower back. Instead, try to imagine that with each stroke, your legs should be doing more than half of the work. But don't let your butt slide back too soon. Straightening your legs too quickly places undue stress on your lower back to bring your torso up into an upright position on the pulling stroke.

The normal pace: It should take less than 1 second to pull and 2 seconds to return. Shoot for 30 strokes per minute.

of how many beats per minute your ticker is pumping.

Another way to tell—start talking as you work out. If you can't even talk, you're probably overdoing it and have a pulse above 80 percent of your MHR. If you could easily speak long sentences without effort, you're most likely taking it easy and have a pulse that's below 60 percent of your MHR. But if you can speak short sentences, but wouldn't be able to sing, experts say you're probably between 60 to 80 percent of your MHR.

4. PLAY WITH THE ZONE

Even though maintaining a range of 60 to 80 percent is considered the standard, it's a gauge that can be tweaked, depending on your goals, or just for variety's sake.

Exercising below 60 percent: Keeping your MHR between 40 to 60 percent may seem like a waste of time, but maintaining a lower intensity makes it easier to work out for longer periods of time, which could help you burn more calories overall in one session.

Exercising above 80 percent: Raising your MHR above 80 percent is perfect if you're looking to improve your performance in a sport, as it helps to boost your maximum VO_2 levels (the highest amount of oxygen your body can take in during exercise).

If sports performance isn't your goal, going above and beyond your MHR is still an effective way to burn off excess body fat. How? Even though your body uses a higher amount of calories from stored fat when your pulse stays between 60 and 80 percent of your MHR, your body utilizes more total calories when you push yourself over the 80 percent mark. However, doing this too often adds stress to your body and can increase your risk of injury.

Rule of thumb: Do it in smaller increments. For example, exercise at a high intensity (above 80 percent of your MHR) for 15 seconds, then exercise at a low intensity (between 40 to 50 percent of your MHR) for 45 seconds. Repeat this 15/45 ratio for the duration of your workout. This type of training—referred to as interval training—will cause your body to blast through even more calories than usual.

Try Out These Workouts For Size
BEGINNER

Warm up by setting the machine at a low resistance and rowing slowly for 5 minutes.

1. Set the machine at a comfortable setting and row for 45 seconds. Rest for 15 seconds, then repeat the cycle for as long as you can. Don't worry if you can't go for that long to start, but try to build up to 20 minutes total.

INTERMEDIATE/ADVANCED

Start with the same 5-minute warmup in the beginner's plan.

1. Set the machine at a comfortable setting and row for 1 minute.

2. Pull the bar as hard and fast as you can for 10 strokes, then perform another 20 strokes at an easy/normal pace to recover.

3. Keep repeating this cycle—doing 10 fast/hard strokes, then 20 easy/medium strokes—for the length of your workout. (If you get to the point where 10 strokes is too hard, do as many as you can, then follow up by doing double the amount of easy strokes to recover. For example: if you can only do 9, do 18 recovery strokes, etc.)

YOUR INSTANT CARDIO COUNTER

Sometimes it's seeing how the numbers break down that decides which machines or activities you use to break a sweat. However, it's the intensity and your body weight that can also decide what cardiovascular activity you pick and, ultimately, what results you can expect to see afterward.

All of the machines described in this chapter are effective at burning calories and excess body fat, as well as strengthening your heart and improving your stamina and overall health. Later on in this book, we'll also be discussing other aerobic options—including classes—that can accomplish the same thing. To take the caloric guesswork out of all of them, this chart is your key.

We've broken down the average amount of calories your body uses per hour with every possible activity you might expect to have access to at your gym. Because your own body-weight acts as extra resistance whenever you work out, the more you weigh, the more calories you'll burn than the lighter person exercising next to you. That's why we've given you three possible body weights to choose from—just find the weight in the chart closest to your own.

Don't think you have enough energy to go an hour? That's okay—just use this fast and easy math on the numbers in this chart to find out what you burn exercising for less than 60 minutes:

- Work out for 20 minutes (divide the number by 3)
- Work out for 30 minutes (divide the number by 2)
- Work out for 45 minutes (multiply the number by 0.75)

MACHINE/CLASS/ACTIVITY	CALORIES BURNED PER HOUR		
	130 LBS.	155 LBS.	190 LBS.
Aerobics (basic)	354	422	518
Aerobics, low-impact	295	352	431
Aerobics, high-impact	413	493	604
Stationary cycling (general)	295	352	431
Stationary cycling (very light)	177	211	259
Stationary cycling (light)	325	387	474
Stationary cycling (moderate)	413	493	604
Stationary cycling (vigorous)	620	739	906
Stationary cycling (very vigorous)	738	880	1078
Boxing (punching the bag)	354	422	518
Boxing (sparring with someone)	531	633	776
Circuit training	472	563	690
Dancing	266	317	388
Martial arts	590	704	863
Racquetball (low intensity)	413	493	604
Racquetball (high intensity)	590	704	863
Rock climbing	649	774	949
Skipping rope (slow)	472	563	690
Skipping rope (moderate, general)	590	704	863

MACHINE/CLASS/ACTIVITY	CALORIES BURNED PER HOUR		
	130 LBS.	155 LBS.	190 LBS.
Skipping rope (fast)	708	844	1035
Stationary rowing (moderate)	378	483	630
Stationary rowing (vigorous)	459	586	765
Running, 5 mph	472	563	690
Running, 5.2 mph	531	633	776
Running, 6 mph	590	704	863
Running, 6.7 mph	649	774	949
Running, 7 mph	679	809	992
Running, 7.5 mph	738	880	1078
Running, 8 mph	797	950	1165
Running, 8.6 mph	826	985	1208
Running, 9 mph	885	1056	1294
Running, 10 mph	944	1126	1380
Running, 10.9 mph	1062	1267	1553
Running in place	472	563	690
Running up stairs	885	1056	1294
Stretching, hatha yoga	236	281	345
Swimming laps (light)	472	563	690
Swimming laps (fast)	590	704	863
Swimming (breaststroke)	590	704	863
Swimming (butterfly)	649	774	949
Swimming (leisurely)	354	422	518
Swimming (sidestroke)	472	563	690
Tai chi	236	281	345
Treading water (moderately)	236	281	345
Treading water (vigorously)	590	704	863
Walking, 2.0 mph	148	176	216
Walking, 3.0 mph	207	246	302
Walking, 3.5 mph	236	281	345
Walking, 4.0 mph	354	422	518
Water aerobics	236	281	345
Weightlifting (light or moderately)	177	211	259
Weightlifting (vigorously)	354	422	518

CHAPTER SIXTEEN

YANK IN THE RIGHT DIRECTION

Understanding and Implementing Stretching Techniques in Your Workout

HERE COMES THAT OBLIGATORY CHAPTER YOU see in most exercise books about the importance of stretching.

No interest in the topic, you say? Don't really care if you can touch your toes or how far you can reach back behind yourself with your arms? Even if staying limber isn't really why you joined a gym in the first place, keeping your joints, ligaments, and muscles as healthy as possible through regular stretching isn't just about helping protect yourself against any future muscle tears, strains, or injuries. Stretching your body every once in a while can make you much stronger in the long run than you would expect.

The more flexible your body is, the greater your range of motion is with each and every exercise we've just shown you. The more range you have, the more muscle fibers you call upon with each and every repetition, making them as strong as possible. Whether your goal is big and strong or lean and firm muscles, knowing the right way to pull on your muscles can help them accomplish their goals a lot faster.

FLEXIBILITY EXERCISES

As we began to explain in a preceding chapter, there are two main types of flexibility to discuss: static and dynamic.

Static flexibility is the type most people are familiar with. That's where you take a muscle into the stretched position and hold it there for 15 to 30 seconds at a time. The objective is to increase the muscle's resting length and improve the range of motion of the joint(s) that muscle acts upon. However, despite the fact that it's been the gold standard for decades, many experts now feel that it may not be a very effective way to improve mobility, which is movement efficiency—how easily you can move about.

Just because you improve the static flexibility of your hamstrings, for instance, doesn't necessarily mean you'll be able to kick higher in your martial arts class. Oh sure, it stands to reason that you would. After all, the hamstrings have increased their length, so the ability to get your leg up in the air must have improved. Or has it? You see, static flexibility increases muscle length by sending a message to the muscles (via the brain and spinal cord) to relax. When you're throwing a kick, your muscles are doing anything but relaxing. So, how do you improve your range of motion while you're in motion? For that you need dynamic flexibility.

Dynamic flexibility simply means flexibility that incorporates movement. Unlike static stretches, dynamic flexibility, or mobility drills as they're commonly known, work by gradually increasing the range of motion your muscles work through, while simultaneously firing them up for activity. That's why mobility drills like the following are the preferred way for both professional and amateur athletes to prepare for competition. Sprinkle them into your workouts between sets, or better yet, use them as part of your preworkout warmup routine. Either way, you're bound to find yourself moving better in no time.

PRISONER SQUAT

(MUSCLES STRETCHED: HIPS, CHEST)

Begin with your feet slightly wider than shoulder-width apart and your hands laced behind your head and elbows back. Begin by pushing your hips back and squatting down as you make sure your elbows stay out of your peripheral view. Pause when your thighs are parallel to the floor, then press back up.

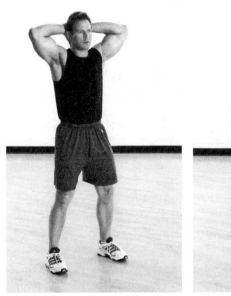

QUAD STRETCH WALK

(MUSCLES STRETCHED: QUADRICEPS)

From a standing position, grab your right instep and and pull your heel toward your butt. Hold for a second, then take a step and do the same with the other leg. Continue this way until you've covered the desired distance.

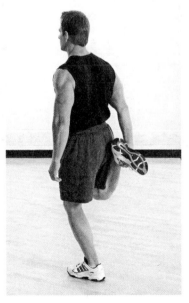
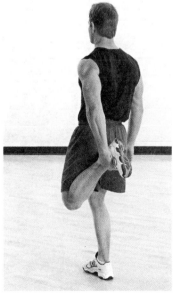

SPIDERMAN

In a pushup position, pick up your right foot and bring it around until it plants softly right next to your right hand. Simultaneously, pick up your right hand and drop your right forearm toward the floor perpendicular to your shin. As you do so, drop your left hip and knee toward the floor. Bring leg back and repeat to the other side.

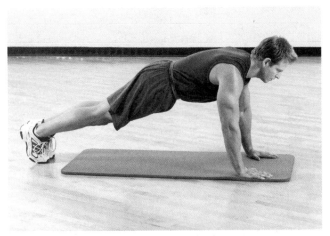
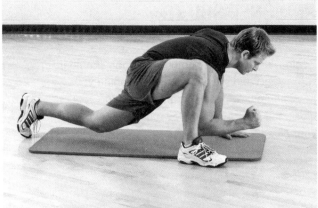

FRANKENSTEIN

With your arms held out in front of you, kick your leg straight up toward your hands without dropping your chest or rounding your back. Repeat with the other leg and continue for the desired number of reps.

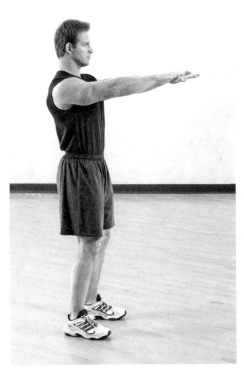
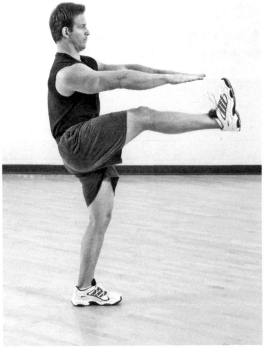

HIP WALK

(MUSCLES STRETCHED: GLUTES, PIRIFORMIS)

From a standing position, lift your right leg across the front of your body and grab your right shin. Once you have it, simultaneously pull up so the shin ends up parallel to the floor and you come up on the ball of your back foot. Lower, step forward, and repeat with the other leg.

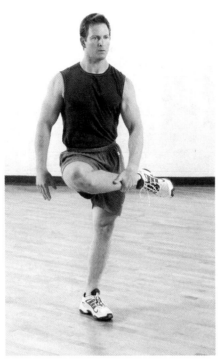
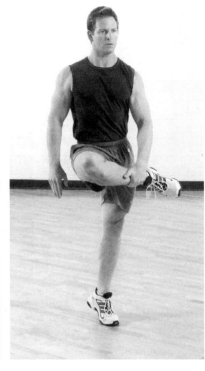

PIKE WALK

(MUSCLES STRETCHED: CALVES, HAMSTRINGS. LOWER BACK)

From a pushup position, walk your hands forward so they're well in front of your head. Keeping your legs totally straight, start walking your feet up toward your hands. Once you've gotten as close as you can, slowly walk your hands back out to the starting position.

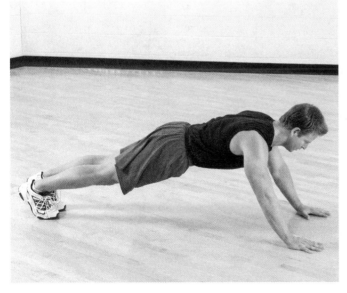
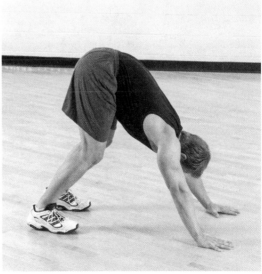

DUCK UNDER

Stand next to a bar set in a rack at approximately hip height. Begin by taking a large step under the bar and then shift your weight as you duck underneath it and come up on the other side. Repeat for the desired number of reps.

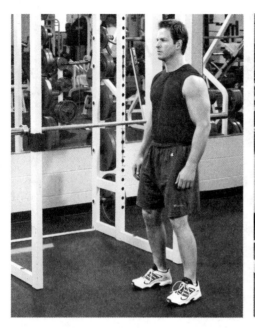 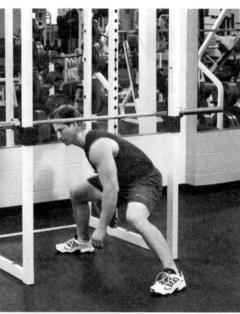

ROTATIONAL LUNGE

(MUSCLES STRETCHED: QUADRICEPS, HIP FLEXORS)

Begin by stepping forward into a lunge so that both knees are bent at approximately 90 degree angles. Once there, rotate your torso and arms as far as you can over your rear leg. Return to the starting position and repeat to the other side.

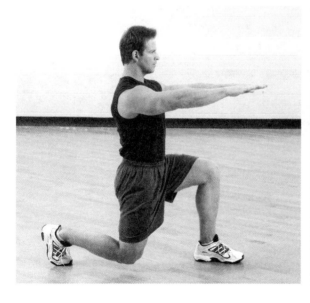 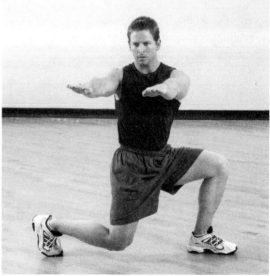

LATERAL LUNGE WALK

Begin by taking a large lunge step out to the side and "sitting" into that hip as you keep the other leg straight. Once the lunging leg is parallel to the floor, push back up to the starting position.

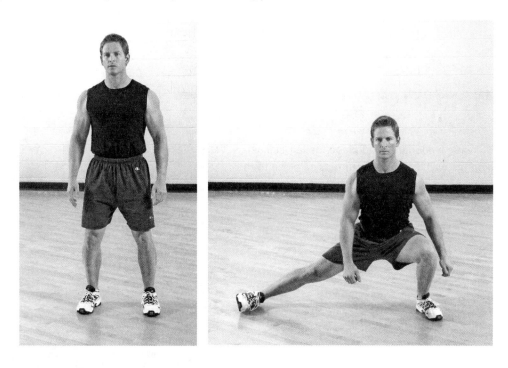

WINDSHIELD WIPER

Lie on your back with your arms out to the sides and legs held up over your hips. Begin by lowering your legs to one side as far as possible without allowing your opposite arm and shoulder to leave the ground. Pause at your lowest point and return to the starting position before repeating to the other side.

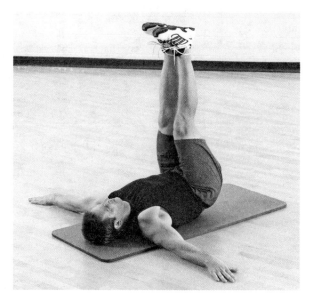
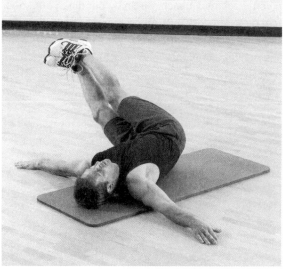

STATIC STRETCHES

Even if they aren't the best way to warm up prior to activity, static stretches aren't completely without merit. After a tough workout, static stretches like the ones we've listed on the following pages can be just the ticket to help restore your muscles to their pretraining state. For best results, hold each stretch for 15 to 20 seconds at a time, doing more repetitions for those areas where you may be a little less flexible.

HAMSTRING STRETCH
(MUSCLES STRETCHED: HAMSTRINGS)

Lie on the floor inside a doorjamb and place the leg closest to the door up on the wall. Try to get your hips as close to the wall as possible while keeping your legs straight.

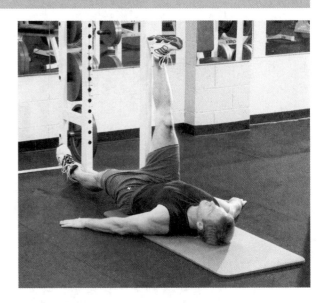

3-POINT QUAD STRETCH
(MUSCLES STRETCHED: QUADRICEPS, HIP FLEXORS)

From a standing position, place your instep on an object that's behind you, such as a bench. Begin by bending your knee until your heel digs into your butt. Once there, bend the supporting leg and reach the leg you're stretching back underneath your body. Hold this position. Optional: lean your torso back while holding the stretch.

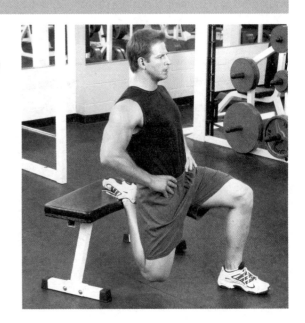

LYING GLUTE STRETCH

(MUSCLES STRETCHED: GLUTES, PIRIFORMIS)

Sit on the floor with your left leg extended and right leg bent at 90 degrees as shown. Lean your torso over your left knee. Switch legs and repeat.

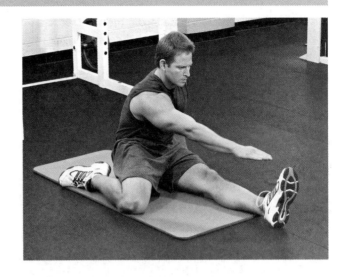

ADDUCTOR STRETCH

(MUSCLES STRETCHED: ADDUCTORS)

Sit with your back to a wall and bring the soles of your feet together. With your back as straight as possible, try to bring your knees as close to the floor as you can.

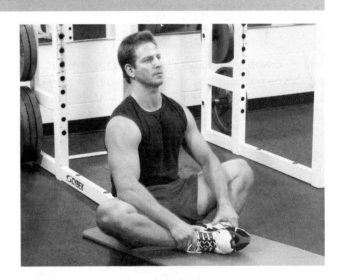

PIKE CALF STRETCH

(MUSCLES STRETCHED: CALVES)

In a pike position, place the ball of your left foot on the floor and rest the other across your left ankle. Next, lower your heel and get it as close to the ground as possible while keeping your right knee straight.

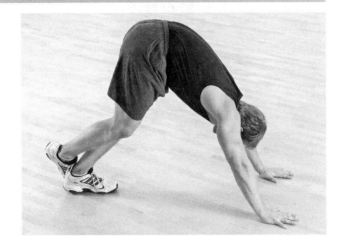

ITB STRETCH

Lie on your back and raise one leg up toward your head as if about to stretch your hamstrings. Once the leg is over your hip, keep it completely straight and reach across with your opposite hand and grab the outside of your knee. Next, gently pull your straight leg across your body as close as you can get it to the floor without lifting the opposite shoulder blade off the ground.

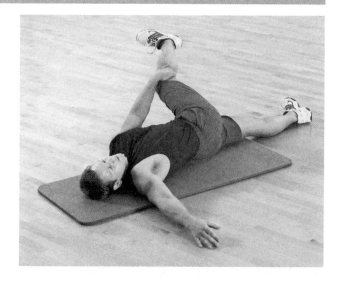

WALL PEC STRETCH

(MUSCLES STRETCHED: CHEST)

Stand sideways next to a wall and place the arm and shoulder closest to it up on it with your palm opened up. Keeping your shoulder and arm completely in contact with the wall, step the same leg across your body and turn away from it.

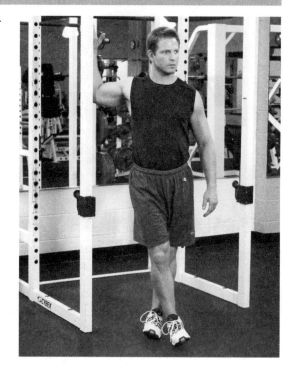

ERECTOR STRETCH

(MUSCLES STRETCHED: LOWER BACK)

Lie on your back and hug your knees into your chest as you simultaneously bring your shoulders off the ground and your head toward your knees.

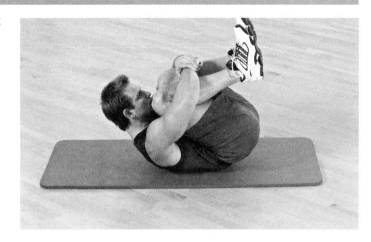

POLE LAT STRETCH

(MUSCLES STRETCHED: LATS)

Stand in front of a sturdy object that won't move and grab it with both hands at about hip level. Next, bend over and sit back into your hips until your arms are completely straight.

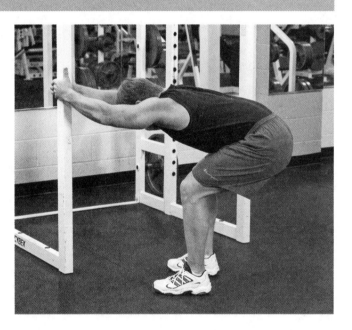

INTERNAL ROTATION STRETCH

Reach over your right shoulder and grab a sturdy object such as a weight rack as shown. Then pull your left hand forward until you feel a stretch in your shoulder.

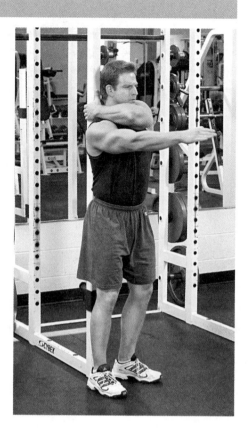

PART THREE

FILLING IN THE GYM GAPS

CHAPTER SEVENTEEN

MEMBERSHIPS MAY RUN OUT ... BUT YOUR RESULTS NEVER HAVE TO!

Advanced Tips for Getting the Most Out of Your Workout

CONSIDERING THE AMOUNT OF INFORMATION WE'VE thrown at you up to this point, you probably figure you know everything there is to know about how to use your gym. We've gone over membership agreements, covered how all of the machines work, and included photos and descriptions of just about every exercise under the sun. With that kind of knowledge under your belt, you're practically guaranteed to get great results well into the foreseeable future, right?

Well, sort of. The thing you have to realize about a successful exercise program is that it becomes a habit. After a while your body becomes accustomed to what you're doing to it. And while a little familiarity can be

nice when it comes to getting to know your fellow gym mates or how to use all of the equipment, settling into too much of a routine often spells doom for your results.

With that in mind, we've compiled a bunch of advanced training tips for getting the most out of your workouts. This is the type of stuff you usually see the biggest or fittest members in the gym doing but are afraid to ask about. It includes everything from little tweaks that can change the feel of certain exercises to ways to get more out of a stretching program. And, just in case we left anything out, at the end of the chapter you'll also find a list of frequently asked questions we've been asked over the years. Consider it your insider's guide to getting in the best shape of your life.

STRENGTH-TRAINING TIPS

The following tips and techniques can help you add some variety and extra intensity to your workouts. Some of them are pretty tough, though, so be sure to follow the guidelines as to how often and how long they should be used.

Negatives

If you hear someone say they're doing negatives, they're referring to the practice of lowering heavy weights under control. Because we're all capable of lowering more weight than we can lift, our muscles really never get worked to their ultimate potential with traditional-strength training exercises. By periodically adding this type of muscle-exhausting technique into your training program, negatives can help you induce a deeper level of muscular fatigue and can often serve as the catalyst to even better gains.

Doing negatives this way can often lead to big improvements in strength by exposing your central nervous system to weights that would otherwise be too heavy for you. That's why negatives are usually best performed with big, compound lifts and require the help of at least one experienced spotter. To do them, load a barbell with anywhere from 15 to 20 percent more weight than you usually use. Begin by unracking the bar and lowering the weight in a slow, controlled manner. Once you've reached the bottom position of the lift, your spotter then helps you get the weight back to the starting position. You then continue for the desired number of reps (usually 3 to 5 per set). The same technique can be applied to non-weight exercises, such as pullups, chinups, pushups, and dips, for example.

Another option is to throw in a few reps of negatives at the end of a tough set when you can no longer lift the weight on your own. You then continue until you can no longer control the lowering phase of the lift. By extending the set this way and keeping your muscles under load for a longer period of time, these types of negatives serve as a great stimulus for muscle hypertrophy (growth). Be mindful that because they're so taxing to your joints, connective tissue (tendons and ligaments), and central nervous system, negatives shouldn't be used too often. Throwing them in for brief 2-week periods a couple of times per year is usually enough to bring about new gains without beating your body up. Try to limit them to one exercise per muscle group and keep the reps on the low side (3 to 5 per set for 3 or 4 sets).

Drop Sets

We have our bodybuilding friends to thank for this grueling maneuver. It's designed to increase muscular size and endurance by tapping into a greater pool of potential muscle fibers than you'd hit with a standard set. To begin, select a weight that allows you to get no more than 4 to 6 reps with good form. As soon as you're done, decrease the weight by approximately 20 percent and crank out anywhere from 4 to 8 more. Finally, drop the weight by another 15 to 20 percent and go for broke. Like negatives, these too should be used sparingly, as they are extremely taxing.

Rest Pause Sets

This advanced technique is great for bringing about increases in strength and size and is best used with compound barbell exercises like squats and bench presses. To begin, load the bar with a weight that would normally only allow you to get anywhere from 1 or 2 reps with good form. Upon completion, rack the weight and rest for a predetermined amount of time before attempting it again (usually about 45 to 60 seconds). Once the rest interval is over, immediately try to crank out another 1 or 2 reps before resting once again. Continue this way until you've done a full set of 10 reps. Then, each week keep the weight the same as you try to decrease the rest interval by 5 to 10 seconds. What makes these different than drop sets is that each time you're working with near-maximal weight, making them much better for strength development.

VARIOUS STANCES AND GRIPS

Depending on the type of stance you adopt or type of grip you take on the bar, it's possible to alter the effect of various exercises.

STANCE

Generally speaking, on lower-body exercises like squats, deadlifts, and leg presses, the wider the stance, where you focus on pushing through the heels, the greater the emphasis on your glutes and hamstrings. The narrower your stance, where you focus on pushing off the balls of the feet, the greater the involvement of your quadriceps. And speaking of increased quadriceps involvement, placing weight plates under your heels during various types of squats (usually done to mask insufficient flexibility in the calves and hip flexors) will also direct more focus to the fronts of your thighs. Finally, turning your toes outward slightly will direct more focus on to your inner thigh muscles.

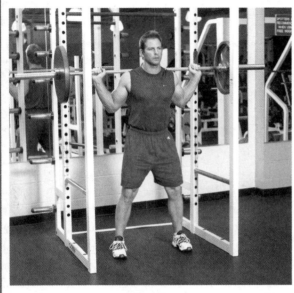

Wide stance

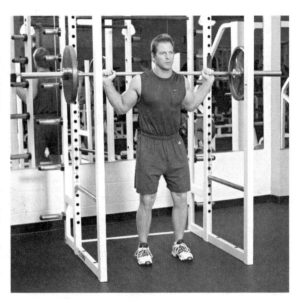

Close stance

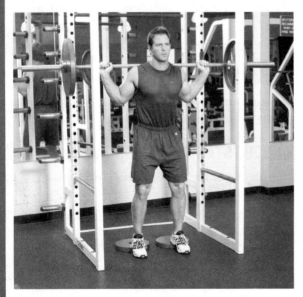

Heels up stance

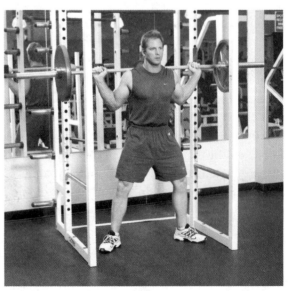

Toes out stance

FOOT POSITIONS

If you watch bodybuilders train their lower bodies, you're bound to notice them turning their feet in certain directions when doing leg extensions, leg curls, and various types of calf raises. This is born out of a belief that altering their foot position will somehow isolate various portions of the quads, hamstrings, and calves. Evidence to support this belief is tenuous at best. What we can tell you, however, is that there are two types of exercises where altering your position at certain key joints can have a significant impact on your results.

The first such exercise is the leg curl. Whether you perform them lying, standing, or sitting, pointing your toes will isolate the hamstrings better by de-emphasizing the contribution of your calves. This is something that should be done often, since your hamstrings and calves work together to flex your knee. Done periodically, though, it can help improve hamstring development by forcing them to work a bit harder than usual. Another variation you can try is called the negative leg curl. With these, pull the weight toward you with your feet flexed, then, at the top of the movement, point your toes and hold your foot in that position as you return the weight to the starting position. This enables you to lift a slightly heavier weight and forces your hamstrings to work harder on the negative portion of the lift.

The other exercise where altering your joint angle can determine which muscles receive more work is the calf raise. Exercises done with straight knees, like the standing calf raise, cause the large, heart-shaped muscle of the calf (the gastrocnemius) to work harder, while bent-knee exercises like the seated calf raise place more focus on the soleus, which lies deep beneath the gastrocnemius.

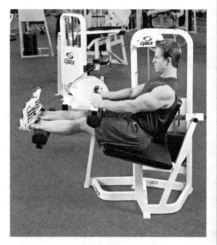

Leg curl

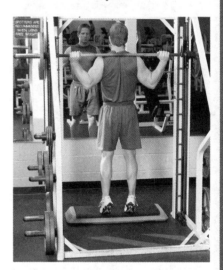

Standing calf raise

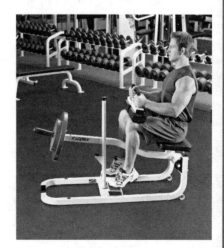

Seated calf raise

GRIPS

As far as your upper body goes, the way you grip the bar can often determine which muscles receive more work. To help you out, we've grouped them into specific body parts for easier referencing.

CHEST

Using a standard grip (slightly wider than shoulder-width) mainly targets the chest, with assistance from the anterior (frontal) shoulders and triceps. Adjusting to a wider grip (twice shoulder-width) decreases the triceps' emphasis and places more focus on the chest and anterior shoulder muscles. Be careful though, as this position is not recommended for those with a history of shoulder problems. Using a closer grip (hands approximately 12 to 18 inches apart) increases the triceps' involvement and is often far less stressful to the shoulders.

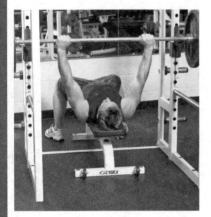

Standard grip

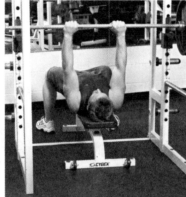

Close grip

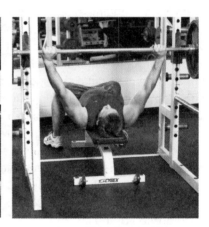

Wide grip

SHOULDERS

Using a pronated grip with either a barbell or dumbbells can be potentially stressful to the shoulders—especially if an underlying condition (such as an impingement) exists. A neutral grip on dumbbell presses frees up joint space and is often more comfortable for the shoulders.

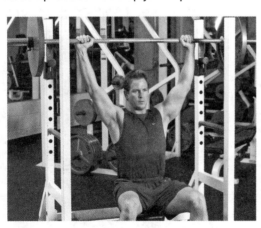

Pronated grip

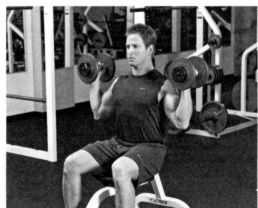

Neutral grip

BACK

With lat pulldowns: A shoulder-width grip with your hands pronated (facing away from you) hits the lats, along with the middle- and upper-back muscles (trapezius, rhomboids, rear deltoids) to a lesser degree, and of course, the muscles that flex the arms (biceps, brachioradialis).

Using a wider pronated grip decreases arm involvement and reduces your range of motion, meaning fewer muscle fibers are stimulated. Neutral grips, where your palms face each other, gives the arms a better angle of pull, allowing for heavier weights to be used. If your grip is shoulder-width or a bit wider, you can slightly increase the range of motion in the exercise. A supinated grip (palms facing you) further increases arm emphasis and is the easiest on the shoulders, but keep in mind that you'll get slightly less back involvement.

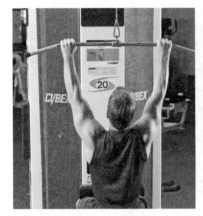
Pronated grip

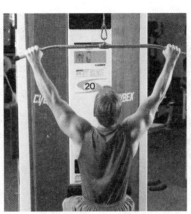
Wide pronated grip

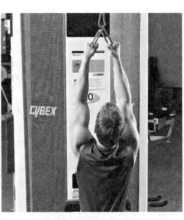
Neutral grip

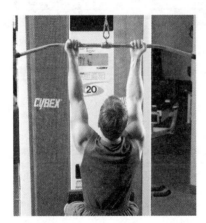
Supinated grip

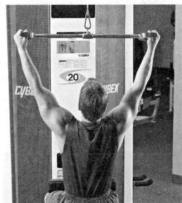
Wide neutral grip

With rowing movements: The big difference between these and lat pulldowns is that they involve a horizontal, as opposed to a vertical, pull. This places more emphasis on the scapular retractors (muscles that pull the shoulder blades together) and less on the lats—especially when using a pronated grip with the elbows held out away from the body. Aside from that, various grip width and hand positions have a similar effect to that of lat pulldown exercises.

TRICEPS

Despite the variety of handles available for doing triceps exercises (see page 190), here it's not so much about grip as it is arm angle. Keeping your arms positioned over your head (as when doing overhead triceps extensions), or angled back slightly when doing lying extensions, places more emphasis on the long head of the triceps, which comprises the back part of your upper arm.

BICEPS

Using a supinated grip mainly targets the biceps, while a neutral, or hammer, grip still recruits the biceps but increases the involvement of the other elbow flexors, such as the brachioradialis. Finally, a pronated grip gives the biceps their worst angle of pull and places the greatest emphasis on the brachialis and brachioradialis. These can, however, be somewhat uncomfortable for the wrists and are best done with an E-Z curl bar.

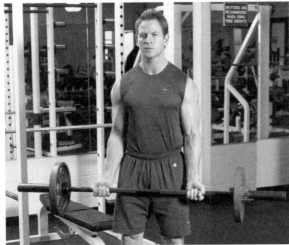

Pronated grip

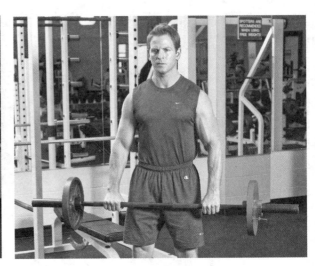

Supinated grip

CARDIO TIPS

Mix things up. Who says you have to stay on one machine the entire time you're doing cardio? One of the best ways to beat boredom and keep your body guessing is to use several different cardio pieces during a single workout. Remember, the faster your body adapts to something, the sooner your results will trail off. Try this workout the next time you're doing cardio and see if it doesn't shake things up a bit.

- Treadmill: 5 to 7 minutes
- Stairclimber: 5 to 7 minutes
- Rower: 3 to 5 minutes
- Elliptical: 5 to 7 minutes

- VersaClimber: 3 to 5 minutes
- Stationary bike: 3 to 5 minutes

Timing is everything. If your goal is weight loss or just general conditioning, it really doesn't make all that much difference when you do your cardio, since it won't have a negative impact on your results. But if you want to build muscle, your best bet is to keep your cardio and strength training as far removed from each other as possible. The last thing you want when you're trying to gain some size is to expend lots of energy doing cardio.

If your schedule allows, try to do your cardio on days off from lifting. If that's just not practical and you have to do everything each time you're at the gym, do your cardio after you lift and try to limit its duration to 12 to 15 minutes at a time. Whatever you do, don't do cardio before you lift, as it might cut into your energy stores and lead to suboptimal gains.

Don't discount a good walk. Walking gets a bad rep with men. Is it true that walking isn't as effective at burning as many calories compared to other high-intensity exercises? Yes. But is it easy on the joints and capable of burning off body fat? The answer is still yes.

If all the cardio machines in your gym are occupied, try this routine. Alternate between walking for 10 seconds at a very brisk, power walking pace—a speed where saying a three- or four-word sentence is doable, but anything longer is out of the question—and walking for 20 seconds at a slow or normal pace. Continue this fast/slow interval for a minimum of 20 minutes, then walk slowly for 3 to 5 minutes to cool down. Trust us—your heart will rev and you'll burn plenty of calories just walking around your gym.

STRETCHING TIPS

Work against yourself. A great way to bring about rapid improvements in flexibility is with a technique known as Proprioceptive Neuromuscular Facilitation (PNF). Although there are several ways you can do it, one of the easiest and most effective ways is something known as the contract/relax method.

To begin, simply take the selected muscle group into the stretched position. Once there, resist with your arms as you contract the muscle group for 5 seconds.

In the example of the hamstring stretch, attempt to bring your straight leg down toward the floor, making sure your upper body is working hard not to allow it to move. After 5 seconds of pushing, take a deep breath in and then exhale as you pull the leg farther back to increase the stretch. You then repeat this procedure 1 or 2 more times, starting from the new stretch position each time you do it. The reason the muscle is able to stretch farther each time is that the preceding contraction forces a greater relaxation and allows the muscle to increase its length to a much greater degree than it can with static stretching.

Stretch between sets. Keeping loose between sets not only makes you feel better, but it also allows for even greater range of motion so you actually end up working more muscle fibers. Keep in mind, though, static stretching is not necessarily the way to go here, because it sends the muscles you're stretching a signal to relax—not exactly desirable when you're getting ready for another tough set. Instead, try some of the mobility drills featured in Chapter Sixteen to keep your muscles limber between sets. For example, doing a Frankenstein walk between sets of leg curls can help free up some

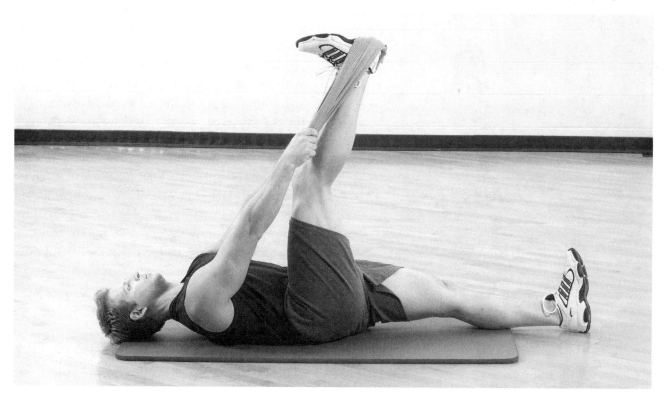

range of motion in your hips and knees, while still keeping your hamstring primed and ready for the next set.

YOU ASK, WE ANSWER

Besides people watching, one of our favorite things to do when we're resting between sets or doing some cardio is listening to some of the questions we hear being asked around the gym. These usually range from the extremely well thought out to the extremely entertaining. The following is a list of what we consider to be among the best we've heard over the years.

Q: With so much equipment to choose from, how do I know what to use?

A: It really comes down to a matter of what you're trying to accomplish. If increasing cardiovascular efficiency and improving flexibility rank high on your list, you won't be doing all that much with the strength-training equipment. If building muscle is what motivates you, obviously then free weights are going to comprise a large portion of your program. Assuming your goals are a little less finite, you may find that a good mix of free weights and machines and using all different types of cardio machines suits you better. In the beginning, that may seem like a bit of an overwhelming proposition given the amount and diversity of equipment most gyms offer.

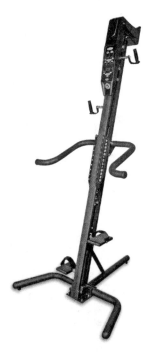

VersaClimber

Remember though, this is something you're going to be doing several times per week, hopefully for many years. Don't sweat it—you'll eventually get around to it all.

Q: What's the best cardio machine for fat loss?

A: The best machine is the one that you like and will use regularly without feeling like you're being tortured in some medieval dungeon. It doesn't matter how effective a given machine is purported to be, the bottom line is: If you don't like it, you're not going to do it—at least not with enough regularity to see any type of noticeable results.

That said, however, the machines that utilize the most muscle mass are the ones that are going to cause the greatest energy expenditure. Among the best are the VersaClimber, rowers, and elliptical machines, because they incorporate the large muscle groups of both the upper and lower body.

Q: When are the best times to work out? The worst?

A: On weekdays, early mornings are usually good. There'll be people there, but by and large this tends to be a pretty no-nonsense crowd since most of them are there to get in a workout before heading off to work. Midmornings are good also, but kind of tough schedule-wise for most working folk. On weekends, early mornings are once again a good choice and the midafternoon to early evening hours are typically pretty dead.

The times you'll want to stay away from, if you can at all help it, are weeknights between 5 and 8 p.m. and midmornings on the weekends. These are the times that seem to work well for most people's schedules, so they're usually the most crowded periods. Depending on what time of year you go, attempting to work out at this time can be an exercise in futility. For instance, go anywhere near a gym between 5 and 8 p.m. on a cold night in January, or on the first truly nice day of spring, and you're bound to see a crowd more appropriate for a Black Friday sale than a fitness center.

Q: How many exercises, sets, and reps should I do?

A: Okay, we seldom hear it phrased like this, but it's easier to explain this way rather than treating them all as separate questions. The truth is, how many of each of these you do is completely dependent on your goals.

GOAL	# OF EXERCISES	# OF SETS	# OF REPS
Strength	3–5	4–6 major muscle groups	3–5
		2–3 accessory muscle groups	8–10
Hypertrophy	6–8	3–4	6–12
Fat Loss	8–10	1–2	8–12
General Conditioning	10–15	1	12–20

Someone who's just interested in general fitness might only need to do one exercise per muscle group while someone more interested in bodybuilding might do better with two or three. The same holds true for the amount of sets and reps you should be doing. The chart above should help clarify things for you.

Q: *How much weight should I use?*
A: This also will be tied in with your goals, along with the number of sets and reps you'll be doing. Remember, though: Whatever weight you do choose, make sure it brings about fatigue in the desired number of reps. Lifting weights that don't offer any kind of a challenge is pretty pointless. Selecting the right weight is basically a process of trial and error. In the beginning, you're going to have to sort of feel things out based on meeting your desired rep range. Once you've figured that out, each successive workout you'll strive to do just a little bit more.

Another factor that ties in with weight selection is rest interval length. Assuming you're doing more than one set of a given exercise, you're going to want to make sure you're resting an appropriate amount of time to be able to repeat that effort. The chart below will provide some guidelines on how long to rest between sets based on various goals.

Q: *What does it mean if someone asks if they can "work in?"*
A: The term working in simply means sharing a piece of equipment. Let's say, for instance, your program calls for you to do 3 sets of 10 reps on a given machine. During your rest interval, someone may come over and ask you if they can work in with you. This doesn't mean they're trying to bully you off the equipment, so there's no need to go running off to report them to the front desk (you'd be surprised how many newbies react that way in this situation). All they want to do is get in a set while you're resting and vice versa.

One thing we'd like to mention here: If you're going to ask someone to work in on exercises like squats, bench presses, or leg presses, make sure the two of you are of comparable strength levels. It's a real pain in the butt to have to load and unload lots of plates every single set.

Q: *What's the proper way to warm up and for how long should I do it?*
A: The main purpose of the warmup is to prepare your body for the more intense training to come. This involves increasing your body temperature and bloodflow to the working muscles, as well as gradually increasing your range of motion around certain key joints. Try performing some sort of low-intensity full-body exercise like walking in place with your arms pumping, running in place, or lightly skipping rope, for example.

You'll also want to do a few lighter sets of some of the same exercises you'll be doing in your workout to help familiarize your body with the specific movement patterns it will soon be doing under heavier loads. To achieve all of this, you'll need to do

GOAL	REST INTERVAL BETWEEN SETS
Strength	2½–3 minutes
Hypertrophy	1–2 minutes
General Conditioning	30–60 seconds
Fat Loss	0–30 seconds

both a general and a specific warmup. General warmups include things like light cardio, various calisthenic exercises, and even some of the flexibility exercises we featured in Chapter Sixteen. All of these things will help increase body temperature and bloodflow, as well as gradually increase your range of motion.

It's important to mention here that although it's long been considered an integral part of warming up, static stretching is one of the last things you'll want to do here. Sending a signal for your muscles to relax prior to intense activity is not the way to go. The only time static stretching should be used during a warmup is if a muscle is so tight that it can't function properly and must first relax before any type of movement can occur.

Here's an example of a good general warmup using some of the mobility drills from Chapter 16. All the mobility drills should either be done with body weight or an unweighted bar.

- Treadmill or stairclimber for 5 minutes
- Overhead Squat × 10
- Reverse Lunge × 20 (10 per leg)
- Frankenstein × 20 (10 per leg)
- Hip Walk × 12 (6 per leg)
- Spiderman × 12 (6 per leg)
- Rotational T × 10 (5 per side)
- Windshield Wiper × 12 (6 per side)

Once you've completed your general warmup, move on to a light warmup set or two of the specific exercises you'll be doing during the workout itself. This will help prep your muscles, connective tissue, and central nervous system for more strenuous lifting. Think of this as sort of a dress rehearsal for your body, with the actual lifts themselves being the main event. Know going in, though, that this whole procedure is quite a bit different from the way most of your fellow gym rats go about warming up, but rest assured, you'll be doing your body a huge service by doing it this way.

Q: *Sometimes after I get warmed up, I can't use a machine right away and have to wait a few minutes—is that okay, or do I need to warm up again?*

A: There isn't an exact science to it, unfortunately. Your body is different than the next person's, and it depends on your physiological makeup, along with how many minutes you warmed up and how intensely. For example, if you've followed the type of warmup explained in the last question, it will probably take your body a good 6 to 7 minutes to cool down. But if you took the path of least resistance and just walked in place for 2 to 3 minutes, your muscles are going to cool down a lot faster.

The thing to remember is it only takes a few minutes of light exercise to get your blood circulating. Similarly, if you don't start exercising right after you finish your warmup, it takes about the same amount of time for it to go right back where it came from.

Best rule of thumb: Always make sure you warm up for 5 minutes, then try to exercise before another 5 minutes is up. If you can't start your exercise in that window, the smarter plan might be to warm up your muscles again.

Q: *How long before I start seeing results?*

A: Actually seeing results is probably a good 4 to 6 weeks down the line. At least, the type of results other people will be commenting on, that is. You'll start noticing some pretty cool changes taking place almost immediately, though. Increased energy levels, tighter, firmer muscles, and clothes that start fitting just a little bit differently are all things that are usually noticeable just a couple of weeks into a new workout program. The great thing is, these little perks are usually enough to keep people motivated until some of the more apparent cosmetic changes take place a little later on down the line.

Q: *Should I use hand weights when I walk or run?*

A: There's a belief that by holding a pair of hand weights adds resistance, so your upper body gets more of a workout—instead of just going along for the ride—and you'll burn more calories. That can be true, but odds are, you could be causing a difference issue that could limit your results.

The truth is, you may end up burning fewer calories and seeing less results. First, the average light hand weight typically isn't heavy enough to build muscle or blast calories significantly. And using a pair that is heavy enough will most likely prevent your arms from swinging freely, which can affect your stride. Too much weight can also cause stress to your rotator cuff muscles and other ligaments and connective tissue throughout your shoulders.

So if you're looking to get more from a walk or run, play with the variables first, such as raising the incline of the treadmill, choosing hillier terrain, increasing the pace at which you're moving, or lengthening how long you exercise. If getting more of your upper body involved during cardio is your goal, try a Nordic ski machine, VersaClimber, or a rowing machine instead. Or, stop walking or running every 1 to 2 minutes and bang out as many pushups as you can muster. Any of these suggestions outweigh the consequences that could arise by relying on a pair of hand weights.

Q: What's the fastest, easiest way to get rid of belly fat and replace it with a "six-pack"?

A: This is probably not what you want to hear, but there's no such thing as a fast or easy way to accomplish this. The fact of the matter is that altering your body composition takes time. Notice that I said altering your body composition—not losing weight. Unless you are clinically obese or need to do so for medical reasons, losing weight should never be your goal. The reason I say this is because when a person loses "weight," along with body fat they also lose water and lean tissue (specifically muscle). I'm all for losing fat, but the latter two are a definite no-no. Losing too much water can leave you in a state of dehydration, and losing muscle will only help accelerate the inevitable slowing of your metabolic rate as you age.

In order to alter your body composition favorably, you need to reduce your body fat content, while simultaneously maintaining or hopefully even gaining precious muscle. These are both time-consuming processes that require tremendous dedication—there is no quick fix. Like it or not, the elusive "six-pack" that so many men seem to covet requires meticulous attention to one's diet and hours upon hours of diligent training. So, despite what you've seen and heard in those late-night infomercials, there is no magical program or "can't miss" training gizmo that will give you the results you're looking for. Don't waste time whittling yourself away with tons of cardio and thousands of repetitions of abdominal exercises. Lift and watch every bite that goes in your mouth, and in several weeks you should see some noticeable improvements.

Q: How can I tell for sure if I'm overdoing it?

A: There are a myriad of signs that can help you determine if you're pushing too hard in your workouts. Perhaps the best indication, though, is a noticeable decrement in performance. Whether you're a runner, a weightlifter, or just a casual fitness enthusiast, your major training objective should be to improve from one workout to the next. Losing a few seconds off your usual time or failing to get the same amount of repetitions with a given load is usually a good indication that you're overdoing it.

Aside from that, other things you can look for are a general feeling of irritability, loss of appetite, difficulty sleeping, and sore, aching muscles and joints. If you're experiencing one or more of these symptoms, it might be time for a rest. Generally speaking, many top trainers and coaches recommend a week of total recovery at least once every 12 weeks. This not only gives your muscles and connective tissue a much-needed break after weeks of intense training, but it also gives your central nervous system a chance to recover as well. Whether you realize or it not, rigorous physical training imposes a tremendous demand on the central nervous system. Failure to allow it to recover adequately can often result in impaired coordination and/or decreased strength and power output.

Q: My gym has a variety of pullup options—which one's the best?

A: They all have their benefits. Like we said earlier in this chapter, changing the placement of your hands matters. With pullups and chinups, the farther you place your hands apart, the shorter your range of motion will be, which reduces the amount of muscle fibers you'll end up using.

But to elaborate on this point, if you use a supinated grip (palms facing you), you'll notice it's easier to pull yourself up to the bar. That's because it places your arms at an angle that allows your biceps to help out your back. The problem is, once your biceps tire out, your back may get cheated out of a thorough workout. If you use a pronated grip (palms facing away from you), it places your arms in a position that minimizes biceps involvement. That may seem great if isolating your back muscles is your goal, but because your biceps aren't there to help out, you aren't able to lift as much weight.

Trying a variety of grips is ideal, but if you only have time in your workouts to do one, use a semi-supinated grip (hands shoulder-width apart, palms facing each other). Using this hand position lets you recruit the most muscle by offering the best range of motion, and letting your biceps help out is just enough to lift a lot more weight without tiring out first.

Q: *Generally speaking, how long should I stick with a particular program?*

A: The truth is, there are no hard and fast rules when it comes to trying to determine an "optimal" exposure to a given style of training. Because we all adapt to physical conditioning at different rates, making widespread generalizations is virtually impossible. While beginners may continue to notice results after several weeks on the same program, more advanced lifters often need to change things up every few workouts or so to keep making gains.

The only way to know for sure when it's time to alter your program is to keep a detailed training log (like the ones we've provided you with in the back of the book). Carefully charting such things as the amount of weight you're lifting, how many repetitions you performed with that weight, or your heart rate at a given level of aerobic intensity will give you the kind of tangible feedback you'll need to continue making progress. Your goal should be to try and improve a little bit from one workout to the next. As soon as you notice an inability to surpass a previous level of effort, it's time to make a change. Don't keep plugging away thinking that you'll eventually be able to push through this plateau. In all likelihood your body has become accustomed to the training stimulus, and further exposure will only result in diminished performance and/or injury.

CHAPTER EIGHTEEN

BRAND MANAGEMENT

Navigating the Innovative World of Exercise Equipment Manufacturers

THERE ARE DOZENS AND DOZENS of commercial exercise equipment manufacturers creating machines for gyms worldwide. If we attempted to write about all of them, this book would look more like a catalog instead of an exercise guide. We want this book to be as useful to you 10 years from now as it is today. That's why—for the purposes of this chapter—we're only going to touch on the more common manufacturers.

Don't see a manufacturer's name that looks familiar on the equipment you're using in your gym? Don't worry. For the most part, most sell their own versions of the machines we've already shown you in an earlier chapter. The only difference might be the type of resistance your muscles may have to push against—or the angle of the machine might be uniquely different—but for the most part, they all work in the same way.

Think of it like knowing how to drive a car, then all of a sudden having to drive a truck or a convertible or a minivan. All four will get you from point A to point B; it's just that the little things you're familiar with may be different—like where you would find the button to adjust the seat or how you would adjust the side mirrors. Your gym may not have the fanciest equipment, but your muscles won't know the difference—for the

most part. Still, there are a few manufacturers whose products are designed differently that may be more comfortable and more effective—if you're lucky enough to belong to a gym that has them.

Odds are, if you see one strength-training machine from one manufacturer at your gym, most—and/or all—of the rest of their strength-training equipment will be from the same manufacturer. That's because gyms get better breaks on the overall cost of their equipment if they buy equipment as a package deal. The following larger manufacturers are some of the more popular companies you might find in your gym.

So why should you care, since you really don't have a choice in what your gym carries and you're basically stuck with what they have? Well, wouldn't it be nice to know the perks about the equipment you're using? Besides, this information might just help end a tiebreaker if you're stuck deciding between two gyms to join.

We've spelled out some of the benefits to each of these brands of equipment. Plus, since some manufacturers have their own company-specific, uniquely patented machines, we've flagged a few standout gems you must try—if your gym was smart enough to buy them, of course. The way we look at it, knowing a little something about the type of equipment you have access to might just help you get a better workout.

CYBEX (CYBEXINTL.COM)

Why your gym probably has it: A leader in the design and manufacture of premium quality cardiovascular and strength-training fitness equipment for 40 years at the time of this writing, Cybex has been revered and widely used by the medical industry, due mainly in part to their equipment's focus on proper biomechanics and body positioning. The company pioneered bringing the sciences of biomechanics and ergonomics to gym equipment. They knew that the more efficiently your body moves as you exercise, the lower your risk of injury and the greater your overall results will be.

Cybex has several lines of premium exercise equipment. Which line your gym carries may depend on its budgetary constraints or whether they cater more to athletes looking for a competitive edge. Some of their product lines include their Eagle NX series, which is their premium line found in more expensive gyms, their Prestige Strength VRS (their Bravo line of functional training equipment), and their VR1 series, which is their more economical and more commonly found line of products, plus a variety of plate-loaded, free weight, and modular, or multistation, machines.

A special piece of equipment to look for: Although Cybex remains renowned for any of their upper-body, duel-axis machines, which let you work each arm separately, the company also has their Cybex SPARC, a cardio machine designed exclusively for HIIT workouts. The modified stepper/elliptical machine features a series of handles that let you change your posture as you exercise and relies entirely on wind resistance—so the harder you move your feet, the harder your workout becomes.

FREEMOTION FITNESS (FREEMOTIONFITNESS.COM)

Why your gym probably has it: FreeMotion's machines use a series of swiveled pulleys and cables—instead of having arms with handles like traditional machines—which let your arms work independently of each other. This gives you more range of motion when using their equipment, hence the name "free motion." Using cables makes it a lot more challenging for your proprioceptive muscles—the tiny stabilizing muscles that help maintain your balance as you move—so you end up developing a better sense of overall balance, stability, and core strength as a bonus. These types of machines don't let you use as much weight as traditional machines do, which is why you generally see this line in more women-friendly clubs, hospitals, sports-specific clinics, and other facilities where getting "healthier" is more important than getting bigger.

Their unique design is appreciated by seasoned exercisers. Why? Trying to do certain exercises with a low or high pulley can be difficult, mainly because you have to pull the handle far enough away from the weight tower so you don't hit your hands on it as you exercise. Some of their machines have a pair of independently adjustable arms that extend "away" from the machine and can be set at different angles. The pulleys come out of the ends of each arm, each set on a swivel that gives you an unlimited range of motion. Because the handles are farther away from the weight stacks, you can pull the cables in more directions than just away from the machine, letting you be as creative as you like with your exercises.

A special piece of equipment to look for: If your gym does have FreeMotion Fitness machines, take a look around the cardio room for their i11.9 incline trainer, a treadmill that lets you raise the belt to as high as a 30 percent incline, and lower it down to a 3 percent decline.

HAMMER STRENGTH (LIFEFITNESS.COM/HAMMER-STRENGTH)

Why your gym probably has it: One of the most popular brands of innovative plate-loaded equipment, Hammer Strength is the maker of the strength-training machines, power racks, and accessories that thousands of world-class athletes, professional sports teams, and the United States military uses and prefers. How come?

Their line of plate-loaded strength-training equipment was originally built and designed for professional athletes with biomechanics in mind—the goal was to develop machines that move in the same way that the human body does. Eventually, their popularity helped them go commercial and spread into gyms worldwide. Their claim to fame is their revolutionary Iso-Lateral technology. Each machine uses a set of dual weight stacks that allow you to work each arm or leg one at a time—or both arms or legs simultaneously—through a range of motion that's more akin to how you actually use your muscles in real life.

Other details that make Hammer Strength equipment groundbreaking include specially designed grip angles that minimize stress on the joints and a counterbalancing system that lets your arms and legs move through a smooth range of motion. Even their exoskeleton structure makes each piece of equipment easier to get in and out of than most conventional machines.

A special piece of equipment to look for: If you hate squats because you find it uncomfortable to have a bar on your shoulders or you have problems maintaining your balance, their V-Squat machine is ideal. Unlike a leg press machine—which lets you train your legs in a similar way to squats, but makes you sit down with your body positioned at a 90-degree angle—the V-Squat machine lets you stand up straight in a posture that's more natural compared to a traditional leg press or hack squat. Just tuck your shoulders underneath the pads, place your feet on the platform and safely squat away. It's also designed to place less strain on your knees and back thanks to a special "curved" arc range of motion—instead of just going straight up and down.

Another classic that's been around for a while, but no one has ever matched is their Gripper. This rarely found station lets you load it with as many weight plates as you need, sit down, and squeeze two sets of thin bars together. By opening and closing your hands, you're able to strengthen your forearms and hands using larger weight loads than traditional exercises that work the forearms will allow you to use.

LIFE FITNESS (LIFEFITNESS.COM)

Why your gym probably has it: The largest commercial fitness equipment provider in the world, Life Fitness's high-quality commercial equipment is distributed in more than 120 countries—which is why it's such a common brand in many gyms. Their claim to fame is their cardiovascular line of Lifecycle exercise bikes, but their strength-training products are just as reliable, effective, and easy to use.

They have several different product lines, but which ones you may come across depends on where you choose to exercise. Their Life Fitness Circuit Series—which lets you push a button to decide your level of resistance—is more commonly found in facilities where there's a higher population of beginners, the aging community, country club goers, or people who may be easily intimidated by exercise. Their Optima Series—as well as their high-end Insignia Series—rely on traditional weight stack resistance and are found in more traditional gyms. Both lines feature easy-to-use incremental weight selectors, placards that show you how to use each machine, and gas-assisted seats that adjust easily for a perfect fit. They're both built to withstand the punishment of high-traffic areas, which is why they are often found in larger, more popular gyms worldwide.

The global leader also recently acquired Cybex, Hammer Strength, and a variety of other gym equipment manufacturers, so don't be surprised if you find other brands mixed throughout your gym or club that may not be Life Fitness.

A special piece of equipment to look for: Every piece of their equipment is newsworthy, but the company continues to build upon its brands. The birthplace of the Lifecycle now has a variety of premium cardio machines—which include a treadmill, both upright and recumbent bikes, an elliptical, and two steppers—that are part of its Elevation Series. All of these machines feature a unique dial that makes it easier to adjust your workout, as well as a touch screen that lets you watch TV, browse the Internet, or track your workout.

NAUTILUS (NAUTILUSSTRENGTH.COM)

Why your gym probably has it: In 1970, Arthur Jones, the founder of Nautilus, designed and sold his first machine. It was the first piece of strength-training equipment to offer variable, balanced resistance, thanks to a special spiral pulley system. By 1984, the company's equipment was in most training rooms and universities, and they had built their own series of more than 3,000 Nautilus fitness centers worldwide.

All these years later, the pioneer of exercise equipment still produces innovative lines of strength-training machines, including their Nautilus EVO and Nitro NOVA series—two weight-stack lines that utilize a patented four-bar linkage system that directs your body through a fuller range of motion than many other machines. Even their plate-loaded equipment—their Nautilus XPLOAD series—offers creative benefits that can make your workouts easier and more effective. Some of their more impressive features include tilt-and-glide adjustable seats and lower-to-the-ground loading points that let you add weight plates without having to lift them up as high.

A special piece of equipment to look for: Anything from the Nautilus ONE series of weight-stack machines. This next-generation model features a single weight tower that's only 4 feet tall, so while it looks unassuming, rest assured that each piece contains a minimum of 250 pounds and up to 445 pounds. The best feature? Instead of messing with a pin or throwing on plates to change the weight, it has a dial. Just turn the knob to the weight load you wish to lift (which you can do while seated at any of their machines), and that's it.

PRECOR (PRECOR.COM)

Why your gym probably has it: Precor's been an innovator and leader in the fitness industry for decades. Since its inception in 1980, the company has been a pioneer and has established new fitness equipment categories (including the elliptical crosstrainer category with the introduction of the EFX Elliptical Fitness Crosstrainer in the mid-1990s) that have become mainstays in the fitness industry. Presently, Precor offers a range of commercial and consumer fitness equipment, from strength to cardio.

A special piece of equipment to look for: While many might be familiar with the Precor EFX elliptical trainer due to its ubiquity in fitness facilities worldwide, the company's AMT Adaptive Motion Trainer is one step beyond. The piece of cardio equipment actually adapts to your unique motion path and lets you exercise using a variety of stride paths, including those similar to elliptical, cycling, walking, and running.

Precor also has the Discovery Series Line, a series of selectorized and plate-loaded commercial strength equipment—as well as benches and racks—that are biomechanically designed to work more efficiently with your body.

PRIME FITNESS (PRIMEFITNESSUSA.COM)

Why your gym probably has it: Use other strength-training machines and you'll generally feel the load is fairly consistent through the entire range of motion of the exercise. However, Prime's equipment features their patented SmartStrength technology, which allows the user to vary the resistance throughout the range of motion. By moving the peak load from the beginning, middle, and end of the exercise motion, users can effectively train the entire stretch of muscle from origin to insertion, ultimately maximizing muscle fiber recruitment.

A special piece of equipment to look for: All of Prime's selectorized machines are versions of the basic machines we discussed in Chapter Twelve. But because of their SmartStrength technology, all of them are worth trying because of how differently and how much harder they make your muscles work compared to traditional machines. With their plate-loaded machines, the most unique piece of equipment that's a must-try is their Extreme Row.

Other seated row machines that strengthen the back muscles have you positioned in an upright position—a posture that makes it easier to cheat by leaning backward to pull the handles toward you. Their Extreme Row machine places your torso at a 45-degree angle (imagine lying backward on an incline bench with your chest on the backrest). All you need to do is grab the handles below you and pull them up to the sides of your body. The slant makes it harder to cheat by making it impossible to lean backward.

TECHNOGYM (TECHNOGYM.COM)

Why your gym probably has it: Offering a complete range of cardio, strength, and functional equipment, Technogym's high-end, state-of-the-art fitness equipment is favored by Olympic athletes (they were the official supplier to five Olympic Games—Sydney 2000, Athens 2004, Turin 2006, Beijing 2008, London 2012, and Rio 2016) and used by more than 35 million people in more than 65,000 wellness centers worldwide.

Besides being both easy to use and aesthetically beautiful (their machines truly are masterpieces in terms of design), users are able to load and track their Technogym workouts on their smartphones, helping them to more easily and effectively achieve their wellness goals.

A special piece of equipment to look for: Their Skill-Mill, the first nonmotorized product that combines power, speed, stamina, and agility training in one product. Shaped like a curved treadmill, it is not found in the cardio section of your fitness facility—most gyms put them near the strength-training equipment. This machine has built-in handlebars—so you can use it like a power sled, among other uses—and sports multidrive technology that lets you select different levels of reactive resistance (from zero to max), all with a simple gearshift, letting you switch from resistance-free running to an all-out sled push instantly.

OTHER EQUALLY NOTABLE MENTIONS TO LOOK FOR

Body-Solid (bodysolid.com): More recognized for their home gym line, Body-Solid equipment is equally common in many gyms, community fitness centers, rehab institutions, and corporate facilities. The company makes everything ranging from cardio equipment (bikes/treadmills/ellipticals), dumbbells and barbells, to compact plate-loaded machines and cable stations. Body-Solid is virtually a one-stop shop of quality equipment, so if you see its logo on anything in your gym, look around—you'll probably see that logo on about 90 percent of everything else.

BodyCraft (bodycraft.com): BodyCraft has been building high quality pieces for gyms and health clubs since 1994. Because their selection isn't extensive, you'll probably come across their treadmills, bikes, rowers, benches, and functional training equipment in smaller facilities—or mixed in with other companies—but their products are built to last and are easy to use.

Hoist Fitness (hoistfitness.com): Hoist Fitness Systems has been producing strength-training products for the commercial and home markets. The company's commercial products can be found all over the world in health clubs, YMCAs, community centers, hotels, personal training facilities, colleges and universities, corporate fitness centers, government facilities, and military bases. Home products can be purchased through specialty fitness retailers throughout the world.

Inflight Fitness (inflightfitness.com): This manufacturer of sleek commercial-grade equipment is often found in schools, gyms, and corporate wellness facilities. Although they don't have as much to offer compared to some of the larger manufacturers, they do offer a full line of weight benches, abdominal benches, counter balanced Smith machines, power racks, and dumbbell racks (among other types of equipment), along with a total-body exercise machine. Just because they're economical doesn't mean they're not quality—their equipment is definitely built to last.

Legend Fitness (legendfitness.com): A staple in the gyms of many professional sports teams and division champion schools, Legend Fitness is renowned for its power cages and racks, selectorized strength equipment, and push/pull power sleds. That's why you'll find their stuff more often in gyms that specialize in functional training or Olympic lifting or any place guys are prone to lifting seriously heavy weight.

Paramount (truefitness.com): Paramount has existed in the exercise space since 1954, designing and manufacturing commercial strength-training products. Being in the industry that long makes Paramount a very common sight in gyms, hotels, schools, corporate facilities, hospitals, and YMCAs worldwide, especially those that have been operating for a while. While their selection is limited, the company was acquired by True Fitness, so your gym most likely has a few pieces of their strength and cardio equipment as well. If so, keep a lookout for their True Stretch—a metal frame that looks like a spider web that lets you perform 30 different stretches.

Star Trac (startrac.com): A market leader in commercial quality cardiovascular, total body, and strength training equipment (particularly weight-training stations, recumbent bikes, and total body elliptical trainers), Star Trac also has a few unique pieces of equipment. Two to look out for: its TreadClimber (a treadmill/stairclimber/elliptical hybrid that feels unlike any other piece of cardio equipment you've tried before) and its BoxMaster, a conditioning machine with 12 striking pads that lets you practice every possible combination of punches through a series of rounds over 30 minutes.

TKO Sports Group USA (tkostrength.com): TKO started out in 1996 specializing in exactly what you might expect—boxing equipment, predominantly heavy bags and speedbags. The company has grown exponentially, branching out into an eclectic mix of home and gym exercise equipment ranging from dumbbells, bodyweight stations, battle ropes, and weight benches to elliptical machines, power cages, selectorized and plate-loaded machines, and even indoor bikes. Odds are, your gym has TKO equipment either because it prefers its atmosphere to look incredible (everything TKO produces is both sturdy and visually stunning) and/or it's a gym that has a heavy focus on sports performance.

Valor Fitness (valorfitness.com): Valor Fitness only has a handful of machines, so don't look for them among the plate-loaded or selectorized equipment. Where you'll probably see them is among your gym's accessories (bars, benches, dumbbells, ropes, slam balls, kettlebells, racks, etc.). Valor Fitness's equipment isn't as showy as some manufacturers—most of their stuff is jet black and/or with a logo that's easy to miss—but what it lacks in flash, it makes up for in function.

York Barbell (yorkbarbell.com): There's a certain nostalgia seeing York Barbell in a gym, since it's been around since 1932. The company revolutionized the design of training equipment, from the early glove barbell designs to today's precision plates, innovative grip plates, finely crafted bars, and residential and commercial free-weight equipment. If your gym has York Barbell, it's probably a facility that takes strength training and powerlifting seriously. And if you're lucky, your gym also has their unique ISO-Grip Olympic Grip Plates. Shaped like a spoke, these barbell plates feature a three-grip design that makes them incredibly easy to grab from all sides—one of the most creative plates on the planet.

CHAPTER NINETEEN

GYM ETIQUETTE 101

Knowing the Rules Can Help You Rule Your Workouts

LOOKING TO RESHAPE YOUR MUSCLES and burn fat faster? Sometimes it's not how you exercise when you go to the gym, it's how you act when you get there that can decide how quickly you see results.

If you're newbie gym goer, the pressure of stepping into a roomful of people who seem like they know what they're doing can be nerve-wracking. It's that kind of pressure that can make it easy to give up sooner than you want to. But knowing the right way to behave can leave you feeling more confident and less intimidated, which many experts agree can help motivate you to try new workouts and even exercise longer.

If you're ready to take your body to the next level, these tried-and-true rules are unspoken—but always appreciated—and work in every gym, no matter what your fitness goals.

ASSESS YOUR HEALTH BEFORE YOU ARRIVE

While you may think you're a trooper to exercise when you're feeling ill, those around you may feel different about your dedication. Can you exercise if your symptoms are limited to "above the neck"—meaning a runny nose, sore throat, and nasal congestion? The answer many experts give is yes. (Anything below the neck, such as coughing, a fever, body aches, or fatigue . . . well, the answer is skip a workout.) But, just because you're okay to

exercise doesn't mean it's always right to bring all those germs to the gym. If doing "the right thing" is your goal, then taking a few days off—or simply working out at home—can be the wiser move.

PLEASE KEEP YOUR HYGIENE IN CHECK

Just because you plan on taking a shower after you work out doesn't mean you shouldn't consider one before you head to the gym. The bottom line is: Think about your stink. Face it, you're not going to smell any better after you exercise. So if you're already ripe beforehand, you're just going to be more offensive to everyone trying to exercise around you. Heading to the gym fresh as a daisy (or at least keeping a few deodorizing body wipes or towelettes in your car for convenience's sake) will spare you any unnecessary embarrassment—and keep your fellow gym members from wishing they weren't downwind from you.

That piece of advice also goes for your clothes. If you're the type who tends to wear the same workout clothes over and over again, those around you will be able to tell. Instead of trying to spray your stinking gym clothes with cologne or rub deodorant on them to create the illusion of being clean, just keep a few extra sets of workout clothes in your car or locker. That way, you'll never be too ripe to work out.

GIVE YOURSELF A QUICK ONCE-OVER

Just having clean clothes isn't a must—they also should be appropriate for the facility. Yes, we get it . . . being in shape makes a guy want to show off all that hard work. But showing too much skin, or wearing baggy clothing that can ride up, may be a turn-off for other members, especially if they end up seeing a little more than they bargained for when you're lying down on a bench or putting your legs in any position that may create an impromptu peepshow of your privates.

Instead, use workout attire that's comfortable, but form-fitting enough so that your chances of exposing parts of you that weren't part of the plan are low. Not revealing too much skin will also minimize your risk of leaving a sweat trail on every machine and bench in the place. So rethink the tank top with the armpit holes that come down to your waist and choose something that can soak up the perspiration.

IF IT'S ELECTRONIC, TURN IT OFF

When was the last time someone's cell phone interrupted your life by buzzing endlessly during a movie or dinner? It's bad enough trying to concentrate on watching a flick or carrying on decent dinner conversation while someone yaks it up a few feet away from you. So imagine what it's like for the poor guy struggling to press twice his body weight when you're doing that!

Serious exercise requires serious concentration, which is why nothing's going to get you more aggravated stares than hearing your cell phone go off in the middle of their set. Being distracted by whatever new ring tone you bought or notification you thought would be cool to blast at full volume every time you received a text or, worse yet, hearing you gabbing on your phone, is just the thing to ruin the focus other lifters need to exercise. So leave your phone elsewhere, turn it off, or at least set it on vibrate, using it only when appropriate. If you need to make a call, do what you would typically do in a restaurant or movie—or at least *should* do—and step outside.

KEEP YOUR ADVICE TO YOURSELF

The book in your hands is filled with useful, easy-to-understand exercise advice guaranteed to give you maximum results. But that doesn't mean other members want to hear all the sage-like fitness advice. The truth is, no one likes a know-it-all, no matter how well informed you may be about exercise. Plus, the person you may be offering advice to may be using a different exercise program than what you're familiar with. Your best bet: Don't offer any unsolicited advice unless someone asks you for it or it looks like someone might be doing something dangerous that could cause them to hurt themselves seriously.

BE PATIENT WHEN SOMEONE'S USING WHAT YOU NEED

You're not the only one with a gym membership, you know. So standing behind, next to, or around someone who's using a piece of equipment you're looking to use next only makes that person feel rushed or uncomfortable, which could possibly put them at risk for injury. If someone's already using the machine or weights you want to use, try to be considerate and either look around for another option—this book is filled with them—wait at a slight inconspicuous distance, or just ask if it's okay to work in with them. Just hold off until they're finished with their set first. Most people will say yes, but if you get a no, just try to respect that they got there first and simply wait your turn.

KEEP A COMFORTABLE DISTANCE

It can be tricky respecting the space of those around you when you're in a crowded gym, but you should always try to avoid working out too close to someone else. With each exercise you do, pick an area that gives others plenty of room to get to things that may be around you. If things are too tight and you're using anything you can pick up safely and use somewhere else (a pair of dumbbells, an exercise mat, etc.), be the better person and just find a less crowded spot.

That same mentality applies to gym lockers and cardio equipment. It doesn't matter if you want to grab the empty treadmill, stepper, or bike next to some cute girl who's sweating away all by herself. If it's the only bike in a crowded gym, then by all means, go for it. But if there are other unused machines around, it's just awkward. So imagine that line of lockers or cardio equipment is a row of empty urinals—and there's only one guy in there using one. Space yourself out accordingly and you'll be fine.

DON'T BLOCK WHAT OTHERS MAY NEED TO USE

Mulling over which exercise or machine you want to try next is fine, so long as you're not unconsciously in someone else's way while you're doing it. Standing in front of the dumbbell rack or positioning yourself in front of a mirror that someone may be using a few feet behind you can keep others around you from getting a decent workout.

The same rules apply to the water fountain. If you're all about staying hydrated and feel the need to consume a gallon of water throughout your workout, then more power to you. But waiting to fill up that super-size jug at the gym may earn you the scorn of those trying to catch a quick sip in between sets. Instead, have your container filled beforehand, so you're not making anyone else wait too long to hydrate.

NEVER LIFT MORE WEIGHT THAN YOU CAN HANDLE

Being around other exercisers makes it easy to fall into the trap of trying to impress them. That's probably the #1 reason why some exercisers often try to use weights that are heavier than they should be using. Trying to lift more weight than you can handle doesn't just increase your risk of injury, but dropping them because you're not strong enough to use them properly makes you look like a novice. Instead, pick a weight load that you can comfortably lift. This will keep the results rolling, instead of the eyes of other gym members.

SAVE THE GRUNTS AND GROANS FOR HOME

Grunting or shouting as you lift weights doesn't just frustrate other exercisers around you, it leaves you looking like you want other people to notice you. And trust us, they will, but not in the way you want them to. If you find yourself making noises unintentionally, try pursing your lips as you lift and breathe properly—exhaling as you raise the weight and inhaling as you lower it.

BE THE PERFECT SPOTTER!

Spend enough time in a gym—especially in or around the weight room—and eventually, you'll be asked for a "spot." If that expression means nothing to you, it basically means that person is asking for you to stand close and watch them during a set of an exercise, so you can help them if they get into trouble during a lift.

Usually, people ask for a spot when they're lifting heavier weights to make sure they don't get themselves stuck or hurt. But sometimes, it's also just to have someone there as a motivator to get them to push themselves a little harder. Either way, follow these tips and you'll always be ready to come to someone else's rescue.

BEFORE THEY START . . .

- If the lifter is using a barbell loaded with weight plates, do a quick check to make sure the weight is the same on both ends.
- **Ask if they want you to "push" them as they lift**—in other words, talk to them as they lift. Some lifters need someone urging them on with a lot of "C'mon, you can do it!" shouts during the last few repetitions of a set, while others may like complete silence so they can focus on what they're doing.
- **Ask for a target rep range.** It's always a good idea to ask the lifter how many reps he or she is aiming for. That way, you'll have an idea of what to expect from them and when your help may be needed. If they've gauged their strength correctly, you shouldn't even have to worry about springing into action until they're a rep or so away from their goal.
- **Position yourself correctly.** You need to be positioned so that if the lifter gets into trouble you can help him or her get the weight safely back on the supports. You also want to do this in a way that doesn't put your own body at risk. For example, say you're spotting someone on a set of bench presses. You wouldn't want to keep your legs fairly straight and bend over at the waist to help them get the weight up, as this could strain your lower back. The right way to spot this lift is to have a healthy bend in your knees and keep your torso upright as you help them guide the bar back up.
- If an exercise requires the person you're spotting to lift a loaded barbell off a set of pins or a rack, such as a barbell chest press, for instance, **you may be asked for a "pop" or a "lift."** This

DON'T LINGER FOR TOO LONG

Don't spend any more time between each set than you have to. Not only will waiting longer than necessary prevent you from getting an efficient workout, but it leaves other people waiting around for you, too. Instead, try timing yourself immediately after you finish each set and make a point to start your next set exactly 1 minute after the last one—or as we recommend in any of the workouts in this book.

This rule goes for sweating it out on cardio machines as well. Many gyms post a time limit somewhere that lets you know how long you can use their cardio machines if others are waiting—typically 30 minutes. If you don't see anything posted, look around at the end of your workout if you plan on exercising longer than 30 minutes. If someone's waiting, then do the right thing and pop off and either go to another machine or try skipping rope or running in place instead.

SHARE AND SHARE ALIKE

In between sets, try to be courteous and look around to see if someone else is waiting around to use the equipment you're using. If they are, then the right thing to do is either ask if they want to work in with you or give them an idea of how many sets you still have to do so they can decide if it's worth the wait.

just means helping them lift the weight out of the racks. To do it right, grab the bar and only offer as much assistance as they need. Pulling too hard or too quickly can be too distracting for some lifters.

AS THEY LIFT . . .

- **Pay attention!** Don't look around or get distracted by other things going on in the gym. All of your attention should be on the person you're spotting so you can assist if and when you're needed.

- **Stay close.** Typically, it's best to stay behind the lifter and close enough so that you can grab the weight from them in case they can't complete a repetition. Don't go pulling weights off someone because they just started training. Nor, by the same token, should you let someone struggle with the weight until they're blue in the face. The key to a good spot is to give the lifter just enough help to complete the rep.

- **Don't touch the bar until it begins to move in the wrong direction.** Helping out too soon can break a lifter's concentration and/or cheat them from getting the most out of a set.

- If you do have to lend a hand, where you place your hands differs, depending on the weights they're using. For barbells, grab the bar with both hands on either the outside or inside of where their hands are. If you're spotting someone who's using dumbbells, don't grab the weights. Instead, place your hands on either of their elbows, forearms, or wrists, depending on the exercise.

- **Don't do too much of the work.** Your objective as a spotter is to keep the weight moving—nothing more, nothing less. Some spotters tend to panic when someone gets stuck raising a weight and immediately lift the weight off them ASAP. Remember, the person you're spotting wants to fatigue their muscles during their set, so unless they're about to drop the weight, help them out, but try to gauge how much help they need. It should be just enough to keep them from going the wrong direction with the weight and that's all.

SAVE THE SELFIES FOR HOME

Yes, there's no better time to take a pic than after a post-workout muscle pump. But even if YOU don't mind the fact that others are probably rolling their eyes as you raise your shirt, flex your pecs, and click away, those same members may not appreciate being part of the background. It's important to remember that some of the people around you may not be as comfortable with where they're at with their bodies. Having you snapping shots from every angle around them could upset or anger some members who may not want to have their image posted online, seen by your friends, or be a part of whatever your plans are for those pictures.

SAVE THE PASSES FOR THE BAR

Sure, you're in a place where everyone around you is sweaty and wearing next to nothing, but that doesn't give you clearance to act like it's happy hour. Hitting on someone—especially when they're stuck on some piece of cardio equipment with nowhere to escape from your pickup lines—is too unfair for words, so leave your game at home. That goes for staring, leering, or anything else that would make you appear creepy anywhere else.

STAY IN CONTROL OF THE EQUIPMENT FROM START TO FINISH

Dropping the weights on the floor after a set—or lowering the weight stacks too quickly so that it slams down—is the fastest way to call negative attention to yourself, especially when everyone turns to see where all the noise is coming from. But worse still, it causes others around you to lose their focus during their sets. This leaves them with less results, and, most likely, more resentment toward you, not to mention it can make other exercisers nervous that you might drop something on them if they exercise too close to you. To prevent you from losing any respect—or toes—try placing the weights on the floor or rack as gently and quietly as you can.

PLACE THINGS BACK WHERE YOU FOUND THEM

Everything in a gym has its place. It doesn't matter if it's a dumbbell, weight plate, or medicine ball. If you've used it, always be considerate and put it right back where you found it when you're finished. Sure, many gyms look like they have plenty of bored staff members standing around with nothing to do, but expecting the gym staff to pick up after your mess won't earn you any points with them. Plus, it just makes it more difficult for other gym members to find exactly what they're looking for.

BRING A TOWEL

A great workout means breaking a good sweat, but no one really wants to see, let alone sit in or lie on, all the hard-earned perspiration you've left behind from machine to machine. That's why a lot of gyms require their members to carry a small towel around during their workouts to wipe away any leftover sweat. Even if your gym doesn't demand this, it's always considerate to do it anyway. If you're too self-conscious to bring your own towel, just use a few paper towels from the gym bathroom instead.

CHAPTER TWENTY

THE 4 QUESTIONS EVERY PERSONAL TRAINER BETTER SAY "YES" TO

If the Answer Is "No"— then It's Time to Go!

HE—OR SHE—HAS ARMS THAT LOOK LIKE LEGS, a set of washboard abs, and a chest you could rest a drink on. And they're claiming they can do the same for your body. But before you commit your muscles to this "Marquis de Sweat," you should know what other exercise secrets they may be hiding.

What few people realize is that personal training is an unregulated industry, one that doesn't require much of an education in order to hang your own shingle. Anyone with great genetics and a few muscles in the right places can pass themselves off as a personal trainer. Deciding which are worth their price takes a little subtle investigation.

Since writing the first edition of the *Men's Health Gym Bible*, there have been a few monumental industry changes regarding the regulation of certification and the fitness industry. That's why for the second edition, we enlisted the help of Anthony J. Wall, MS, ACE-CPT, director of strategic partnerships, education/professional development at American Council on Exercise, who offered us even more in-depth details that may help you pick not just someone who's highly qualified, but also the right fit for you.

That said, you don't have to know about exercise to vet the right candidate. All you really need are a handful of questions that only decent trainers can answer correctly. The next time that trainer you're considering is busy posing in front of the mirror, try posing the following four queries. If he or she flinches at any one of them, you may want to spend your workouts with someone else.

CAN YOU GIVE ME A FEW REFERENCES?

Just because trainers are affiliated with your health club doesn't mean they know what they're doing. Some health clubs aren't as careful as they should be when screening the trainers that work in their gyms. Asking trainers to cough up a few references can reveal a few things, especially if they can't provide you with any references to begin with.

Asking your trainer for three clients similar to yourself in terms of goals will do more than allow you to run a background check. It also reveals whether they have ever trained someone with your particular needs. They may be great at getting high school softball players in shape, but they might not know anything about helping you lose 20 pounds. If you can't find your equal in their clientele list, they're most likely going to have a tougher time meeting your fitness needs.

Wall's advice: "With testimonials, it's also important to remember that no one gives bad references voluntarily. But keeping that in mind, testimonials can still be powerful.

"As you listen to them, ask yourself what you're hoping to get from your experience with the trainer. Are you looking for someone that's very instructive in nature—someone who comes in and tells you exactly what to do—or do you want someone who's more of a coach and makes it feel like you're both working together toward success? Think about what would be the ultimate experience for you, and ask yourself if it sounds like that fitness professional is going to make that happen.

"A few questions to ask include: 'If you were unable to come into the gym one day, did he/she follow up with you?,' 'Have they ever followed up with you after a workout to see how you felt?,' 'Are they always on time?', 'What happens if you have to cancel?', and 'What happens if they have to cancel—do they give you a break or a free session, when they inconvenience you?'"

CAN I TRY A ONE-SESSION DEMO?

Your body is too valuable to risk on a trainer who only claims to know the business, which is why taking your trainer for a test-drive can help see if you like his or her style before you sign. During your workout, ask questions such as, "What muscles am I working?" "Is there another way to do this exercise?" or "What does that machine do?"

This simple grilling will force the trainer to prove just how creative and knowledgeable he is about exercise without having the time to pull big words or programs from some magazine stuffed in his locker. A good trainer will always try to answer your questions, giving you at least five different ways to do basic exercises. Trainers who lack creativity or any exercise sense will always either dodge these questions or give vague answers that all sound the same. Not being imaginative on the fly could be a sign of how dull your workouts will be down the road.

Wall's advice: "During the workout, ask yourself if the trainer is creating an environment where you feel that one day, you won't need their services? A good fitness professional doesn't need people to come back to them. Instead, they want to give the tools to somebody so they can be successful on their own. Some people like that dependency and want that, and that's fine. But if a trainer can educate you to the point where you can go to the gym on your own, understand the types of things you want to do, and be able to do them correctly, then over time, you're going to be a lot more successful."

THE "MY WAY OR THE HIGHWAY" MISTAKE!

"Nobody comes into a gym saying that they want to put on body fat and lose muscle," says Anthony J. Wall, MS, ACE-CPT. "Everybody wants to lose fat and gain muscle, but a good trainer will ask you many questions to get to the heart of 'why' you want to lose weight, especially within the first 15 to 30 minutes of meeting them. They should be focused on finding out about 'your' goals, and seeing how they can personalize and tailor what they can do to meet your needs.

"For example, if a fitness professional insists you should train with them 3 days a week because that's how they train all their clients, that's like walking into a doctor's office and having the doctor say they treat everybody the same way, regardless of their ailment. So having a trainer tell you right out of the gate that they have a 'certain way' they train demonstrates a lack of flexibility.

"Maybe you don't have the financial means or the time to work out with them 3 times a week. So you need to always feel—not only at the start but at every session—that the trainer is focused on you, and that they're always trying to both understand you and find out what motivates you."

THE "ASK THE PACK" TRICK

"If you step into a gym with 10 trainers and you're interested in one, walk around and ask the other nine what they think about that person," suggests Wall. "What you're going to get back are two things—one, a very good understanding about the level of that fitness professional, and two, you'll be able to tell if the culture of that gym is a 'team culture.'

"If everybody tells you that trainer's an idiot (and okay, maybe he or she is one!), it speaks volumes about the level of professionalism that exists within that gym, since there is always a right way and a wrong way to say things. But, if everyone you speak with handles the question in the same professional manner, you will get a better understanding about the culture of the gym you're going to be training in."

CAN I SEE YOUR CERTIFICATION DIPLOMA?

Getting a glance at their diploma makes it easier for you to compare them to others in the field. Even if they have one to show you, some trainers still get nervous revealing where they got their exercise education. That's due to the fact that earning a personal training certificate can require anywhere from several days' to several years' worth of study.

A lot of trainers get theirs from 2-day workshops that anyone with cash and a weekend to blow can buy. According to Wall, "there are over 100 organizations that 'certify' trainers in the United States. Of those hundred organizations, they range greatly in how they issue their certifications. For some, it can be as easy as going online, downloading a test, and taking it using a manual; if they decide they want to buy a certification, they can pay afterward."

A decent certification typically requires trainers to reach a specific score by taking an exam made up of both written and practical application questions and comes with the expectation that trainers will pursue continuing education credits in order to remain certified.

Look for a certification from one of the larger, more reputable certification organizations, such as ACSM, ACE, NASM, AFAA or NSCA. (Each requires longer periods of study and follow-up classes to renew licenses.) If you don't recognize the organization from this list, then search the Web to see what it would take for you to get the same degree yourself. If you get yourself one by sending 5 dollars to a post office box in Tallahassee, you may want to reconsider.

Wall's advice: "Look for a trainer with an NCAA-accredited credential, which is considered the gold stan-dard not only in the fitness industry, but also in a lot of medical-based occupations. These organizations rely on a third-party testing center and are held up to the highest standards possible in their field.

"In fact, simply asking them how they 'upskill' themselves can be very telling. If a person is continuously building upon their education, they should be able to tell you which workshops they've recently attended, what programs they've pursued, etc. If they can't give you an answer, then they definitely do not have an NCAA-accredited credential, since it's mandatory to do professional development in order to maintain an NCAA-accredited certification.

"Another tip: Know that a 'degree' is not the same as a certification. Just because your trainer has a PhD in exercise physiology doesn't mean they know anything about creating exercise programs for someone. It may mean that they understand all of the physiological details about why the body works a certain way and how the body may react to certain types of exercise, but that's on a practical level—and a degree does not give you the right to train somebody. But when you have a 'credential' in personal training, in theory, it means you should be able to start training someone."

DO YOU HAVE INSURANCE?

You're paying good money to entrust this person with your health. The least she can do is make sure your medical bills, lost wages, and other financial concerns are covered in case she drops a weight on your head.

"If someone doesn't have insurance, then they're probably not a reputable fitness professional anyway," says

DON'T KNOW WHERE TO START?

Every large certification organization, such as the American Council on Exercise, the American College of Sports Medicine, the National Strength and Conditioning Association, and others, give you the option through their Web sites both to validate a trainer's credentials and to find a trainer—all you need to do is type in your zip code and they can recommend trainers in your area.

Wall. "Not having insurance is a good indication that they don't value your safety or are unconcerned because they are not taking steps to ensure that they're covered."

Trainers hired through a health club are generally covered by the gym's insurance policy. However, bringing in a trainer that's not affiliated with your gym places the responsibility into the hands of your personal trainer. Since liability insurance costs a trainer (on average) between $22 up to $90+ a month (depending on their deductible), not having any makes a statement about just how unprofessional they are.

Insured trainers may still hate this question, since it may also get you asking about what emergency procedures they have at the ready. A professional should be CPR-certified and always have a cell phone handy, in case they need to call 911. The less prepared a trainer is, the more at risk you and your health will be.

Wall's advice: "Don't just ask if they're insured; make the next question you ask, 'What type of insurance do you have?' That will give you the opportunity to look up exactly what type of coverage they are offering. The type of insurance a trainer is required to have depends on different factors, such as if they're an independent operator, if they work in a gym or club, if they're working indoors versus outdoors, if they are working as an individual or part of a group, etc. Understanding what type of coverage a trainer has will give you the peace of mind of knowing that if you're injured, their insurance company will be able to deal with any issues that might arise."

HOW TO MINE FOR GOLD

The gold standard of certifications in the fitness industry, that is.

According to Wall, "the United States has always done things differently from the rest of the world when it comes to regulating the fitness industry. Overseas, there are a number of registries in which, if you want to work in the country as an exercise professional, you need to be registered."

The United States wasn't regulating the industry when we published the first edition of the *Men's Health Gym Bible*—but they sort of do now in an attempt to raise the benchmark of fitness professionals. Today, there's the United States Registry of Exercise Professionals (or USREPS), an internationally recognized registry of exercise professionals in the United States created by a number of fitness certification organizations (including the American Council on Exercise, the American College of Sports Medicine, the National Strength and Conditioning Association, the Cooper Institute, the National Council on Strength & Fitness, and several others).

So what's that mean to you?

"It means you can go to usreps.org, type in the name or organization of a trainer you're thinking about, and see if that person has credentials," says Wall. "If they're not on that registry, it doesn't mean they don't have credentials, because not every NCAA-accredited organization is part of it. There can also be extenuating circumstances where even if a trainer is certified by a participating organization, they may not want their personal information out there. But if they're in the system, you'll be able to learn about that trainer and instantly validate that they have the credentials they claim to have."

CHAPTER TWENTY-ONE

THE INS AND OUTS OF EXERCISE CLASSES

Get the Lowdown on Every Class So You Can Get Even More Results

LOOKING FOR NEW WAYS TO LOSE FAT doesn't have to be so limiting, you know?

If you're a guy, most likely you can count the few "calorie-burning" options available to you in a gym on one hand. If it's not the treadmill, stationary bike, or rowing machine, you could always pop on a stairclimber, elliptical machine, or Nordic ski machine if you felt comfortable enough to do so. Beyond that, all that's left is that lonely jump rope in the corner of the gym that no one ever seems either in shape—or coordinated—enough to use.

Oh sure, there are plenty of other ways to burn calories in the gym, but those options usually mean signing up for some sort of exercise or fitness class. For most guys and many women, that whole notion may be one that's entirely out of the question.

For some people, it's the fear of looking silly or stupid—or believing they may lack the coordination required to pull off some of the moves. For others, it's not knowing if the class they're interested in is the best way for them to get the results they're personally looking for. For many others—and this is generally a male issue—it's the disproportionate amount of women to men that makes it too nerve-wracking to try.

That's too bad, because joining a group exercise class can be a fun, effective way to blast fat that's not as monotonous and repetitive as using traditional machines. It's also perfect for people that need the higher level of motivation that exercising in a group can bring to their workout regime.

If fear is what's always held you back from joining an exercise class, you're not alone. Even if you're ready to start, just trying to select a class from the hundreds to choose from out there can be excruciatingly intimidating. That's where we can help.

Did you know that most of those unrecognizable exercise classes you see on your gym wall—you know, the ones with all the fancy trademarked names that sound more painful than promising—aren't as unique as you think. Most classes are just offshoots of about a dozen basic types of classes. The moves, instructors, and music may be different, but the kinds of exercises they use and the intensity of the workouts are usually the same. Some may even incorporate exercises you're already familiar with in your weight-training routines.

If you've ever had any interest in trying an exercise class—or just want to understand why so many people flock to them in your gym—we've taken a look at the most common ones and broken them down into what they have to offer. Once you know what to expect from each of these classic exercise classes, you can decide which ones are worth your time and which may waste it.

ABS CLASS

Other nicknames or examples: Core training class, core class, 10-Minute Abs (or any amount of time for that matter), etc.

The gist: A specialized exercise class that focuses strictly on improving your abdominal muscles. Some traditional-style classes use a variety of different crunches, leg raises, and situps, while others may rely on a series of different stability challenges, movements, and/or exercises that rely on your core muscles to stabilize your body when performing them.

Positives: If you know only a handful of exercises to work your abs, these classes can be a great way to pick up a few dozen unique ways to train them. Most people use crunches when they focus on their abs—a move that only targets the upper portion of the rectus abdominus. Even an average instructor will still run you through a mixture of moves that should hit all of your core muscles, including the lower portion of your rectus abdominus as well as your transverse abdominus, obliques, and lower back.

Negatives: If your master plan is thinking this type of class is all you need to burn off all your belly fat, think again. Most abs classes are great at strengthening all of the abdominal muscles, but it still takes watching your diet and using other forms of cardiovascular activity to burn excess calories to get rid of all the fat in front of that six-pack.

Typical male/female ratio: 50/50

AEROBICS CLASS

Other nicknames or examples: Cardio class.

The gist: A traditional aerobics class is basically a choreographed set of body movements designed to strengthen your cardiovascular system led by an instructor. The rule-of-thumb guide to the three types of aerobic classes is fairly simple:

Low-impact aerobics—typically preferred by those who are overweight, elderly, or not in the best of shape—are about as difficult as a brisk walk and involve low-intensity exercises and movements that always keep one foot in contact with the floor. Water-based aerobic classes also tend to fall into this category because they are nonimpact movements that don't put excess stress on your joints.

Medium-intensity aerobics is a combination of both low- and high-impact aerobics.

High-impact aerobics—better suited for those already in some semblance of shape—are high-intensity classes, typically performed at a continuous nonstop pace to keep the heart rate high in order to boost cardiovascular health and burn as many calories as possible.

Most of the varieties you'll find in this chapter are more creative versions of a traditional aerobics class. The truth is, most gyms or clubs tend to shy away from using the word "aerobics" any more because it seems outdated and not as energizing, which is why "cardio"—or more often, some crazy trademarked name of a specific aerobics-based class, many of which you'll see in this chapter as examples—is usually preferred.

Positives: These choreographed classes—usually set to some sort of high-energy music—are terrific at improving your overall fitness and feeling the solidarity of being a part of a group.

Negatives: The typical aerobics class usually doesn't use weights, bands, or any form of resistance to strengthen your muscles—you'll see other versions in this chapter that do use resistance training tools in their programs to maximize their results. Because of this, don't expect to build much muscle, unless the muscle you care most about is your heart.

Typical male/female ratio: It really depends on the class.

BARRE CLASS

Other nicknames or examples: Barre3, the Bar Method, Pure Barre, etc.

The gist: This ballet-inspired exercise class is a mix of dance, Pilates, yoga, and functional training moves—sometimes requiring props including small hand weights and exercise balls—but mostly performed using only your body weight as resistance. Instead of performing exercises through a full range of motion, you'll perform high reps and only move in tiny, 1-inch increments, which engages your muscles by placing them under a lot of isometric tension. Even though the movement is slight, you'll feel all of your muscles firing from head to toe just to maintain your balance through certain movements.

Positives: Because the movements are very small and subtle, Barre classes are nonimpact and incredibly joint-friendly. They also do a thorough job of developing core strength, improving your spine's range of motion, and teaching your mind and muscles to work together.

Negatives: Because the intensity is much lower than an average cardio class, Barre classes never rev your heart rate quite as high, so they aren't the best if cardiovascular conditioning is your goal. Also, because the movements are body weight–based, as you progress, certain exercises may become easier to perform as your muscles become stronger and weigh less.

Typical male/female ratio: 5/95

BODY SCULPTING CLASS

Other nicknames or examples: Les Mills BODYPUMP, group strength class, etc.

The gist: Picture an aerobics class, only imagine that the class gets your heart racing by having you run through a series of resistance exercises instead of just body movements. That's a body sculpting class. Depending on the gym or studio, you may rely on hand weights, light dumbbells, a light barbell or body bar, resistance stretch bands, a stability ball, medicine balls, kettlebells, sandbags, or any mix of strength-training equipment to accomplish this.

Positives: Not only does it help elevate your heart rate, but it allows you to train your muscles at the same time as you burn fat.

Negatives: Because these exercises are typically done using light weights for higher repetitions, you won't build strength as effectively as training using the routines we've shown you in this book. Still, if muscular size and strength aren't your primary interest, this type of class is a great way to sneak weight training into the routine of someone who doesn't usually weight train.

Typical male/female ratio: 15/85

BOOT CAMP CLASS

Other nicknames or examples: Military aerobics, Barry's Bootcamp, Totally Fit Boot Camp, etc.

The gist: Mix together the exercises you would do in your average phys-ed class with the exercise moves you might encounter in the military and you have the underpinnings of this high-intensity class. You'll do a lot of running—usually in place—squats, pushups, situps, lunges, and coordination exercises, either to music or a trainer impersonating a drill instructor (or both).

Positives: Because most of these classes incorporate a lot of body weight exercises, this is one of the few cardio classes that can actually build substantial muscle. It also requires less coordination, since many of the exer-

cises are ones you'll remember from your childhood.

Negatives: These classes use a lot of strength-building exercises compared to your average cardio class. If you're already serious about your weight training and lift weights, this may overtax your muscles by never giving them the time they need after a weight-training workout to heal and rebuild themselves.

Typical male/female ratio: 30/70

BOSU CLASS

Other nicknames or examples: BOSU Cardio, BOSU Circuit, etc.

The gist: This cardio class family uses a BOSU—a piece of exercise equipment that's a cross between a balance board and a stability ball. With the help of an instructor, you'll be asked to perform a variety of balance exercises that challenge your stability from head to toe.

Positives: Unlike many cardio options, this type of class provides both an aerobic and muscle-strengthening workout. Because of its rounded shape, the BOSU challenges your balance and agility, causing all of the muscles from your midsection down through your legs to contract just to keep your body steady. The benefit to you: a terrific core workout while you sweat it out.

Negatives: The BOSU can drastically improve your sense of balance, but if you lack any coordination from the start, you may be too busy losing your balance instead of gaining the benefits.

Typical male/female ratio: 30/70

BOXING CLASS

Other nicknames or examples: Boxing aerobics, Boxercise, Aerobox, etc.

The gist: You'll quickly run through a mix of typical boxing exercises and drills like skipping rope, pushups, and ab exercises using a medicine ball. You'll also be asked to quickly throw combinations of all the basic punches—jab, cross, hook, and uppercut—to raise your heart rate and break a sweat.

Positives: This is one of the better classes for isolating the muscles of the upper body. It's also a great stress reliever for people who enjoy working out their anger or frustrations by firing off a few punches. Plus, all the twisting that comes from throwing punches works your core muscles indirectly.

Negatives: There's not much for the lower body to

do when boxing, so your legs may not get as much of a workout, depending on your instructor. Also, even if your instructor may be a former Golden Gloves champ, don't believe you'll walk out of a few classes a better fighter.

Typical male/female ratio: 40/60

CARDIO KICKBOXING

Other nicknames or examples: Martial arts aerobics, Cardio Kick, Turbo Kick, Tae Bo, Hit It!, etc.

The gist: These classes have you run through a mix of traditional martial arts moves—kicks, punches, and blocks—in a fast-paced workout that provides an aerobic and muscle-strengthening workout.

Positives: You don't have to be that flexible to get started in most classes, so if you've stayed away from the calorie-burning benefits of trying a real martial art out for size, this can be a good alternative. Because many of the moves require balancing on one leg as you kick, it's also great for improving your stability and balance, developing core strength, and working your glutes.

Negatives: Just like a cardio boxing class, if you're looking to learn to defend yourself, this isn't the place. The routines in these classes are aimed to burn fat, not break boards. Overzealous exercisers may also be more prone to injury. Even though instructors typically have students kicking only the air, this can sometimes strain your knee or groin if done incorrectly—so be careful.

Typical male/female ratio: 50/50

CIRCUIT-TRAINING CLASS

The gist: Similar to a body-sculpting class, but structured differently, circuit-training classes consist of an instructor who selects a variety of free weights, plyometric exercises, and/or weight machines and has you move from station to station with little to no rest in between exercises.

Positives: This rapid pace of moving from exercise to exercise challenges your cardiovascular system while giving your muscles a thorough strength-training workout.

Negatives: If you're looking to build larger, powerful muscles, this type of class won't accomplish it. The exercises are generally done for higher repetitions using less weight, so it can define your muscles, but it won't get them as big as traditional weight training.

Typical male/female ratio: 40/60

DANCE FITNESS CLASS

Other nicknames or examples: Zumba, QiDance, Jazzercise, Cardio Funk, Bollywood Funk, Cardio Capoeira, Hip Hop, etc.

The gist: These choreographed classes mix dance steps and aerobic moves into a routine that gets your heart pumping. The music can vary from class to class, ranging from rock, pop, hip hop, jazz, salsa, etc.

Positives: These types of classes can improve your stamina and burn off as many calories as an average aerobics class. The unique musical tie-in is also better for people who hate aerobics classes because of the typical "nightclub" beats they generally blare. One final perk: You'll not only lose fat and gain energy, but you also may even learn a few moves that could impress at the next wedding you're asked to attend.

Negatives: Some of the higher-intensity classes can expect a lot of flexibility at the start, and the constant jumping and stepping required can aggravate your knees and ankles if you're prone to bone, joint, or ligament problems. Also: Although no one will admit it, if you lack any sense of rhythm, you'll find it much harder to get into the flow of the class, which can minimize what you yield from it, leaving you more frustrated than fulfilled.

Typical male/female ratio: 10/90

INDOOR CYCLING CLASS

Other nicknames or examples: Spinning, Schwinn, SoulCycle, LeMond, etc.

The gist: Imagine a roomful of cyclists, each perched on a specially designed spin bike—a sturdier version of the traditional stationary bike. As you pedal, fast-paced music blares around you while an instructor changes the tempo and intensity by ordering you when to speed up, slow down, and change the resistance on your bike. Certain parts of the ride may even have you standing up in your seat.

Positives: Unlike traditional stationary bikes, indoor cycling bikes are far sturdier, letting you shift your body without tipping it over. This lets you train your legs from both sides, so you can work your hamstrings just as hard as your quadriceps. It's also a great—and less embarrassing—way to work the inner and outer thigh and the glutes.

Negatives: Although you can burn a lot of calories while strengthening the muscles of the lower body, your upper body never really gets a "true" full workout.

Typical male/female ratio: 30/70

PILATES

Other nicknames or examples: Pilates Mat, All-Levels Pilates, Cardiolates.

The gist: Originally developed for dancers, Pilates uses a series of slow, graceful movements that strengthen and stretch your muscles, especially the core muscles. These moves are typically balance-challenging poses that use your own body weight as resistance. You're likely to do them on a mat, but some advanced classes may have you use a Pilates machine known as a reformer.

Positives: Pilates is one of the pioneering activities for strengthening the core muscles. Done regularly, it can improve your posture, increase your muscular endurance, and make your body less prone to injury.

Negatives: The exercises are amazing for improving your core muscles, but it's not a huge calorie-burning activity—even though it may leave you feeling exhausted afterward. If you're really looking to lose the pounds, adding a little extra cardiovascular activity to your workout week is recommended.

Typical male/female ratio: 20/80

POWER YOGA

Other nicknames or examples: CorePower Yoga.

The gist: This more intense version of yoga ties a series of yoga poses together into one long sequence. You'll hold each pose from 15 seconds up to 3 to 4 minutes, pushing your sense of balance and muscle endurance to the limits more so than traditional yoga.

Positives: The poses in power yoga also strengthen and stretch your muscles simultaneously and offers the same posture-improving perks as its passive predecessor. However, power yoga's higher intensity pushes your aerobic threshold a bit further for more of an aerobic experience.

Negatives: Although it punishes your muscles in many ways, the lack of movement limits how many calories you actually burn. This makes power yoga's promise to shave away fat a bit less impressive than what you may expect from another exercise class.

Typical male/female ratio: 30/70

STEP CLASS

Other nicknames or examples: Step aerobics.

The gist: This type of aerobics class has you burn calories by performing a series of step and dance movements, using a plastic step that you can adjust in height.

The higher you set the step, the harder your workout.

Positives: Having to rapidly move on and off the step mimics stair climbing. Your own body weight acts as added resistance, giving your legs—and your heart—a more intense workout than just staying put on the floor.

Negatives: If you suffer from knee pain, this type of class uses a lot of step-up movements that some people can find aggravating to their knees.

Typical male/female ratio: 10/90

TAI CHI CLASS

Other nicknames or examples: None—what you "chi" is what you get.

The gist: A traditional class will have you move fluidly through 108 intricate—yet passive—martial arts sequences (or poses). The pace is deliberately slow, making the experience more of a mind-body relaxation exercise by forcing you to focus on every movement you make, as well as meditate and control your breathing as you go.

Positives: Tai chi is said to improve muscular strength, coordination, and mental focus. It also improves your balance, lowers high blood pressure, improves blood circulation, and lubricates your joints. Plus, it's one of the few classes that's meant to relax you instead of rev up your heart.

Negatives: Even though tai chi can improve your health on multiple levels, building muscle and burning fat really aren't on the menu. The only sweat you'll break doing this class is trying to remember all the moves.

Typical male/female ratio: 35/65

WATER AEROBICS

Other nicknames or examples: Aqua Fitness, Splash Dance, etc.

The gist: These classes use many of the same movements and exercises you would typically see in the average aerobics and body sculpting classes. But instead of doing them in the gym, you'll do them in a pool.

Positives: You get all the fat-burning perks of an aerobics class, but by doing them in water, there's less impact on your joints. In fact, the added resistance of the water helps you burn a few extra calories than you would on dry land.

Negatives: Many gyms don't have pools, so it's not always as easy to find a class to join. Getting ready for a class also takes a little more prep time, so just jumping into a class at the last minute is a lot harder to pull off.

Typical male/female ratio: 20/80

YOGA

Other nicknames or examples: Bikram Yoga, Prana Flow Yoga, AntiGravity Yoga, etc.

The gist: An instructor will calmly guide you through a series of different poses that stretch and strengthen your body simultaneously. You'll also learn how to control your breathing and focus your concentration. Many yoga movements are slow and controlled, but there are some classes—like Power Yoga—that use a faster pace to add an aerobic element to your workout.

Positives: Yoga uses a gentle approach to passively improve muscle strength, lower your blood pressure, and increase flexibility. Some of the body-weight resistance poses help you develop your muscles without being as stressful to your joints as other body weight exercises like pushups and pullups can be.

Negatives: Again, if big muscles or losing a lot of fat are your goals, yoga isn't as effective as other forms of exercise.

Typical male/female ratio: 15/85

CHAPTER TWENTY-TWO

DON'T RECOGNIZE IT? DON'T WORRY!

Becoming Familiar with Some of the Lesser-Known Equipment in the Gym

OKAY, WE ADMIT IT.

Even a couple of seasoned gym rats like us occasionally stumble across a piece of equipment we're not quite sure about. Given the ever-evolving nature of the fitness industry and gym owners' desires to stay one step ahead of the competition, continually being presented with new and unique training aids is par for the course. Besides, it keeps things interesting, as many of the newer pieces often represent a dramatic improvement over their predecessors. As our understanding of biomechanics continues to grow, equipment manufacturers are becoming more adept at developing pieces that more accurately mimic the way our bodies move.

Not that brand-spanking new machines with lots of bells and whistles are the only ones capable of raising an eyebrow. Over the years, we've noticed plenty of people looking at even some of the most low-tech pieces of equipment ever developed in apparent bewilderment. Therefore, in addition to all of the other bars, benches, machines, and assorted paraphernalia we've already

introduced you to, we felt it necessary to throw some of these lesser-known pieces into the mix. So, whether it's state-of-the art, or just induces a state of confusion, this chapter will help you figure it out.

45-Degree Back Extension: Think of this as sort of a kinder, gentler version of the regular back extension. Because it's easier to get into and out of and doesn't force you to overcome the force of gravity to the same degree, it's not as difficult to perform the exercise on this one. To begin, set the adjustment so that your belly button is just above the top of the support pad. After that, lock your feet into place and allow your torso to descend over the front of the bench. You then simply reverse direction as you extend your spine back to the starting position.

Airdyne Exercise Bike: Even though this classic piece of cardio equipment has been around for quite a while, it's not as common in many gyms—although it's made a major comeback as a staple in many Mixed Martial Arts (MMA) gyms and studios. The bike uses a unique form of wind resistance where the faster you pedal, the more resistance you have to push against. It also has an attached pair of oscillating handlebars that you can pull and push forward and backward against resistance to work your upper body. The pedals and handlebars can each be used independently or simultaneously.

The reason it's popular is that when you get your arms and legs moving, it burns a lot of calories compared to an average stationary bike. But because you control the resistance by deciding how fast or slow you go, it makes it a lot easier to pull off a high intensity interval training (HIIT)-style workout without having to push any buttons. It's common to see riders alternating between pedaling and moving the handles as fast as possible for 15 seconds, then quickly shifting to a slow leisurely pace for 45 seconds.

Butt Blaster (or Donkey Kick Machine): Although not just for ladies, you'll seldom if ever catch a guy on this machine. It's designed to target that all-important gluteus maximus. After selecting your weight, begin by getting down on all fours (get your mind out the gutter) and placing one foot up on the force plate. From there it's just a matter of pressing the weight up until your leg is just about straight. Hold, lower, and repeat.

Donkey Calf Raise: Another machine that puts you in a rather precarious position, this is one of the best calf developers you'll find. Once you've selected a weight, simply position your lower back under the pad, with only the front part of your feet on the footplate. Resting on your forearms, keep your back as straight as possible as you rise all the way up onto the balls of your feet. Pause for a second at the top and then lower the weight back down until your heels are below the level of the footplate. Repeat for the desired number of reps.

Glute-Ham Bench: Not many gyms have these, so if yours does, consider yourself lucky. This is quite simply one of the best lower back/glute/hamstring exercises you can do. Begin by positioning yourself in the machine with your knees either directly on or slightly behind the pad, your feet firmly on the platform, and the back

of your calves gently pressed against the upper ankle hook.

Your torso should be perpendicular to the floor, arms folded across your chest. Begin by squeezing your hamstrings, glutes, and abs as you slowly lower your body until your torso is perpendicular to the floor. From there, press your toes into the footplate and pull yourself back into the starting position using your hamstrings.

Knee Raise/Dip Station: These usually look like big old high chairs, only adult-sized and minus the seat. Depending on your gym, they might come with a pullup bar across the top, but they can also stand alone. This multipurpose piece can be used for doing knee lifts to work the abs, dips to work the chest, shoulders, and triceps, and if it's got a pullup bar, pull-ups to work the upper back and biceps.

Power Plate: This unique piece of exercise equipment is reportedly used by three-quarters of the teams in the NFL, NBA, and MLB and uses a patented vibration technology that stimulate your muscles to move 30 to 50 times every second. How's it work? As you perform certain exercises on it, such as squats, planks, lunges, etc., the vibrating Power Plate moves up/down, forward/backward, and side-to-side, all at the same time. What this does is boost the intensity of whichever exercise you're performing by simultaneously activating every single muscle in your body. The machine is proven to improve balance and circulation, increase metabolic demand to help in weight loss, and even reduce the appearance of cellulite—even though that's not really a guy issue (but it's certainly nice to know).

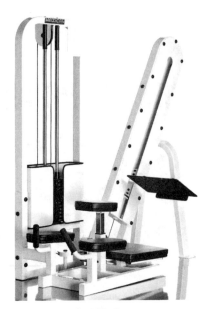

Butt Blaster

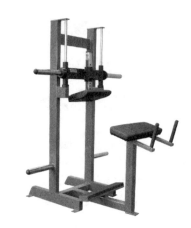

Watson Plate Load Donkey Calf Raise

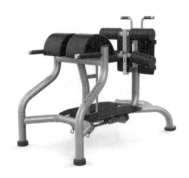

Glute-Ham Bench

To use it, the control panel on a Power Plate is always located front and center on the machine—all you do is press the start button. You can adjust the amount of time the vibration will last and the vibration level. If you're a beginner, try some basic exercises to start—such as squats or lunges—at a lower vibration level to get a feel for it. In addition to doing body-weight exercises on it, other workout tools can be incorporated easily, such as wrapping resistance bands around the platform or placing a foam roller on the platform—the vibrations may actually help boost the effectiveness of your massage therapy.

Spider Row: Pretty much the same idea as the T-Bar Row except for the fact that your upper body is supported by the pad, easing strain on the lower back. The only adjustment to make here is to the footplate. Make sure it's positioned so that the pad hits you right in the middle of the chest. Then you simply select your grip and pull the weights up until your elbows slightly pass your torso. Hold, lower, and repeat.

T-Bar Row: Even though this is technically a machine, the fact that it's plate-loaded usually makes it a staple in the free-weight section. It's much like a bent-over row, but slightly easier to perform due to the leverage advantage it gives you. It allows you to use a variety of grips to target different areas of the back. Whichever grip you choose, the execution is pretty much the same. Stand on the platform with your feet shoulder-width apart and lean forward at the waist, keeping a slight arch in your lower back. Select your grip and keeping your knees bent and torso fixed almost parallel to the floor, pinch your shoulder blades

together and pull the bar up to your chest. Pause, lower, and repeat.

Tibia Dorsi Flexion Machine: You may notice this rather odd-looking contraption on the floor over by the calf machines. Its purpose is to strengthen the oft-overlooked tibialis anterior muscle, which is located on the front of your shin. Strengthening this seemingly insignificant little strip of muscle can help stave off shin splints, as well as improve the stability of your ankle joints. To use it, simply load the weight on the side (careful, it won't take much) and from either a seated (using both feet) or standing (using one foot at a time) position, slide your foot in under the pad and pull your toes up toward your shin(s). Hold for a second, return the weight back down, and repeat.

Upper Body Ergometer (or Upper Body Cycle): Another hard-to-find cardio piece, this one relegates its torture to just your upper body. To begin, position the seat so that when one arm is extended it still has a little bit of bend in the elbow as you're grasping the handle. You'll also want to set the seat height so that your shoulder is basically even with the rotational axis of the machine. Having your shoulders set higher, or especially lower, than this position could cause some discomfort. From there it's as simple as cycling your arms either forward or backward until you've completed your workout.

VersaClimber: Those of you who are old enough to remember Rocky IV may remember Rocky's opponent, Ivan Drago, pumping away on this futuristic climbing machine. Well, decades later, equipment manufacturers still haven't been able to top this consummate calorie burner. Because

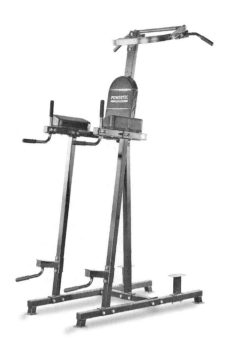

Knee Raise/Dip Station

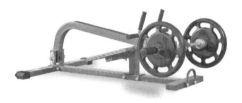

T-Bar Row

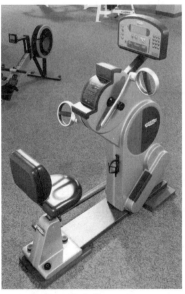

Upper Body Ergometer

it mimics the act of climbing and engages both your upper and lower body simultaneously, the Versa-Climber is one of the toughest cardio-vascular machines around. Simply strap your feet into the foot pedals, grab the handles, and away you go.

Vertical Leg Press: This somewhat intimidating piece is actually one of the best there is for developing strong, powerful legs. To position yourself in the machine, simply lie on your back and place your feet up on the force plate. (Placing your feet higher up will increase glute and hamstring emphasis, while placing them down low will increase the onus on the quadriceps.)

Once in position, just press the weight up off the supports and unlock the sled by simply turning the handles. Lower the weight down until your thighs are parallel to the force plate before pressing it back up to the starting position. You can also use this machine to work your calves by placing only the balls of your feet at the bottom of the platform and keeping your legs straight as you raise and lower the weight.

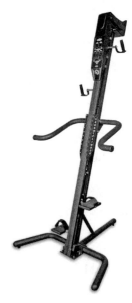

VersaClimber

CHAPTER TWENTY-THREE

BOUTIQUE GYMS: THE NEW APPROACH TO FITNESS!

How to Find Your Way around the Gyms of Today!

THERE ARE A LOT OF NEW types of gyms emerging out there—gyms that don't look a thing like your average health club.

They aren't massive complexes where just walking from one end to the other to find the locker room can be a workout in itself. They aren't always teeming with the usual strength-training and cardio equipment you would expect to see in a place with the word *gym* or *club* attached to its name. In fact, most don't even use the words *gym* or *club* at all, oftentimes substituting the word *studio* or *box* in their place.

They're called boutique gyms, a term that's been coined in recent years for small personalized fitness centers that are more intimate in nature. In 2014, boutique facilities made up more than 20 percent of the market—a number expected to continue to rise with every passing year. More important, in that same year, research conducted by IHRSA found that of all health club members in the United States, 42 percent were members of a studio or boutique facility .

Unlike medium-size or large gyms or clubs, where you're pretty much left on your own to do whatever you wish, these smaller specialized facilities tend to differ from the big boys in other unique ways besides size. You see, most boutique gyms focus on a specific style of niche exercise that can range from functional training, indoor rowing, and new-age spinning to Pilates, plyo dancing, boot camps, and anti-gravitational yoga. These sessions are oftentimes guided by instructors, which is why most boutique gyms are also typically more expensive, compared to a traditional big-box gym or club.

Keeping classes small enough so that instructors and trainers can keep members accountable and engaged is one of the top reasons why many people prefer them. But not every boutique studio shares the same goals and strong sense of community. To get a sense of what you may be in for, here's what you need to know.

BOUTIQUE STUDIOS (IN GENERAL)

At the start of this chapter, we already defined what a boutique fitness studio is, but know there are hundreds of hundreds of different brands to choose from. Some of the more popular ones presently include: SoulCycle (presently the biggest indoor cycling chain in the United States), Title Boxing Club, Pure Barre, CorePower, Flywheel, Physique 57, Solidcore, and CrossFit.

Because a boutique studio can range from a single facility to an entire franchise, trying to list them all would fill this chapter, although in the time it takes you to read this chapter, one studio will most likely close down while another one will be proudly opening its doors. That said, this trend continues to evolve, but here are a few general things you can count on, no matter which one you're considering.

Their Strengths
THEY AREN'T SO OVERWHELMING

Stepping into a big box gym can be intimidating, due to its sheer size and the variety of equipment. Is this book designed to guide you through the process of figuring out how to fit in at a gym and understand how to use all the equipment? Absolutely! But truth be told, if you're still the type that, despite being armed with know-how and the need to get in shape, you're still skittish about stepping into a large gym, then a boutique gym can be a great starting point.

YOU MAY FIND MORE PEOPLE LIKE YOURSELF

Maybe you tried out a boutique studio because it specialized in jujitsu, boxing, or some other cool sport because you love the MMA. Well, guess what? Odds are, that's the same reason many of the other members sweating shoulder-to-shoulder with you did as well. Step into a big box gym and those around you may have different interests than yourself. But with boutique gyms, there's a higher chance that you'll meet like-minded people who, even if they don't share your interests, still may share your same curiosity with the class.

YOU COULD GET A BETTER EXERCISE EDUCATION

Being specialized in one specific area of fitness means the instruction you'll get through a boutique will typically be top-notch. Think of it like the difference of a general family doctor versus a specialist. The trainers you might find in a traditional gym typically need to know a little about everything, and some may focus on a handful of specialties on top of that. But in a boutique gym or studio, the instructors not only tend to have a better understanding (and many times more credentials) regarding whatever style of fitness they're teaching, but they've

also logged a lot more miles just by teaching that style eight times a day.

YOU'RE MORE FREE TO EXPERIMENT

Most boutique studios are a month-to-month or class-by-class commitment, so there's no pressure to sign up for a year. Instead, that can give you the freedom to play the field a lot easier than being tied down to a year-long (or longer) commitment to a big box gym.

Their Weaknesses
THEY MAY NOT BE CONVENIENT

Many boutique studios are set up no differently than an ordinary exercise class. Each day, classes start at a specific time and end at a specific time. So, if that time doesn't work with your schedule, well, that's just too bad. With a traditional gym, you at least have the freedom to start and stop your workout at any time (so long as no one is hogging the equipment you're hoping to use, of course). Throw in the fact that many don't even offer a place to shower and that alone may make you think otherwise.

THEY MAY COME WITH LIMITATIONS

One of the biggest complaints is how some boutique gyms only allow you to come in and take a certain amount of classes per week. That's done in order to maintain their "intimate setting" and keep classes from becoming overcrowded, so that's acceptable. But, if you're the type who needs to work out more often than what a boutique gym may allow, make sure you read the fine print first.

THEY ARE USUALLY MORE EXPENSIVE

All that personalized attention comes at a price, which ranges depending on the facility or chain—but is generally more than you would spend investing in a typical gym membership. Many charge by the visit or class (ranging from $20 to $40+), although others do charge a monthly fee. Just know that the monthly fee can sometimes be (on average) $10 to $40 higher than an ordinary gym membership and may not allow you unlimited access like a traditional gym membership would.

THEY CAN BE TOO ONE-SIDED

In order to stand out, many boutique gyms and studios focus on being as different as possible from other boutique studios and gyms. That can lead to them catering to a niche activity such as kickboxing, cycling, or a certain type of dance. Sometimes, that can lead to having an imbalanced body—let's say, if the studio only focuses on cycling, for example—or it can limit you from being able to target certain areas of fitness that may be more beneficial for you.

DON'T EXPECT MUCH ONE-ON-ONE TIME

In an average gym, you have the freedom to ask someone for help or hire a personal trainer to give you some instruction. But because of the business model of most boutique gyms, which is teaching a group of individuals simultaneously, the option to request a little "me and you" time with a trainer isn't always available and/or convenient.

YOU MAY FEEL OUTNUMBERED

Outnumbered by the opposite sex, that is. More women tend to gravitate toward boutique studios for various reasons, including the lack of intimidation, the fact that they may have never tried a traditional gym in their youth (which more men typically have), and the fact that a lot of studios typically arrange activities that are more interesting to women, such as ballet or dance-themed workouts. Point being, if you need to be around more testosterone to feel inspired, even though you'll probably get a fantastic workout if you stick it out, you may have to find the right boutique gym to feel like you're not the only guy in the room.

CROSSFIT

It's almost hard to conceive that when the first edition of the *Men's Health Gym Bible* was being compiled back in 2005, there were only 13 CrossFit affiliated gyms—called boxes in CrossFit speak. Today—or at least around the time this second edition was written—the company has exploded to well over 13,000 boxes worldwide, with a new box probably opening its doors in the time it took you to read this paragraph.

Started by former gymnast and gymnastics coach Greg Glassman, CrossFit is a high-intensity interval training (HIIT) style program that incorporates powerlifting, Olympic weightlifting, gymnastics, sprints, calisthenics, and other unique moves—such as box jumps, kettlebell swings, flipping huge tires, and rope climbing, just to name a few—into a short, intense workout. A typical workout lasts between 10 and 20 minutes and

has been shown to elevate your metabolism considerably, so you burn calories and fat hours afterward even when resting.

It's that "more results in less time" philosophy that has attracted millions and millions of people to CrossFit, especially those looking to get in the fittest shape possible. It's also revered for making members compete with each other—as well as support each other—toward a common goal. That common goal is completing the Workout of the Day (WOD).

Each time you exercise, you're told what the WOD is. That workout dictates exactly which exercises you'll need to do, as well as how many reps, sets, and even how much weight you need to use per exercise. You're encouraged to race to finish a certain number of reps in a certain amount of time or do as many rounds as you can of that mix of exercises. However, if you can't do a specific exercise in the way it's prescribed, you can "scale" it, which means you can alter it to suit your physical abilities.

Its Strengths
THEY MAKE YOU FEEL LIKE FAMILY

One of CrossFit's greatest appeals is the built-in community it comes with. Members tend to be not only devoted to the program, but also equally devoted to each other and highly supportive. Whether at a box or online, the camaraderie among CrossFitters is contagious, in that others around you are quick to encourage you to not quit and persevere. There's a team mentality among members of a box and among anyone who does CrossFit, that you generally never experience at most gyms or clubs.

YOU'LL SEE RESULTS—GUARANTEED!

Because of its high-intensity design, you will find it difficult to find anyone that does CrossFit consistently (so long as they haven't pushed themselves too hard) that isn't in better shape than when they first started. One classic study out of the University of Wisconsin-LaCrosse found that men using a typical CrossFit workout burned 20.5 calories per minute on average, while women burned roughly 12.3 calories a minute.

IT WORKS EVERY MUSCLE FROM HEAD TO TOE

Unlike some boutique-style facilities that may specialize in a certain type of exercise that only works a portion of your body—such as a cycling-specific class—CrossFit workouts rely on a wide range of multijoint exercises that involve several muscles at once. After a workout, odds are, you'll have hit every major and minor muscle group at least once, if not several times.

IT DEVELOPS REAL-WORLD FUNCTIONAL FITNESS

When was the last time you needed to bench press 300 pounds off your chest or curl anything heavy up to your shoulders when you weren't in the gym? Exactly! Even though some of the exercises found in a typical CrossFit routine may include some weight-training staples, most of the moves focus on functional movements that force (and teach) your muscles to work together.

THEY MAKE IT IMPOSSIBLE TO BE BORED

Because CrossFit changes the WOD every single day, it's never the same workout twice. So if you're the type who hates the monotony of lifting weights and hopping on a treadmill to build muscle and burn fat, the constant "every day is different" atmosphere will keep your mind and muscles always guessing.

Its Weaknesses
IT WON'T BUILD MASSIVE MUSCLES

If your main goal is to experience maximum muscular hypertrophy—meaning, you want to make your muscles as large as humanly possible—then sticking with a traditional gym may be a better fit. Although CrossFit implements certain compound exercises that are ideal for putting on size—such as pullups, push presses, and deadlifts, for example—the high-speed, high-rep pace of a CrossFit workout may be ideal for burning more calories and training everything at once—strength, speed, coordination, and endurance—but it's not the best climate for building serious muscle mass.

IT ENCOURAGES FAST OVER FORM

Trying to perform technically complex lifts—such as deadlifts, squats, or clean and jerks, for example—for a high number of reps, as fast as possible, and/or when you're extremely fatigued is frowned upon by some experts. That's due to the fact that any—or all—of those situations can cause you to sacrifice proper form, which could increase your risk of injury. Also, because of the competitive spirit in a box, you may find yourself taking shortcuts in your form to eke out a few more reps to impress your fellow CrossFitters, which not only could

rob your muscles of a more thorough workout, but increase your chances of injury as well.

IT'S NOT BEGINNER-FRIENDLY

If you're new to exercise, CrossFit's high-intensity pace could make you more susceptible to quitting because of how tough it is. Some—if not many—of the exercises typically recommended also tend to be more complex moves that require time to perfect their form. To avoid this, you might want to come in with a little more experience under your belt or ask a CrossFit instructor about taking a 6- to 8-week beginner's program that can walk you through the moves using little to no weight.

TOO OFTEN MAY BE TOO MUCH

Being obsessed with pushing yourself as hard as possible in every workout isn't always best.

CrossFit workouts are a form of high-intensity interval training (HIIT), which is a style of training that's incredibly effective at burning fat and strengthening the cardiovascular system, but shouldn't be used in excess according to experts.

Doing any form of the HIIT program too often without giving your body time to recover takes its toll on the central nervous system and could have other negative effects on the body depending on the activity. Those effects range from joint pain, hormone depletion, a rise in cortisol (which can promote fat gain, particularly around your waistline), insomnia, depression, and an increased risk of getting injured, among many others. Listen to your body when trying CrossFit—and know when you may be overdoing it—to minimize those risks.

EXPRESS GYMS

You've driven past them, most likely in your local strip mall, tucked between eight or nine other stores in a row. Pop your head inside and you'll most likely see a room about 1,000 to 2,000 square feet with 8 to 14 pieces of exercise equipment spread along the outer walls. Take a few extra seconds to listen to their sales speech and that's when you'll learn they can promise you a strength-building, fat-burning workout in 30 minutes or less.

That said, what exactly is an express gym?

Most are simply a room or two with about a dozen or so pieces of fitness equipment inside. These pieces of equipment differ depending on which express gym you're in, since each franchise has its own unique program of machines and exercises that they use. Each piece of fitness equipment is generally numbered for convenience, so you'll know which exercise to start with.

As a member, the plan is simple. When you walk in, you immediately start on machine #1 or the first exercise, depending on which express gym you're in. From there, you work out continuously until an instructor or a prerecorded voice over the stereo system tells you to move to the next machine/exercise. You'll keep jumping from machine to machine—usually every 30 to 60 seconds—until you finally run through all of the machines/exercises in the room. You may have to repeat the cycle once or twice more—again, depending on the express gym—but that's the gist.

No thinking required. No waiting in line for exercise equipment, since the person using the next machine you need to use next also has to move to the machine when the instructor commands you to. No excuse to not exercise, right?

Well, that's entirely up to you. Is an express gym really for you? That depends on where you see yourself—or more important, what you expect from your body—in the long run.

Their Strengths
THEY CAN BE MORE CONVENIENT

Not requiring as much space or equipment makes it easier for these smaller-size gyms to set up shop in more locations than a typical larger gym. Because of that advantage, most people find they most likely have an express gym somewhere around them that's easier to get to, which is ideal if hating to travel is the main reason you don't exercise as often.

THEY CAN BE LESS INTIMIDATING

This book is designed to teach you how to handle yourself in any gym. But if the thought of walking into one still feels unnerving for some reason, an express gym could be a smart way to ease yourself into exercise. You're pretty much told what to do and which machines to use throughout the entire workout, so there's less danger of feeling awkward or confused. Plus, most express gyms typically attract a same-sex clientele that fall within a certain age range, which makes it easier to find one with clients who are just like you.

THEY KEEP YOUR HEART RATE ELEVATED

If you're the type who tends to waste time lingering between exercises in a regular gym or even when you work out at home, you're in luck. The pace that an express gym enforces—by making you move from machine to machine—trains your muscles in a circuit-training fashion. This edge helps keep your heart rate up and your body burning more calories than you might burn if left on your own.

THEY CAN FEEL MORE PERSONAL

In larger gyms, it's sometimes easy to feel lost among all the machines. Throw in a few staff members who ignore you, plus a few dozen members too focused on their own workouts to speak, and a crowded gym can still feel like a lonely place. If you need to feel part of a community when you work out, the smaller size of an express gym forces more interaction with other members and staff. Plus, the whole "musical chairs" aspect of their circuit-training routines can make your workout feel more social, as if you're participating in an exercise class.

THEY CAN BE A CHEAPER ALTERNATIVE

Although some express gyms may rank right up with larger gyms with their fees, most are slightly cheaper in price. If you're new to exercise, this can feel like a safer gamble to invest your money in, just in case the whole "working out" thing doesn't catch on with you.

Their Weaknesses
REGULAR GYMS CAN STILL BE JUST AS FAST

Most express gyms promote how time-saving their routines are because of the ease of being able to sit down and instantly begin your workout by moving from machine to machine. In fact, seeing them situated in strip malls, juxtaposed to other types of stores known for their convenience, may even help perpetuate the feeling that these types of gyms MUST be faster to use. But the main reason you can just "walk in and work out" is because you have no choice—most don't offer showers or a locker room. By coming to their gym in your workout clothes and leaving without a shower, you automatically chop 10 to 15 minutes off your workout time, but that has nothing to do with the gym's program.

You can still accomplish a "30 minutes or less" routine, if that's what you're looking for, in any gym. So long as you're disciplined enough to jump from machine to machine without needing someone else to tell you when to move or wasting too much time between sets. Come prepared and skip the showers and watch how fast you'll get a workout without any of the hype.

THEY OFFER LESS VARIETY

As you read earlier in the book, the more ways you can challenge a muscle, the more you force it to adapt, change, and grow to its full potential. The variety of machines used in an average express gym ranges between 8 and 16 pieces of equipment. Using them all typically works all of the major muscle groups in your body, but when you do the math, it turns out you end up challenging each muscle group with only one or two different machines/exercises and that's all. Even a basic gym equipped with nothing but free weights can offer you hundreds of different ways to strengthen each muscle group—and you know how to use them, thanks to this book.

IT CAN GET OLD . . . QUICKLY!

Express gyms rarely bring in new equipment to use or change their routines around. For you, that means repeating the same workout, in the same order, at the same pace, with the same machines, for the length of your membership. That can leave you feeling more like you're showing up for work at an assembly line, instead of going out to get a great workout.

YOU MAY BE THE ONLY GUY IN THE ROOM

Just like some boutique gyms, if you're looking for the camaraderie of other guys, you may not find it as easily, since pretty much all express gyms and clubs tend to cater toward the interests of women. That's not to say that trying one on for size won't be a challenge or get you in shape—quite the contrary. If it's a reputable studio, you can expect to see results. However, if you need an even mix of men around to feel motivated, you may have to investigate the ratio ahead of time.

YOU WON'T BUILD AS MUCH MUSCLE

If your goal is to build bigger, stronger muscles, you're in the wrong kind of gym. In most express gym workouts, you do each exercise quickly for as many repetitions as you can, using light weights, before having to move to the next station. This type of lightweight, high-repetition training—12 to 20 repetitions or more per set—stimulates only slow-twitch muscle fibers. This is fine if you're looking to build up your muscular endurance. However, to increase muscular strength and size, it's necessary to activate fast-twitch muscle fibers. These come into play when you use heavier amounts of weight and do fewer repetitions—from 3 to 12 repetitions per set.

THEY MAY LIMIT YOUR OVERALL GOALS

Like we said before, with an express gym, you're stuck doing the same workout at the same intensity with the same machines. Just because you might be able to do the same workout every day without getting too bored doesn't mean your muscles share the same opinion. In fact, studies have shown that your muscles can adapt to the same workout within just five or six times of repeating it. After that, unless you change some variable of the workout you're doing (such as the weight you're using, increasing the number of repetitions and/or sets, or adding a different exercise or two), your muscles stop seeing the need to improve themselves, resulting in less effective workouts.

CHAPTER TWENTY-FOUR

GYM RESOURCES

WE TOLD YOU IN CHAPTER TWO that most experts agree that picking a gym that's farther than 15 minutes from where you live reduces your chances of staying committed to exercise. But just because you're partially limited to what you'll find on your smartphone doesn't mean you can't explore your options.

Here are some of the best sources to use to help you choose when you're finally ready to put everything we've shown you throughout this book to good use.

HEALTHCLUBS.COM

International Health, Racquet & Sportsclub Association (IHRSA) has its own consumer Web site that lets you search for all of IHRSA's 10,000+ member health clubs in the United States, Canada, and more than 67 countries. The site lets you handpick a gym that has every amenity you might be looking for, including personal training, group cycling, group exercise, a running track, a pool, on-site massage, a sauna, physical therapy, childcare, and other features. After that, it shows you a local map with all of your gym options located on it. You can click it to get their gym-specific information and driving directions.

Other Similar and Helpful Resources:

- gymlocator.com
- usgyms.net
- fitnesszone.com
- gymticket.com
- gymsandfitnessclubs.com

Some of the More Popular National/International Gym Chains Include:

24HOURFITNESS.COM

24 Hour Fitness is the world's largest privately owned fitness center chain, with more than 4 million members worldwide. Their multisport exercise facilities are reasonably priced and ideal for exercisers of all levels. As their name implies, all of their 450 clubs located in 18 states and overseas at the time of this publication are open 24 hours a day, 7 days a week.

ANYTIMEFITNESS.COM

With more than 2 million members and 3,000 gyms located in over 20 countries worldwide, Anytime Fitness dominates the health club industry. The co-ed fitness club franchise offers 24-hour access and security, lets you try their facilities free for a week, and is ideal for everyone from the first-timer to the serious exerciser, offering a huge selection of free weights, racks, selectorized equipment, cardio machines, and classes no matter which facility you visit.

CRUNCH.COM

Founded in 1989, Crunch serves more than 600,000 members with over 150 gyms worldwide, including 120 franchise locations in 17 different states, Puerto Rico, and Australia. Their philosophy since opening has always been about "making serious exercise fun" by fusing fitness and entertainment. So in addition to having an impressive selection of weights, cardio machines, and studio space, they are equally known for their unique exercise classes

AIRPORTGYMS.COM

Looking to take your gym workout on the road? Or more important, while you're stuck on the road? Now you don't have to waste time waiting around the next time you know you'll be laid over on a long flight. Airport Gyms lists a wide array of gyms, fitness centers, and exercise clubs for free, all available either inside or around many popular airports in North America (both the United States and Canada). The Web site has a stellar reputation and is updated frequently, which is why health conscious travelers have relied on its accuracy since 2002.

(Hip-Hop Aerobics and Co-Ed Action Wrestling, for example) and "everyone's welcome" mentality.

EQUINOX.COM

This pricey upscale fitness club chain isn't huge in numbers—it only operates 77 full-service clubs in prestigious areas of New York, Chicago, Los Angeles, San Francisco, Miami, Boston, New Jersey, Texas, and Washington, DC, as well as international locations in London and Toronto. It frequently ranks among the top ten health clubs for its luxurious ambience and many uniquely branded programs, services, and products. To maintain their reputation for having an impressive offering of highly specific strength and cardio training, studio classes, personal training, spa services, and products, Equinox goes above and beyond to hire only the best trainers, teachers, and facility managers to keep their gyms running at peak performance.

GOLDSGYM.COM

Gold's Gym, 3 million members strong and one of the most widely known gym chains, is one of the largest coed gym chains in the world, with more than 700 exercise facilities in 38 states and 23 countries. Once known as more of a bodybuilder's gym for men, they've broken that stereotype with their mix of state-of-the-art cardio equipment, more female-friendly equipment, and group exercise classes including Spinning, Pilates, and yoga. Serious bodybuilders still have a home at Gold's, though, with some of the best strength equipment and racks of free weights to build from.

LAFITNESS.COM

LA Fitness, founded in 1984, remains one of the fastest growing health club chains in the United States and presently has more than 660 locations in 28 states, Washing-ton, DC, and Canada. Its nationwide network of health clubs offers its members one of the widest ranges of amenities available and a comfortable unisex, all ages environment that makes it a welcoming choice for those looking for less intimidation and more perspiration.

LIFETIMEFITNESS.COM

Life Time operates more than 120 healthy living, healthy aging destinations in 26 states and Canada and in 35 major markets. With more than one million members, Life Time goes well beyond the traditional health club in providing a high-end experience for every age group. In addition to what you might expect to find, the destinations include indoor and outdoor aquatic centers, basketball and racquet sport courts, a Kids Academy that includes everything from yoga to Spanish immersion, a full-service LifeSpa salon, spa and medispa, and Life Café.

MYSPORTSCLUBS.COM

Step into any of Town Sports International's health clubs and you'll wish you had one in your neighborhood (presently, they are only based in eight states). Still, their Sports Clubs Network of clubs—which include New York Sports Clubs, Boston Sports Clubs, Washington Sports Clubs, and Philadelphia Sports Clubs—make them the largest health club chain in the northeastern United States, with more than 150 health clubs and a half million members. Each of their spacious facilities features ample weight training equipment, state-of-the-art cardio equipment with personal TVs, plenty of group classes, and other services, including babysitting and kids programs.

PLANETFITNESS.COM

Founded in 1992, Planet Fitness presently has more than 1,000 fitness centers in 47 states, the District of Colum-bia, Puerto Rico, Canada, and the Dominican Republic. The inexpensive franchise takes the act of providing its members a welcoming, nonintimidating environment (what they call their Judgement Free Zone) very seriously. So if you're looking to access ample strength and cardio equipment but prefer a less intimidating atmosphere, it's a great choice for beginners through advanced exercisers.

POWERHOUSEGYM.COM

Since 1975, this classic institution has grown into 300+ locations in 40 states nationwide and more than 20 countries, with well over 1.5 million members. Both male and female gym goers of all fitness levels enjoy the rows and rows of dumbbells and mirrors, dozens of fitness classes, and high-tech strength-training equipment.

WORLDGYM.COM

Another legendary gym chain, World Gym facilities have more than 200 locations around the globe. The iconic brand is where bodybuilding greats including Arnold Schwarzenegger, Lou Ferrigno, and Dave Draper developed their physiques in the '70s. Today, it's less hardcore and caters more to men and women of any fitness level. Their gyms have everything from aerobics classes, private training, nutritional advisement, and hundreds of pieces of strength-training equipment to choose from.

XSPORTFITNESS.COM

Although this fitness club has fewer locations, its 330,000 members get to enjoy a mind-blowing number of perks, thanks to the size of their facilities (about 50,000 square feet each!). You can expect to find unique exercise opportunities ranging from TRX stations to climbing walls, along with an enormous selection of cardio, mind/body, strength training, aqua, cycling, dance, and Les Mills classes.

YMCA.NET

Over 22 million men, women, and children in more than 10,000 communities are members of the 2,700+ YMCAs throughout the United States. Although they aren't usually packed with the top strength-training equipment, they always have the basics you need to get in shape. They are the most convenient gym option in most American towns, as 64 million households are located within 3 miles of a YMCA.

Some of the More Popular Boutique Gyms Include:
9ROUND.COM

9Round currently has more than 100,000 members located throughout 335+ gyms worldwide in 38 states, Canada, Mexico, Australia, New Zealand, Saudi Arabia, England, and Jordan. The specialized fitness center blends boxing and kickboxing fitness training into a 30-minute, full-body circuit format. Members perform rounds that involve cardio, weight training, abdominal exercises, kicks, and punches. Every gym is equipped with two 100-pound bags, a double-end bag, an uppercut bag, a speed bag, jump ropes, kettlebells, medicine balls, free weights, and a free motivational trainer.

BARRE3.COM

Founded in 2008, barre3 has more than 100 studios nationwide and over 250 body-shaping, do-anywhere online workouts ranging from 10 to 60 minutes. Inspired by yoga, Pilates, and ballet barre work, barre3 incorporates large-range movements with low-impact cardio to build strength, improve balance, jump-start the metabolism, and re-oxygenate the body. Clients are encouraged to "find their edge" by taking barre3 moves to the next level with free weights, resistance bands, and the barre3 core ball or by following the instructors' modifications that best suit their body.

BARRYSBOOTCAMP.COM

Since its founding in 1998, Barry's Bootcamp boasts to offer *The Best Workout in the World* to a legendary following, including A-list celebs, models—even Olympic athletes. The brand's signature hour-long workouts include 25 to 30 minutes of interval cardiovascular treadmill routines and 25 to 30 minutes of strength training utilizing free weights, resistance bands, medicine balls, and other equipment. Trainers, muscle groups, and even workout segments vary throughout the week so that no one class is ever the same, and the chain currently has 22 locations in major US cities as well as overseas.

FITBODYBOOTCAMP.COM

Founded in 2009, Fit Body Boot Camp is best known for its specialized Afterburn workouts, which uses a combination of high intensity interval training (HIIT) and Active Rest Training to get the body to burn more fat and calories than traditional workouts in only 30 minutes.

The indoor fitness boot camp presently has over 50,000 members at 400 plus locations across 41 states. Every program they offer is personalized to provide clients the best possible results and cater to an individual's fitness level—as opposed to using a cookie cutter, one-size-fits-all approach.

KOKOFITCLUB.COM

Koko FitClub opened its first studio in Massachusetts in 2008. Since then, it has grown to over 100 locations in 30 states and Canada, serving more than 100,000 clients. The chain is actually an individualized coaching gym that provides clients of all abilities with customized strength and cardio conditioning—as well as functional training—using the company's patented, tech-driven Smartraining equipment. The Koko Smartrainer is a full-body strength-training machine that acts like a virtual personal trainer, guiding you through every step of your workout via an interactive touch screen. As you go, the screen shows you how to do each exercise properly. Workouts take around 45 minutes or less and include a dynamic warmup, a little circuit training, and 15 minutes of cardio HIIT or functional training.

ORANGETHEORYFITNESS.COM

Since opening its first studio in Fort Lauderdale, Florida, in 2010, Orangetheory Fitness is up to 400 studios and nearly 300,000 members. The company currently has locations in seven countries, including the United States, Canada, the United Kingdom, Australia, Mexico, Dominican Republic, and Colombia. The franchise is known for its 60-minute workout, which is broken into intervals of cardiovascular and strength training, led by highly skilled coaches using a variety of equipment including treadmills, rowing machines, TRX suspension training, and free weights.

RETROFITNESS.COM

Since 2004, Retro Fitness has evolved from a regional northeastern gym concept into a national fitness system that serves more than 500,000 members nationwide in its 140-plus franchise locations in 16 states (the company plans to add 200 more locations by 2019). The low-cost franchise offers members access to all clubs nationwide, and each facility has at least 60 to 100 pieces of circuit and weight-training equipment, a variety of cardio machines (all with personal flat-screen TVs and iPod hookups), and other amenities including full-service locker rooms, a supervised children's playroom, certified personal trainers, and group classes.

SNAPFITNESS.COM

Founded in 2003, Snap Fitness has grown into a 2,000+ club franchise that—at the time this book was written—extends across 18 countries. Offering fewer amenities than higher-priced clubs—meaning, don't expect a pool, sauna, or even lockers, for that matter, although they do have a few changing rooms and cubbies for your stuff—the no-frills chain is open 24-7 and has a fair amount of traditional cardio machines, free weights, plate-loaded strength equipment, and typical exercise equipment, such as stability balls and medicine balls.

TITLEBOXINGCLUB.COM

TITLE Boxing Club is a boutique fitness studio specializing in boxing and kickboxing fitness classes. The nonintimidating unisex club presently has more than 175 facilities in 33 states and 70,000+ members, with another 250 clubs under development nationwide and in Mexico. Their POWER HOUR workout is designed to challenge individuals of every fitness level and is split into three sections: an intense 15-minute cardio warmup, 30 minutes on heavy bag work, and a final 15-minute core workout and cool down.

UFCGYM.COM

UFC GYM, a brand extension of the UFC that started in 2008, can be found throughout half of the 50 states so far and currently has 100,000 members (although with the UFC's popularity growing each year, you can expect those numbers to be much higher as time passes). Packed wall to wall with what you might expect a gym to have (free weights, cardio equipment, medicine balls, etc.), the chain also offers mixed martial arts training, functional fitness classes (ranging from TRX to a "family boot camp"), and a wide range of exercise classes that will surprise you (including a BOSU circuit, a total body barbell class, restorative yoga, and a high intensity 30- to 60-minute jump rope interval session).

SAMPLE WORKOUTS AND TRAINING LOGS

THE FOLLOWING WORKOUTS AND ACCOMPANYING LOGS will allow you to keep track of your training so that you can accurately gauge your progress. The workouts contained in this section vary depending on your workout goals (fat-burning/total fitness, muscle building, or strength) and current fitness level (beginner/intermediate or advanced). There is also a special section on functional fitness using the exercises from Chapter Thirteen.

Use these logs to keep track of the number of exercises you do, as well as your sets, reps, rest intervals, and training loads. As a general rule, remember that anywhere you

see exercises grouped with specific letters and numbers (A-1, A-2 or B-1, B-2, etc.) they are to be performed as supersets, where you do one exercise, rest, and then do the other, repeating the sequence if necessary.

Anywhere you see the exercises listed by themselves, perform them as straight sets, do each exercise and then rest for the prescribed time interval before repeating as many times as necessary. Also, keep in mind that some of the workouts contain no specific core exercises and none of them list any cardio. Feel free to add those in according to the guidelines we set forth in earlier chapters.

FAT-BURNING/TOTAL-FITNESS WORKOUTS

BEGINNER/INTERMEDIATE LEVEL [WORKOUT A]

MUSCLES	EXERCISE	SETS PER EXERCISE	TARGET REPS	REST BETWEEN SETS	DAY 1		DAY 2		DAY 3	
					WEIGHT	REPS	WEIGHT	REPS	WEIGHT	REPS
Lower body	A-1 Dumbbell Squat	1-2	10-12	30 seconds						
Upper back, biceps	A-2 One-Arm Row	1-2	10-12	30 seconds						
Lower body	B-1 DB Lunge	1-2	10-12	30 seconds						
Chest, front shoulders, triceps	B-2 DB Bench Press	1-2	10-12	30 seconds						
Lower abs	C-1 Incline Reverse Crunch	1-2	10-12	30 seconds						
Upper back	C-2 Lat Pulldown	1-2	10-12	30 seconds						
Upper abs, obliques	D-1 Russian Twist	1-2	10-12	30 seconds						
Lower body	D-2 DB Stepup	1-2	10-12	30 seconds						

BEGINNER/INTERMEDIATE LEVEL (WORKOUT B)

MUSCLES	EXERCISE	SETS PER EXERCISE	TARGET REPS	REST BETWEEN SETS	DAY 1		DAY 2		DAY 3	
					WEIGHT	REPS	WEIGHT	REPS	WEIGHT	REPS
Upper back, biceps	A-1 Cable Row	1-2	10-12	30 seconds						
Lower body	A-2 DB Split Squat	1-2	10-12	30 seconds						
Shoulders, triceps	B-1 DB Shoulder Press	1-2	10-12	30 seconds						
Hamstrings, glutes	B-2 Leg Curl	1-2	10-12	30 seconds						
Lower body-hip dominant	C-1 DB Romanian Deadlift	1-2	10-12	30 seconds						
Chest, shoulders, triceps	C-2 Pushup	1-2	10-12	30 seconds						
Lower abs	D-1 Vertical Knee Raise	1-2	10-12	30 seconds						
Lats, chest, triceps	D-2 DB Pullover	1-2	10-12	30 seconds						

ADVANCED LEVEL (WORKOUT A)

MUSCLES	EXERCISE	SETS PER EXERCISE	TARGET REPS	REST BETWEEN SETS	DAY 1		DAY 2		DAY 3	
					WEIGHT	REPS	WEIGHT	REPS	WEIGHT	REPS
Lower body	A-1 Barbell Squat	2-3	8-12	30 seconds						
Chest, front shoulders, triceps	A-2 Machine Chest Press	2-3	8-12	30 seconds						
Lower body	A-3 DB Lunge	2-3	8-12	30 seconds						
Upper back, biceps	B-1 Pullup	2-3	8-12	30 seconds						
Lower body	B-2 Leg Press	2-3	8-12	30 seconds						
Shoulders, triceps	B-3 Military Press	2-3	8-12	30 seconds						
Abdominals	C-1 Stability Ball Jackknife	2-3	8-12	30 seconds						
Lower back	C-2 Back Extension	2-3	8-12	30 seconds						
Calves	C-3 Standing Calf Raise	2-3	8-12	30 seconds						

ADVANCED LEVEL (WORKOUT B)

MUSCLES	EXERCISE	SETS PER EXERCISE	TARGET REPS	REST BETWEEN SETS	DAY 1		DAY 2		DAY 3	
					WEIGHT	REPS	WEIGHT	REPS	WEIGHT	REPS
Upper back, biceps	A-1 Bent-Over Row	2-3	8-12	30 seconds						
Lower body	A-2 Hack Squat	2-3	8-12	30 seconds						
Chest, front shoulders, triceps	A-3 Incline DB Press	2-3	8-12	30 seconds						
Upper back	B-1 Lat Pulldown	2-3	8-12	30 seconds						
Lower body	B-2 Reverse Lunge	2-3	8-12	30 seconds						
Chest, front shoulders, triceps	B-3 Dip	2-3	8-12	30 seconds						
Lower abs	C-1 Reverse Crunch	2-3	8-12	30 seconds						
Calves	C-2 Seated Calf Raise	2-3	8-12	30 seconds						
Rotators	C-3 Cable External Rotation	2-3	8-12	30 seconds						

MUSCLE-BUILDING WORKOUTS

BEGINNER/INTERMEDIATE LEVEL (WORKOUT A)

MUSCLES	EXERCISE	SETS PER EXERCISE	TARGET REPS	REST BETWEEN SETS	DAY 1		DAY 2		DAY 3	
					WEIGHT	REPS	WEIGHT	REPS	WEIGHT	REPS
Upper back	A-1 Lat Pulldown	2-3	6-8	60 seconds						
Lower body	A-2 DB Stepup	2-3	6-8	60 seconds						
Shoulders, triceps	B-1 DB Shoulder Press	2-3	6-8	60 seconds						
Lower body	B-2 DB Lunge	2-3	6-8	60 seconds						
Lower back	C-1 Back Extension	2-3	6-8	60 seconds						
Chest, shoulders, triceps	C-2 Close-Grip Bench Press	2-3	6-8	60 seconds						

BEGINNER/INTERMEDIATE LEVEL (WORKOUT B)

MUSCLES	EXERCISE	SETS PER EXERCISE	TARGET REPS	REST BETWEEN SETS	DAY 1		DAY 2		DAY 3	
					WEIGHT	REPS	WEIGHT	REPS	WEIGHT	REPS
Lower body	A-1 Leg Press	2-3	6-8	60 seconds						
Chest, front shoulders, triceps	A-2 DB Bench Press	2-3	6-8	60 seconds						
Hamstrings, glutes	B-1 Leg Curl	2-3	6-8	60 seconds						
Upper back, biceps	B-2 One-Arm Row	2-3	6-8	60 seconds						
Calves	C-1 Standing Calf Raise	2-3	6-8	60 seconds						
Upper abs	C-2 Cable Crunch	2-3	6-8	60 seconds						

BEGINNER/INTERMEDIATE LEVEL (WORKOUT C)

MUSCLES	EXERCISE	SETS PER EXERCISE	TARGET REPS	REST BETWEEN SETS	DAY 1		DAY 2		DAY 3	
					WEIGHT	REPS	WEIGHT	REPS	WEIGHT	REPS
Lower body	A-1 DB Split Squat	2-3	6-8	60 seconds						
Upper back, biceps	A-2 Prone DB Row	2-3	6-8	60 seconds						
Hamstrings, glutes	B-1 Stability Ball Leg Curl	2-3	6-8	60 seconds						
Shoulders, traps	B-2 DB Upright Row	2-3	6-8	60 seconds						
Upper abs, obliques	C-1 Russian Twist	2-3	6-8	60 seconds						
Calves	C-2 Seated Calf Raise	2-3	6-8	60 seconds						

ADVANCED LEVEL (WORKOUT A)

MUSCLES	EXERCISE	SETS PER EXERCISE	TARGET REPS	REST BETWEEN SETS	DAY 1		DAY 2		DAY 3	
					WEIGHT	REPS	WEIGHT	REPS	WEIGHT	REPS
Chest, front shoulders, triceps	A-1 Bench Press	2-3	6-8	60 seconds						
Upper back, biceps	A-2 Cable Row	2-3	6-8	60 seconds						
Chest, front deltoids	B-1 Incline Fly	2-3	6-8	60 seconds						
Upper back, trapezius, biceps	B-2 Face Pull	2-3	6-8	60 seconds						
Lats, chest, triceps	C-1 DB Pullover	2-3	6-8	60 seconds						
Upper abs	C-2 Weighted Situp	2-3	6-8	60 seconds						

ADVANCED LEVEL (WORKOUT B)

MUSCLES	EXERCISE	SETS PER EXERCISE	TARGET REPS	REST BETWEEN SETS	DAY 1		DAY 2		DAY 3	
					WEIGHT	REPS	WEIGHT	REPS	WEIGHT	REPS
Lower body	A-1 Leg Press	2-3	6-8	60 seconds						
Lower body	A-2 Lunge	2-3	6-8	60 seconds						
Lower body-hip dominant	B-1 Romanian Deadlift	2-3	6-8	60 seconds						
Hamstrings, glutes	B-2 Leg Curl	2-3	6-8	60 seconds						
Calves	C-1 Standing Calf Raise	2-3	6-8	60 seconds						
Calves	C-2 Seated Calf Raise	2-3	6-8	60 seconds						

ADVANCED LEVEL (WORKOUT C)

MUSCLES	EXERCISE	SETS PER EXERCISE	TARGET REPS	REST BETWEEN SETS	DAY 1		DAY 2		DAY 3	
					WEIGHT	REPS	WEIGHT	REPS	WEIGHT	REPS
Upper back, biceps	A-1 Pullup	2-3	6-8	60 seconds						
Shoulders, triceps	A-2 DB Shoulder Press	2-3	6-8	60 seconds						
Chest, front shoulders, triceps	B-1 Dip	2-3	6-8	60 seconds						
Shoulders, traps	B-2 Upright Row	2-3	6-8	60 seconds						
Shoulders	C-1 Lateral Raise	2-3	6-8	60 seconds						
Shoulders	C-2 Cable Crossover	2-3	6-8	60 seconds						

STRENGTH WORKOUTS

BEGINNER/INTERMEDIATE LEVEL (WORKOUT A)

MUSCLES	EXERCISE	SETS PER EXERCISE	TARGET REPS	REST BETWEEN SETS	DAY 1		DAY 2		DAY 3	
					WEIGHT	REPS	WEIGHT	REPS	WEIGHT	REPS
Chest, front shoulders, triceps	Machine Bench Press	5	5	120 seconds						
Lower body	Split Squat	5	5	120 seconds						
Shoulders, traps	Upright Row	5	5	120 seconds						

BEGINNER/INTERMEDIATE LEVEL (WORKOUT B)

MUSCLES	EXERCISE	SETS PER EXERCISE	TARGET REPS	REST BETWEEN SETS	DAY 1		DAY 2		DAY 3	
					WEIGHT	REPS	WEIGHT	REPS	WEIGHT	REPS
Lower body-hip dominant	Dumbbell Deadlift	5	5	120 seconds						
Upper back, biceps	Assisted Pullup	5	5	120 seconds						
Hamstrings, glutes	Leg Curl	5	5	120 seconds						

BEGINNER/INTERMEDIATE LEVEL (WORKOUT C)

MUSCLES	EXERCISE	SETS PER EXERCISE	TARGET REPS	REST BETWEEN SETS	DAY 1		DAY 2		DAY 3	
					WEIGHT	REPS	WEIGHT	REPS	WEIGHT	REPS
Shoulders, triceps	Military Press	5	5	120 seconds						
Lower body	Leg Press	5	5	120 seconds						
Chest, front shoulders, triceps	Dip	5	5	120 seconds						

ADVANCED LEVEL (WORKOUT A)

MUSCLES	EXERCISE	SETS PER EXERCISE	TARGET REPS	REST BETWEEN SETS	DAY 1		DAY 2		DAY 3	
					WEIGHT	REPS	WEIGHT	REPS	WEIGHT	REPS
Lower body-hip dominant	Deadlift	5	5	120 seconds						
Upper back, biceps	Pullup	5	5	120 seconds						
Shoulders, back	Military Press	5	5	120 seconds						

ADVANCED LEVEL (WORKOUT B)

MUSCLES	EXERCISE	SETS PER EXERCISE	TARGET REPS	REST BETWEEN SETS	DAY 1		DAY 2		DAY 3	
					WEIGHT	REPS	WEIGHT	REPS	WEIGHT	REPS
Lower body-hip dominant, upper back	Power Clean	5	5	120 seconds						
Chest, front shoulders, triceps	Bench Press	5	5	120 seconds						
Upper back, biceps	Bent-Over Row	5	5	120 seconds						

ADVANCED LEVEL (WORKOUT C)

MUSCLES	EXERCISE	SETS PER EXERCISE	TARGET REPS	REST BETWEEN SETS	DAY 1		DAY 2		DAY 3	
					WEIGHT	REPS	WEIGHT	REPS	WEIGHT	REPS
Lower body	Squat	5	5	120 seconds						
Chest, front shoulders, triceps	Dip	5	5	120 seconds						
Traps	Shrug	5	5	120 seconds						

FUNCTIONAL FITNESS MUSCLE BUILDING WORKOUTS

As mentioned in Chapter Thirteen, any of these functional fitness exercises can be added to your existing workouts. After all, innovative tools like these are capable of breathing life into just about any training program. If you're looking for a bit more of a challenge, though, you could try some of the workouts featured below, which are an amalgam of many of the drills contained in Chapter Thirteen and specifically designed to meet certain goals.

For instance, if you're looking to put on a little size, check out the upper- and lower-body muscle building workouts. Or, maybe you're more interested in burning fat. Not to worry, our array of functional firepower will help you burn off that belly in no time. A grueling core workout? Improved sports performance? You can check them off the list, too, as we have a couple of killer workouts that address those needs as well.

No reason to stop there, though. Once you get the hang of how to use this stuff, feel free to start experimenting on your own. Before long you'll be a regular "functional phenom" who'll have other gym rats coming up to you and asking for advice!

Upper Body

Perform as supersets, going from A-1 to A-2 without rest and then taking the prescribed break before completing the rest of the sets and moving on to the B exercises and so on.

EXERCISE	# OF REPS	# OF SETS	REST INTERVAL
A-1 TRX YTW	x 6 of each	2-3	None
A-2 Sandbag Bent-Over Row	x 8-10	2-3	60-90 seconds
B-1 Slideboard Fly	x 10-12	2-3	None
B-2 Prowler Press	x 8-10	2-3	60-90 seconds
C-1 KB Bottom Up Press	x 8-10 per side	2-3	None
C-2 Pullups	x 6-10	2-3	60-90 seconds
D-1 TRX Triceps Extension	x 8-10	2-3	None
D-2 TRX Biceps Curl	x 8-10	2-3	60-90 seconds

Lower Body

EXERCISE	# OF REPS	# OF SETS	REST INTERVAL
A-1 Slideboard Reverse Lunge	x 8-10 per side	2-3	None
A-2 TRX Leg Curl	x 8-10	2-3	60-90 seconds
B-1 Sandbag Zercher Squat	x 8-10	2-3	None
B-2 KB Turkish Get-Up	x 5-6 per side	2-3	60-90 seconds
C-1 Slideboard Lateral Squat	x 8-10 per side	2-3	None
C-2 Sandbag Rom. Deadlift	x 8-10	2-3	60-90 seconds

Fat-Burning Workout

Perform as a circuit, where you go from one exercise to the next with no rest and then break once you've completed the entire circuit. Then take the prescribed amount of rest and complete 1 or 2 more times.

EXERCISE	# OF REPS	# OF SETS	REST INTERVAL
KB Swing (2 Arms)	15-20	2-3	None
TRX Atomic Pushup	10-12	2-3	None
Tire Sledgehammer Hit	10-12 per side	2-3	None
KB Reverse Lunge & Press	x 8-10 per side	2-3	None
Battle Rope Slam	x 30 seconds	2-3	None
Prowler Push	x 15-30 yds.	2-3	None
TRX Row	x 10-12	2-3	None
Sandbag Shoveling	x 8-10 per side	2-3	None
Slideboard Mountain Climber	x 30 seconds	2-3	None
BOSU Squat	x 10-12	2-3	90-120 seconds

Core Workout

Here you have the option of using either format: You can do the exercises as paired supersets, by completing all of the A's first and then moving to the Bs, etc. Or, you can treat the workout as one giant core circuit and do 2 or 3 full rounds.

EXERCISE	# OF REPS	# OF SETS	REST INTERVAL
A-1 KB Turkish Get-Up	x 5-6 per side	2-3	None
A-2 Plank Body Saw	x 10-12	2-3	30-60 seconds or None
B-1 Battle Rope Cyclone	x 30 seconds	2-3	None
B-2 Sandbag Lunge with Rotation	x 8-10 per side	2-3	30-60 seconds or None
C-1 KB Windmill	x 8-10	2-3	None
C-2 KB Renegade Row	x 5-6 per side	2-3	30-60 seconds or None
D-1 Slideboard Pike	x 10-12	2-3	None
D-2 Sandbag Front-Loaded Good Morning	x 8-10	2-3	30-60 seconds or None

Sports Performance

Perform all of the exercises in this sports-themed movement workout as paired supersets, by doing all of the A drills and then moving on to the Bs, etc.

EXERCISE	# OF REPS	# OF SETS	REST INTERVAL
A-1 Tire Flip	5-6	3-4	None
A-2 Tire Jump In and Out	6-10	3-4	90-120 seconds
B-1 KB Single Arm Snatch	3-5 per side	3-4	None
B-2 TRX Side Plank	x 30 seconds per side	2-3	90-120 seconds
C-1 BOSU Lateral Bound	x 6-8 per side	3	None
C-2 Slideboard Skater	x 30 seconds	3	90-120 seconds
D-1 TRX Pistol Squat	x 8-10 per side	2-3	None
D-2 KB Halo	x 6-8 per side	2-3	None
D-3 Battle Rope Hip Flip	x 30 seconds	2-3	90-120 seconds

INDEX

Boldface page references indicate references indicate photographs. <u>Underscored</u> references indicate boxed text.

U

Unanchored Situp, 36, **36**
Unilateral Bench Press, 126, **126**
Unilateral Deadlift, 41, **41**
Unilateral High Cable Fly, 92, **92**
Unilateral Low Cable Fly, 93, **93**
Unilateral Romanian Deadlift, 41, **41**
Unilateral Scarecrow, 103, **103**
Unilateral Shoulder Press, 105, **105**
Unilateral Stability Ball Leg Curl, 46, **46**
Unilateral Standing Calf Raise, 114, **114**
Unilateral Triceps Extension with a Lean,
    142, **142**
Upper back
    bench exercises, 121–33
    body-weight exercises, 38–40
    cable exercises, 92–99
    free weight exercises, 53–55
    squat rack and power cage exercises,
        160–61
Upper body, functional fitness workout for,
    317
Upper body ergometer, 297, **297**
Upright Row, 100, **100**

V

Valor Fitness, 279
VersaClimber, 270, **270**, 297–98, **298**
Vertical leg press, 298
Vests, weighted, 17
V-Leg Raise, 119, **119**
Vocalizations, gym etiquette and, 282
VO$_2$ max, 4

W

Walking
    calories burned per hour, 249
    fast/slow interval, 269
    hand weights used with, 272–73

Wall Pec Stretch, 258, **258**
Warm up, 239, 271–72
Water aerobics class, 293
Water fountain etiquette, 281–82
Weight collars, **16**, 16–17
Weighted Crunch, 49, **49**
Weighted Russian Twist, 50, **50**
Weighted vests, 17
Wide grip, 266–67
Windmill, Kettlebell, 193, **193**
Windshield Wiper, 255, **255**
Wobble boards, 19
Woodchopper, 50, **50**
Woodchopper: High to Low, 90, **90**
Woodchopper: Low to High, 90, **90**
Workout of the Day, 301–2
Workouts
    anatomy of, 30
    elliptical trainer, 245
        beginner, 245
        intermediate/advanced, 245
    fat-loss workout, 6-week, 232–33, 233
    functional fitness, 317–19
        core workout, 318
        fat-burning, 318
        lower body, 317
        sports performance, 319
        upper body, 317
    gym etiquette, 280–84
    muscle-building workout, 6-week, 233–35,
        235
    overtraining, 273
    planning, 29–34
    rowing machine, 247
        beginner, 247
        intermediate/advanced, 247
    samples, 309–16
        fat-burning/total-fitness, 309–11
        muscle building, 311–14
        strength, 314–16
    stairclimber, 244
        advanced, 244
        beginner, 244
        intermediate, 244

stationary bike, 242–43
    advanced, 243
    beginner, 242
    intermediate, 242–43
strength-building workout, 6-week,
    235–36, 236
terminology, 30
time of day for, 270
total-fitness workout, 8-week, 236–37,
    237
training logs, 274, 309–16
training tips, 262–74
    cardio, 268–69
    flexibility, 269–70
    strength-training, 262–63,
        264–68
treadmills, 240–41
    advanced, 241
    beginner, 240
    intermediate, 240–41
warm up, 239, 271–72
Wrist Curl
    Barbell, 149, **149**
    Barbell Reverse, 149, **149**
    Dumbbell, 148, **148**
    Dumbbell Reverse, 148, **148**
    Standing, 110, **110**
    Standing Barbell, 69, 69
Wrist rollers, 18

Y

Yoga
    exercise classes, 294
    power yoga class, 293
York Barbell, 279
YTW, TRX, 216, **216**

Z

Zercher Squat, Sandbag, 199, **199**
Zottman Curl, 70, 70